On Suffering

Beverley M. Clarke

On Suffering

PATHWAYS TO HEALING & HEALTH

Dartmouth College Press
Hanover, New Hampshire

DARTMOUTH COLLEGE PRESS
An imprint of University Press of New England
www.upne.com

Manufactured in the United States of America
Designed by Eric M. Brooks
Typeset in Quadraat and Quadraat Sans by
Passumpsic Publishing

University Press of New England is a member of the
Green Press Initiative. The paper used in this book meets
their minimum requirement for recycled paper.

Library of Congress Cataloging-in-Publication Data appear
on the last printed page of this book.

5 4 3 2 1

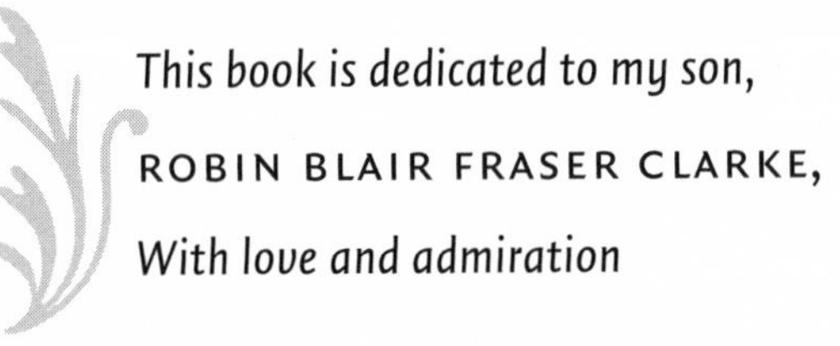

This book is dedicated to my son,

ROBIN BLAIR FRASER CLARKE,

With love and admiration

CONTENTS

PART III. CARING FOR THOSE WHO SUFFER

When the World Is Too Much with Us

FOREWORD

Professor Beverley Clarke is a pioneer in the investigation and understanding of the concept of suffering. She has collected large amounts of clinical data on epilepsy, rheumatoid arthritis, migraine, and spinal cord injury. Professor Clarke has demonstrated that suffering should be considered distinct from pain. She has combined information from clinical, research, philosophical, and legal areas in showing the importance of suffering in all these areas. This book is the product of a comprehensive and thoughtful analysis of available literature and information from many sources.

In my opinion this book provides an assembled text on many complex issues, and it represents many years of work on such an important subject.

DR. ADRIAN R. M. UPTON,
M.A., M.B., B.Chir., LRCP, MRCS, FRCP(C), FRCP(E), FRCP(G), Professor of Medicine—Neurology, Director of Neurology and Epilepsy Clinics, and Director of Diagnostic Neurophysiology, McMaster University Medical Centre, Hamilton, Ontario, Canada

PREFACE

The impetus for writing this book comes from my early experiences as a physiotherapist treating two young, injured military men in a veteran's hospital. (The stories of these two young men, Dan and Roger, like other stories in this book, are imaginative conglomerations of events inspired by my many experiences as a clinical physiotherapist. These stories are not real-life reports.) The first patient, "Dan," was a soldier who, on a particularly hot summer day, dived into a lake to cool off and broke his neck. (I use the term *patient* here because it is specific to those who are receiving medical care.) Prior to his injury, Dan was a vigorous, fun-loving, intelligent family man who enjoyed a beer or two with his pals. After the accident, he was physically helpless and in a constant rage, lashing out at everyone. Dan and I worked together several times a day for over seven months in the rehabilitation hospital. Ours was the typical physiotherapist–patient relationship. I pushed him as hard as I could to achieve everything that was humanly possible, and he tried with all his heart and soul to help himself. Sometimes he called me "Bubbles" and sometimes I was the battleaxe from hell. But we worked hard together. Dan made some improvements, but it soon became apparent that he would never become the person he once was. Eventually Dan was discharged to a long-term care facility. Three months after his discharge, I heard that Dan had committed suicide. I cried.

"Roger," the second patient, was a young airman whose plane crashed on an icy mountaintop. Roger was paralyzed from the waist down, and both his arms had to be amputated because of frostbite. My first encounter with Roger occurred on the day his mother died. Roger and I started the long and difficult process of rehabilitation, and once again I was sometimes "Bubbles" and most of the time I was the "devil's handmaiden." Roger and I worked, argued, talked, laughed, and worked some more, day after day. After several months Roger was discharged from the hospital. For a long time, I never knew what had happened to him. One day, I had a phone call from a friend of mine who was a nurse working in the United States. She told me about a patient of hers by the name of Roger who had asked her to give me a message. She said Roger was an outpatient at her hospital. She said he seemed happy, was involved with a wheelchair sports team, was living independently, and self-managing minor health problems. He asked her to say "hi" to Bubbles and tell her "I'm doing okay." Those two patients and countless others troubled me throughout my professional life. Why did one person survive suffering while another did not? The psychologically pat answers of medicine only explained medicine's need to fight disease and death. I could not dishonor my patients by giving such explanations. I pursued my clinical career, assumed the responsibilities of academic life, and continued to explore the question of suffering in medicine. This book is the result of twenty-five years of treating those who suffer and another twenty years of scientifically exploring the issue of suffering and health. This book argues that suffering is a life experience that is separate from, and only sometimes caused by, pain. Individuals suffer when there is a perception of threat to the idea of self and how this self should act in the face of adversity. Failure to incorporate suffering into clinical treatment plans results in a loss of human potential and an escalation of health care costs.

ACKNOWLEDGMENTS

Suffering in medical practice has long been recognized and addressed in the area of palliative care, but suffering outside the context of terminal illness is often not recognized. In 1986, in the Department of Clinical Neurology at McMaster University, our team of clinical researchers began to explore suffering as an entity separate from pain in patients with chronic illnesses. The projects were originally supported by the De Groote Foundation for Epilepsy Research under the auspices of Dr. Adrian Upton, professor of medicine, McMaster University, Hamilton, Ontario, Canada. I would like to thank all the patients and their families who helped advance the understanding of suffering in contemporary medicine.

I am very fortunate to have the support of Dr. Upton, whose broad knowledge base and expertise in neurology, psychology, the law, and the humanities has provided a stimulating academic and creative milieu for the development and testing of new ideas about suffering and the care of patients in contemporary medicine.

My association with Rev. John O'Connor, a longtime chaplain at McMaster University who continues his work in the Republic of Guyana, has contributed a great deal to my understanding of the power of the human spirit. Reverend O'Connor has extensive experience in palliative care and bioethics. I have a deep admiration for all my colleagues who help those who suffer recover their lives. Reverend O'Connor has shown me that suffering, per se, is the responsibility of all health care professionals, and this perspective is the foundation of this book. I would also like to thank Reverend O'Connor for his contribution to chapter 13.

Because McMaster University is committed to a small-group, problem-based education model, my students come from all areas of health care delivery. I admire their dedication to lifelong learning and the pursuit of optimal care for those who suffer. I feel privileged to have been part of their educational journey.

Claudia Castellanos, our research assistant, has been an invaluable member of our team. Ms. Castellanos has a degree in psychology, and her contribution to the chapter addressing the difference between sadness and depression was invaluable. Not only has she participated in our numerous research projects, she has tirelessly typed and retyped this manuscript. I am very grateful to Claudia for her dedication to these projects, and I appreciate her intelligent questions and discussions of the issues.

This work is respectfully offered to all my fellow health care professionals who work tirelessly and unceasingly to help those with disease and/or injuries face adversity with a sense of nobility and the ability to hold their heads high without fear or prejudice.

On Suffering

Introduction

The dynamic of suffering is complex and rarely addressed outside the context of palliative care both in medicine and in the society at large. Linguistically, the word *suffering* is nonspecific and is used to describe many experiences, such as hardship, adversity, pain behaviours, discomfort, anxiety, and even religious devotion. Some believe that suffering is inevitable, immeasurable, the secondary component of pain, and that if pain is eliminated, suffering stops. If pain is treated and suffering does not stop, then either the pain intervention is ineffective or the individual is not being truthful. Clinical practice and research evidence refute these viewpoints. I argue in this book that the experience of suffering is an entity separate from pain; has universal, measurable characteristics; and is only sometimes directly related to pain. Further, it is the expression of suffering that is idiosyncratic, not the experience per se. Failure to recognize suffering as a phenomenon separate from pain results in incomplete problem identification of patient complaints, ineffective treatment interventions, inappropriate referrals to psychology, increased health care expenditures, and an escalation of human misery. Suffering is not a pathological experience.

Current research studies of persons with chronic pain provide evidence that suffering occurs only when individuals perceive a threat to their idea of self and their personhood.* Some perceptions are the result of physical and/or emotional limitations due to impairments, disability, loss, workplace challenges, upset family systems, and sometimes pain intensity and/or chronicity. Cultural, religious, and societal beliefs about suffering may be associated with social values that can impact on treatment outcomes. For example, in cases involving automobile accidents, personal injury claims, or workplace accidents, the outcome of suffering and pain may be monetary gain. There are many legal and administrative processing pressures on patients to maintain the status quo with regard to their health. The fear that legal claims may not be successful may increase suffering. Health professionals' lack of understanding of basic legal principles of tort law may add to patient fears because patients may be labeled as malingering when behaviours are inconsistent with the natural history of the illness or disorder. If health professionals have a basic understanding of the legal system, they can help patients improve their health status even though litigation is still in progress. In situations

*E. Cassell, *The Nature of Suffering and the Goals of Medicine*, 2nd ed. (Oxford: Oxford University Press, 2004).

involving terminal illness, bereavement, or chronic disability, those who suffer may be regarded as role models. Becoming a symbol of bravery is isolating to the individual and may also result in further deterioration of health. The challenge to health care providers is to identify those who suffer and to develop best methods of practice to resolve patients' concerns. To achieve this goal requires a clear working definition of suffering as an entity distinct from pain, and a valid and reliable measurement tool to identify those who suffer. Further, clinicians must have an understanding of how cultural, religious, and societal factors may affect suffering. Suffering-specific strategies must be developed and incorporated into treatment plans.

This book begins with a poem written by a patient that depicts the powerful impact of suffering on a person's idea of self. The following chapters clarify the issues mentioned here by presenting a working definition of suffering, a discussion of factors that contribute to further suffering, a method of identifying those who suffer and key elements of their suffering, as well as strategies to relieve suffering.

The book is divided into three parts. Part One, "Suffering: What Man Has Made of Man," consists of seven chapters that introduce current theoretical perspectives of suffering in contemporary society. Universal characteristics of suffering are identified. The dynamics of the relationship between suffering and health are outlined, and the scientific rigor required to assess the construct of suffering is described.

Part Two, "Identifying Those Who Suffer: Now Is The Time to Know," contains four chapters that describe a measurement tool, the "Measurement and Assessment of Suffering Questionnaire" (MASQ); the statistical results of reliability and validity testing of the tool; methods of clinical application, data scoring, and data collation; and the usefulness of the questionnaire in clinical decision making. While it is recognized that factors contributing to an individual's dream of self are highly individual, issues relating to personhood are more universal. Consequently, normative data scales are of critical importance in determining the impact of suffering on personhood. Personhood encompasses every aspect of an individual's lifestyle and how the individual believes he or she should manage adversity. The importance and limitations of developing normative standards of care are fully explored, and key components of suffering in chronic illness are delineated. Part Two concludes with guidelines for treatment. Specific end-of-life issues in palliative care are beyond the scope of this work.

Part Three, "Caring for Those Who Suffer: The World Is Too Much with Us," consists of five chapters that explore how patients can be helped to resolve suffering. Information is provided about the roles of various health care professionals who assist patients from onset of suffering to survival and reentry into the community at large. A brief history of the origins of the professions of nurses, physicians, chaplains, physiotherapists, and social workers are explored. The scope of practice and the constraints imposed on each professional who assists those who suffer are illustrated. Issues relating to professional autonomy, ethics, and responsibility are outlined so that individuals who seek help have knowledge about the type of assistance available to them.

In Part One, the first chapter, "Suffering in Medicine: A New Aspect to an Old Problem," shows that traditional definitions of suffering and contemporary societal understandings of suffering are in conflict. A clear, concise definition of suffering is presented, free from psychological and spiritual/religious bias. The universal characteristics of suffering, in which there is a loss of central purpose, increased self-conflict, and impaired interpersonal relationships, are delineated. It is argued that suffering is a phenomenon that is unique and only sometimes related to pain.

The problem of suffering in contemporary medicine is portrayed through a letter from "Marlene," a young woman who has severe kidney disease, and the story of Mr. Whitehead, a patient with advanced Parkinson's disease. "Marlene" has dreams of a future, but she suffers because she believes her dreams will not come true. Her story is one of loss of the idea of self and personhood. Marlene reaches out to anyone in cyberspace who may be able to help her understand her suffering because health care professionals and her family, while well intentioned, do not understand suffering from her perspective. The story of Mr. Whitehead is about a man who is distraught because of the loneliness and anger he feels because his friends have labeled him a "hero." His story shows the power of self-conflict in suffering. The chapter concludes with a brief overview of the challenges to clinical decision making when suffering is understood as a phenomenon that is only sometimes related to pain. The problems of diagnosing versus assessing suffering, the challenges in assisting those who suffer, and the difficulties surrounding the development of suffering-specific treatment strategies are outlined. These issues are explored more fully in later chapters.

Chapter 2, "Suffering Is Not Pain: The Evidence," provides objective data to support the theory that suffering and pain are separate phenomena and are only sometimes related. This research evidence was obtained from over 350 patients with epilepsy, arthritis, migraine headache, and spinal cord injuries. The chapter focuses on incorporating these research results into clinical practice. The significance of recognizing suffering as a distinct construct is explored through examples of the resolution of medical legal issues that are based primarily on tort law. The importance of acknowledging suffering as an entity separate from pain is discussed from the perspective of health care reform in which escalating health care delivery costs are of paramount concern. The story of Neil illustrates this point further and shows the impact of suffering on an individual's life.

Chapter 3, "The Power of Religious and Spiritual Beliefs," focuses on traditional spiritual/religious teachings about health and suffering and the power of these beliefs on those who suffer. Judeo-Christian, Hindu, Buddhist, Confucianist, North American and African aboriginal, and Islamic traditions illustrate the diversity of beliefs about suffering and the challenges these beliefs present to the management of chronically ill patients in culturally diverse societies. This chapter presents the argument that even in contemporary societies, where people may state that they have no spiritual beliefs, clinical studies show that when illness occurs people often refer back to early childhood teachings. Health care delivery is most cost effective and humane if health care professionals are aware of the basic tenets of their patients' spiritual lives.

Chapter 4, "Suffering and Culture," reviews common understandings of culture, ethnicity, and nationality in contemporary society and illustrates the differences between individuals' ideas of self and self-identity. The importance of understanding the ethos or characteristic spirit of a culture or community is critical to effective health care delivery to those who suffer, particularly if power differentials between health care professionals and patients are to be eliminated and when suffering is addressed as an entity separate from pain. The dynamics of xenophobia (i.e., the undue fear of strangers) in dominant cultures and minority cultures within a pluralistic society are examined because of the impact of these issues on suffering. A discussion of the importance of health care providers being knowledgeable about the differences between assimilation and acculturation in multicultural, pluralistic societies shows the challenges patients currently face when they try to resolve the experience of suffering. The importance of cultural sensitivity and how attitudinal shifts may be accomplished when addressing suffering are explored through the story of Marron, a young woman of aboriginal heritage who suffered a severe spinal cord injury. Marron's story illustrates the fact that for some patients successful treatment outcomes are the result of combining both scientific methods and culturally specific health care practices. In Marron's case, her need to be freed from her belief that she had been "cursed" by paranormal spirits is explored from the perspective of cultural traditions rather than psychological pathology. The systemic challenges to the health care system and the demands placed on individuals and health care providers are illustrated.

Exploration of developmental psychosocial tasks in chapter 5, "Crises of Suffering across the Life Span" shows how failure to accomplish these psychological tasks can escalate the process of suffering in chronic illness. This chapter also shows how various understandings of what constitutes a family impact on the achievement of psychosocial development tasks. Family dynamics are very briefly reviewed both from a family systems and an ecosystem approach to care. Challenges to family systems and individuals who suffer are illustrated through the story of Robbie, a young child who despite severe handicaps was able to maintain an intact idea of self and personhood. Health care organizational policies may also be in conflict with the life tasks of patients and their families. Failure to consider the importance of these issues and the potential for serious harm to patients and their families is illustrated through the story of Mr. Cjenchuck and his relationship with his very ill adolescent daughter. In this story, the father and daughter's relationship was thought to be improper by some health care professionals who did not understand the psychosocial tasks of father and daughter over the life span or the cultural demands on the family.

Chapter 6, "The Language of Suffering," presents the story of Laura, a young woman who was severely injured in a car accident that took the lives of her family. Through examples of Laura's poems and the story of Laura's experience in a rehabilitation facility we learn about the language that is sometimes used to express the universal characteristics of suffering and about the effect that current medical practice has on escalating the process of suffering. Key contributors to suffering in clinical practice are the loss of patients' personal power and the fact that autonomy has become simply an act of obtaining permissions to avoid legal litigation. The concept of autonomy is examined from its historical roots and its social ramifications both in contemporary society and, more specifically, in clinical practice. The challenge that changed social beliefs presents to the goals of ethical health care delivery is explored, with emphasis on the effects the lack of autonomy has not only on those who suffer but also on their health care providers.

"Medical-Legal Disclosure of Suffering," chapter 7, argues that both medical and legal discourse may contribute to suffering. Without a clear understanding of the historical origins of legal systems, the purpose and process of the law may be misunderstood by clinicians and inadvertently result in harm to the patient. Examples of the mechanisms of the legal system that can contribute to suffering are traced from the British legal system to current American or Canadian law, because both the American and Canadian systems have evolved from the British system. A brief history of the origins of the law shows that contrary to common belief the law is a process with origins based on contracts and monetary restitution. Justice is often regarded in those terms rather than in the ethic of caring for the sick and curing ailments of the individual. That is not to suggest that the ethics of law are immoral, but rather that its tenets have origins that are different from those of "care and cure" of medicine. Differences between medical and legal definitions of suffering and similarities between medical and legal discourse and loss of patients' autonomy are considered. A critique of current justifications for the loss of personal power due to medical and legal discourse explores the ethical considerations critical to the effective management of suffering and health in a pluralistic, multicultural society. The failure of health care professionals to have at least a basic understanding of the purpose and limitations of legal systems can result in an escalation of suffering.

In Part Two, chapter 8, "Power Differentials and Suffering" argues that restoration of the personal power and autonomy of patients who suffer because of chronic illness may be restored if health care providers have objective measurement tools to identify those who suffer and provide patients with the information and organizational mechanisms to achieve these objectives. Suggestions to achieve these goals are presented through examples of patient information packages and consent forms that are designed based on the moral imperative of personal responsibility, both in clinical practice and clinical research. These examples show that it is possible to obtain individuals' consent in ways that are not based solely on contractual permissions. In addition, the importance of collecting both objective and subjective data from those who suffer is discussed. Examples of pertinent data collection from patients with arthritis, epilepsy, migraine headaches, and spinal cord injuries, based on results from research studies that identify components of suffering, show that suffering is not disease specific.

The purpose of chapter 9, "How to Assess Suffering," is to illustrate a valid and reliable, self-administered questionnaire, the MASQ. The MASQ not only identifies those who experience suffering but it also delineates key items for further exploration by clinicians. Raw data may be collated in either a long- or short-form format. The long format is most useful in cases where therapeutic interventions are applied. The short format is most useful in cases where determinations of monetary compensation for workplace accidents or other insurance claims require specific objective data of an individual's suffering. Examples of patient raw data scores are given and interpreted to show the usefulness of raw data scores in clinical practice.

Chapter 10, "Standards of Care," demonstrates the need to have comparative data critical to the development of standards of practice. Normative data results obtained from a sample of 166 patients with arthritis and 100 individuals with epilepsy are reported for suffering and pain items. Methods of calculating normative scores from raw data are illustrated, and examples of the clinical interpretation of normative data show the usefulness of normative data to clinicians who must make referrals for treatments. The availability of normative data is particularly important in the management of suffering if reports of individuals' idiosyncratic expressions of suffering are not to be confused with the universal characteristics of the experience.

Chapter 11, "Key Components of Suffering in Chronic Illness," provides a brief description of the natural history of arthritis, epilepsy, migraine headache, and spinal cord injuries. These descriptions delineate research studies done on groups of patients who, although they all had chronic illnesses, experienced vastly different impacts on ideas of self and personhood from these illnesses. In spite of these differences, individuals identified the same items as factors contributing to their suffering. These data refute the common opinion that suffering cannot be assessed and that the process of suffering is disease specific and idiosyncratic. Further, they show that the arguments presented in this book are not merely speculative theories but ideas supported by objective evidence. A call is made for more research to be done in this area to test these hypotheses. The chapter concludes with a discussion on the value of effective communication skills of both individuals and health professionals and the necessity of marrying objective data with subjective clinical communication competencies, factors essential to the care of those who suffer.

In Part Three, chapter 12, entitled "The Resolution of Suffering," begins with a poem written by a health care student and describes the conflicts of individuals who suffer when they ask the question "Who am I?" A variety of methods of identifying suffering through the analysis of common types of stories patients tell clinicians about the process of suffering are given. Key story types explored are restitution, chaos, and quest stories. Analyses of these story types show how the dynamics of storytelling relate to ideas of self, personal power, and autonomy. Guidelines are given to assist clinicians in addressing the issue of suffering as it relates to restoration of the self and personhood in everyday practice. This chapter shows how medicine's current belief that science is the answer to all of humankind's problems can cause or enhance suffering. The current practice of third-party interpretations of patients' stories is particularly harmful to those who suffer because this process robs people of personal power. Specific steps to restructuring the self are given. The focus of the chapter is to show how restoration of the self and personhood can occur through interactions with health care professionals involved in the individual's care. Even slight changes in methods of clinical listening and assessing patients will aid in the restoration of the self, and at least prevent the process of suffering from escalating.

While chapter 12 explores the care of those who suffer from a theoretical perspective, the thrust of chapter 13, "The Roles of Health Care Professionals," is to illustrate the nature and challenges of contemporary health care environments on health care professionals and the impact these factors have on those who suffer. Professional responsibility and the power of personal and professional autonomy in suffering are examined. The specific roles of physicians, nurses, and chaplains, who are usually the first frontline health care professionals that those individuals who suffer meet, are described and illustrated through the story of Rev. John. The profession-specific challenges and the barriers to effective care are outlined. The argument presented is that the resolution of suffering demands that patients have realistic expectations of their health professionals, and this objective can only be achieved if individuals have at least a basic understanding of both the organizational and external professional constraints placed on their care providers.

"Habilitation and Rehabilitation" is the title of chapter 14. The environmental constraints of health care professionals who assist patients in the restoration of personhood as they reenter their communities are explored through analysis of the roles of the physiotherapist and social worker. Issues of professionalism, professional autonomy, and ethical practice are once again examined, but this time, within the context of rehabilitation and reentry into the community at large. The role of the physiotherapist in suffering is illustrated through the story of Eric, a crusty old soldier and gentleman, who was in acute respiratory distress, and his relationship with Clare, a "sassy" young physiotherapist assigned to his care. This story clearly demonstrates the need for all health care professionals to address suffering and shows how effective team work, directed in part by the patient, can help restore patients' dreams, idea of self, and personhood.

Chapter 15, "The Wounded Spirit: Reclaiming Personhood," involves the problem of patients who have suffered and are left with a wounded spirit. Both surviving and the hope of thriving after suffering require an understanding of the concept of a wounded spirit. Examples from the poetry of the patient Laura, whose family was killed in a car accident in which she was also severely injured, show the difficulties individuals experience when they try to find a new rhythm for their lives. Patients are often bombarded by the resurgence of memories from the past, and it is important for families and health care clinicians to realize that such occurrences are normal life events and not usually indicators of pathological emotional illness. The wounded spirit is explored also from the perspectives of those patients who have developmental disorders as well as those patients who have acquired injuries and/or chronic illnesses. The variety of understandings about the nature and value of work in contemporary society show that work is one method through which personhood is reestablished and the ability to thrive after suffering can be achieved. Work, either for monetary gain or solely for emotional restoration, is a method of achieving reentry into the world at large.

Chapter 16, "Surviving and Thriving," focuses on barriers to surviving suffering that can occur when health care clinicians fail to recognize the differences between sorrow and depression and the power of fear, anxiety, and loneliness on an individual's fragile new ideas of self and personhood. Sorrow is often a common and prolonged expression of suffering, but it is not a psychological illness. Depression is identified as an emotional illness with distinct characteristics. While some individuals who suffer may also have depression, this experience is not a given. Surviving and ultimately thriving after suffering are shown to occur when health care providers acknowledge the differences between the above factors and ensure that problem identification is accurate. The chapter presents for consideration the value of facilitating the innate human creativity all people possess as an effective approach to the care of those who suffer. This chapter shows that to thrive after suffering, individuals must be able to define and redefine their problems and be able to choose appropriate strategies to resolve difficulties.

The care of those who suffer and the maintenance of health demand that health care professionals and patients understand that the process of suffering in medicine falls outside the specific contexts of religious and spiritual teachings. That is not to say that these teachings are not to be respected and valued, for they are integral to the individual's beliefs about self and personhood, but in the restoration and maintenance of health, medicine must be clear about identifying the problem at hand. It is not the role of medicine to determine the value of suffering, as may be the case in some spiritual traditions. In health care, suffering has no intrinsic value. The objective of medicine is the maintenance and restoration of health. Not only information, but also knowledge and objective evidence about suffering are needed to provide ethical, client-centred, cost-effective, evidence-based care. The challenges are many in multicultural, pluralistic societies. This book provides a framework to address the complexities of managing suffering in clinical practice outside the realm of palliative care. In addition, health care practitioners and others are given a useful tool, the MASQ, to identify those who suffer and to determine the nature of their suffering. Guidelines for practical, empathetic, and compassionate treatments are outlined. Understanding suffering from the perspective of an individual's felt experience, outside the construct of the world politic, is a critical first step towards humane care of those who suffer. Many examples throughout the text are from patients' expressions of suffering. These clinical scenarios show that it is the patient who "knows" the felt experience of suffering, and the health care practitioner who must "serve."

All case stories presented for clarification are imaginary conglomerates of events inspired by my many experiences as a clinical physiotherapist. They are not real-life reports. Names and details of incidents do not refer to specific individuals alive or deceased. The authorship of the patients' poetry presented is anonymous at the request of the poet.

1 Suffering

WHAT MAN HAS MADE OF MAN

1 Suffering in Medicine

A NEW ASPECT OF AN OLD PROBLEM

Suffering in contemporary society has many meanings based on religious, legal, cultural, and secular societal belief systems. While it is important to understand the origins of individuals' beliefs about the nature of suffering, it is not useful to combine suffering and pain as one entity in medical practice. Clinically, it has been observed that some individuals who suffer experience little pain and others who experience considerable pain report little suffering.

The purpose of this chapter is to present an overview of the problems of suffering in modern medicine. The chapter begins by: (a) examining definitions and characteristics of suffering as an entity separate from pain, (b) delineating the process of clinical decision making in patients who suffer, and (c) illustrating the differences between diagnosis and assessment. These issues and other factors contributing to the power of the experience of suffering and its relationship to health are explored in more detail in the following chapters. The chapter concludes with a summary of the key issues of suffering and an outline of the theoretical differences in approach to treatment.

Defining Suffering

The *Oxford English Dictionary* defines suffering as "being subjected to something bad or unpleasant" (1). Common usage and understandings are more complex. Traditional interpretations of suffering range from religious teachings, in which suffering has a moral and ethical value, to societal attitudes that consider suffering to be a heroic act. Some religious teachings are that good people endure suffering and are rewarded in an afterlife and bad people experience trials and tribulations for all eternity. Sociological perspectives of suffering occur within the contexts of human misery, poverty, illness, and political and social reforms. Sociological evaluations of human suffering are within the context of social resources rather than individual needs.

A more useful definition of suffering, and the one explored in detail throughout this text, states that suffering is a process that occurs when some vital part of a person's "idea of self" and "personhood" is perceived to be threatened (2). "Idea of self" refers to those qualities and attributes that an individual believes are critical to personal existence.

Past medical beliefs embraced the idea that suffering is the secondary component of pain and that if pain is eliminated, suffering stops. Recent research studies refute this view and provide evidence to support the hypothesis that suffering and pain are separate entities that are only sometimes related. Suffering was also thought to be idiosyncratic and not measurable, but again, research findings support the argument that it is only the expression of suffering, not the process per se, that is unique to a given individual (3).

Some contemporary definitions of suffering tend to focus on the idea of an individuated self. For example, some analyses differentiate among many "selves." It is argued that there is a "neurological self" representing the body, or "body self"; an "agent self," which interacts at a behavioural level with the environment; and a "cognitive self," which operates at a cognitive level to encompass an awareness of the person's past, present, and future. In addition, a "dynamic self" is identified that seems to relate to a developmentally emerging sense of being (4).

Others argue that individuals develop a strong sense of self in childhood that is a critical determinant of human behaviour (5). As the child develops, this sense of self is undermined or lost due to negative societal and cultural attitudes. As a result, individuals begin to lose their sense of an authentic complete self and develop "safety zones" in an attempt to maintain a sense of wholeness. These fragmented "safety zones" take many forms. An example of a safety zone may be the belief that if one earns more money or is always pleasant or helpful, then personal safety is assured. Proponents of this theory argue that suffering is a process in which an individual's incomplete self begins to reemerge in concert with a deep longing for the nonintegrated parts of the self. The therapeutic task is to help the patient unify the self (5).

Such theories are firmly rooted in pathophysiology, and while they are very important in special circumstances such as mental illness, clinical depression, or terminal illness, suffering per se is usually considered to be a normal life experience outside the realm of mental and/or emotional incapacity or impairments. None of the above theories are incompatible with the classic work of Cassell and others, who view suffering as a perception of threat to self and personhood, but rather they provide additional insights into suffering, particularly, when patients are unable to manage adversity (2, 6–8). To be of assistance to those who suffer, the concepts of "idea of self" and personhood must be understood clearly.

MARLENE'S STORY

Several years ago, I was asked to prepare a talk for a group of professional mental health care workers on the topic of suffering. In preparation for this meeting, I remembered a conversation I had with a friend who was upset about all the people who write to chat rooms for support when their lives are in crisis. My friend was concerned about a young woman whom I will call Marlene. It seems that Marlene had chronic kidney disease and posted a message on an Internet chat room about the fear she was experiencing. She wrote, "Please, please help me. Can anyone help me? I've had kidney disease problems for years. A couple of months ago, my doctor sent me to see a kidney specialist who said I have chronic renal failure. They did a lot of tests and last week when I went back to get the results from my tests, the kidney doctor walked into the room with a whole bunch of doctors and the first thing he said to me was 'you are going to need a kidney transplant.' He then started to ask me questions such as 'are your parents and sister healthy?' He and another doctor then started talking about dialysis or a kidney transplant donor. They were using all kinds of doctor language that I didn't understand. My heart started beating so fast that the room was spinning. I thought I was going to pass out. I'm so shocked that I don't even think that I even heard it all. It is starting to hit me now and to be honest, I'm terrified. I have no one to talk to. My mother is great but I don't think she really understands what I am feeling from that scared inside-me place. When I start to talk about my feelings, she starts crying and then I just want to run away and hide. No one seems to hear me when I try to tell them that all my dreams and hopes are lost forever. They keep telling me that I'm strong and everything will be OK but it won't! Nothing will ever be the same. I feel that I am crying inside myself all the time. Can anyone help me?"

As I read this message, I paused because it occurred to me that this young woman was writing not only about a perception of the threat to her idea of self but also about the threat to her dreams of self and personhood. Marlene seemed to believe that she would not be able to live a "normal" life.

Marlene continued: "I used to have dreams of falling in love and meeting someone special, being a beautiful bride and eventually having a family, but now I can't really see that happening. Is there anyone else who has these feelings, or am I all alone with these awful fears?" Marlene continued to ask her anonymous cyberspace companions about various treatment options she had heard about. Questions were about her overwhelming fear that treatments were painful and wouldn't work. She kept asking, "How does it feel to have the kidney of someone who has died in you?" She kept saying, "I feel alone." Marlene concluded the letter with "It's hard to explain what I am feeling right now. Sometimes I just want to scream and scream until my bad thoughts stop. Am I the only one who has these terrible thoughts? When I talk to my family, I feel so guilty. . . . I know they want the best for me and are scared too. I just wish there was someone who knew how I feel from deep inside me. If anyone can relate to what I'm saying, please help me with my questions so that I don't feel like I'm trapped alone in a long dark tunnel. Thanks Marlene."

As my friend and I talked about this Internet posting, I expressed the opinion that I thought that it showed how suffering is often separate from pain and that suffering involves a process in which individuals perceive a threat not only to their physical self but also to the dream or idea of self that they believe is critical to their survival. It was extremely distressing to read this message because, to me, it highlighted the failure of health care professionals to address the issue of suffering in the management of patients with chronic illness.

Within the construct of suffering, an individual's idea of self is a cherished ambition or fantasy about what he/she believes is an acceptable way of managing not only life but also adversity. Personhood encompasses all aspects of an individual's life. Interpersonal relationships; workplace performance and the emphasis on skill levels; communication competencies; and the personal qualities of honesty, integrity, and compassion are all key issues. Individual expectations of acceptable personal behaviour in avocational activities with family, friends, and others are also aspects of the whole person. Personhood is intrinsically linked to the idea of self and involves all aspects of an individual's life, ranging from past performance to future expectations. This approach encompasses the whole person in society at large (9). People suffer when they believe that the dream of self and personhood cannot be realized (10–12). Cassell effectively argues that suffering must be regarded within the context of the patient's personal and social history (2). The advantage of the early work of Cassell and others is that suffering can be understood in less convoluted but more comprehensive terms than theories based on pathophysiology (2–16).

Proponents of this classical definition of suffering argue that relief of human suffering, in medicine, is dependent on what is deemed to be acceptable both from an individual and societal viewpoint and is based not only on religious and spiritual teachings but also on cultural and societal belief systems. Because the goal of clinical practice is to help those it serves achieve their maximum human potential, it is critical to have a clear understanding of what suffering means to the individual and how religious, sociological, and societal attitudes impact on beliefs and clinical outcomes.

In modern medicine, a useful working definition of suffering must be one in which the entity of suffering has universal, measurable, characteristics. Management of suffering in clinical practice involves knowing the patient as a unique individual and clearly understanding the patient's internal and external environments.

Characteristics of Suffering

There are three major characteristics defining the process of suffering. The first involves a perception of threat to personhood and ideas of self, followed by self-conflict and loss of a central purpose in life (12).

Ideas of Self and Personhood

Individuals have a sense of separateness from others. In Marlene's story she speaks of the goodness of her family but is distressed because they don't understand her suffering from "that scared inside-me place." An individual's belief of self is private and is dependent on a belief in the integrity of his/her own experience. People have a sense of "me" in the world, and world events are interpreted in relationship to the self.

Individuals believe that circumstances change but they as individuals remain the same. Each of us possesses a life now and in the future. How individuals interpret their history is central to their sense of self. Marlene seemed to be saying that with a kidney transplant she would no longer be herself. She was concerned because she believed that with surgery she would be a damaged person. Her personhood desires involved meeting a man who would be her husband. Her fear was that no one would want to be a partner with a woman who Marlene believed was no longer whole. This last point is critical to understanding suffering. Often suffering occurs because of an inability to interpret life events and histories in a manner acceptable to oneself. For example, if an individual has been taught to present a brave face regardless of circumstances, and suddenly the person is faced with a catastrophic event in which presentation of a brave face is not possible, the patient may perceive his/her response to the present situation as a failure. The end result may be feelings of guilt and shame. Interpretation of past teachings (bravery at all costs) becomes one of failure and shame. Suffering occurs because the individual has become a victim of a belief that he/she has exhibited unacceptable behaviour.

No one is ever fully able to predict what he/she may do in any given set of circumstances, and while people may, at times, be surprised by their own behaviour, the belief that one "knows oneself" persists. It is possible, however, to change our idea of self. Behavioural scientists report that in order to change the self (13) individuals must be able to imagine what they will be like once they have changed. Often this does not seem possible in the face of illness or disability. The severity of illness becomes so omnipresent that it seems impossible to see how to survive. The second challenge is to try to behave in a way that this new self might behave. This task may be impeded by the expectations of others, individual self-criticism in relation to others, and the belief that we have specific social roles that we believe can no longer be fulfilled. Early family experiences teach people how to negotiate a view of themselves and of others. Conscious awareness of the power of past teachings may prevent the rejection of views that may no longer be relevant. Individuals become attached to past ideas of self and suffer because these ideas are no longer true. However, if clinicians and family members know not only that the idea of self can change, but also what factors impede change, they may be able to help those who suffer a loss of idea of self.

Changing the idea of self requires the removal of a previous belief while simultaneously replacing this old belief with a new one. Further, pivotal to a comprehension of the phenomenon of suffering is the understanding that suffering is an issue of personhood and not a problem of the body. People have character, personality, have lived a past, and hope for a future. Individuals live in relationship with family, friends, community, and the environment. We live in a society, have a culture, and construct a world often through our work. Personhood also involves our spiritual dimensions and the desires of our inner world. Suffering occurs when any component of personhood is perceived to be threatened. Patients often speak of suffering in language that expresses "how much concern or worry" they have about the perceived negative impact that their illness or injury is having or will have on personhood issues.

Loss of Central Purpose

All persons have a central purpose in their internal life even if the nature of that purpose is unknown, unplanned or incoherent (15). In suffering there may be such decentralization of purpose that people feel they have lost their idea of self and how this self would/should act. They become focused solely on removing the cause of the suffering. Personal autonomy, interpersonal dynamics, and the central guiding purpose of life may disappear. Patients may feel that they are lost, that they are on the sidelines watching their lives unfold without any passion or involvement. They may express feelings of isolation and fear and/or have a sense of being disconnected from society.

Experiences of Self-Conflict

Persons who suffer may experience considerable emotional conflict. They may not be able to respond to expectations of behaviour, their own and those of others, even though they continue to try to meet these expectations. If they do defeat the limitations of illness, they may be perceived as "heroic" and experience the social isolation of the hero. The following story is an example of how the designation of "hero" can lead to social isolation and an escalation of suffering.

MR. WHITEHEAD'S STORY

One afternoon, a courtly gentleman with a high-browed face and intelligent blue eyes lumbered into my office displaying the typical unsteady gait of a person who has had Parkinson's disease for a long time. In a quiet, controlled, slurring voice, interrupted only by periods of laboured breathing, he slowly told me of a conversation he had had while playing cards with friends. As I listened, I watched his trembling hands and noticed the little specks of spittle that collected at the sides of his mouth, which were quickly dispersed by uncontrollable jabbing aimed in the general direction of the offensive moisture. Mr. Whitehead had been a renowned electrical engineer who had presented countless scientific papers at international meetings. Today, he was struggling to tell me how sad and hurt he felt because a good friend had called him a hero. The comment was well intentioned but Mr. Whitehead told me that it made him feel like an outsider in the real world. "I am not a hero;" he protested bitterly, "I am just trying to do the best I can. I need my friends to see me, not this rotten disease. I am not a disease! I need to be part of this world, not some saintly hero."

Mr. Whitehead's story is not uncommon. Many patients experience the hurt of being isolated from the world they once knew. We talked about why a dear friend would express such views, but Mr. Whitehead said he was tired of understanding others' fears. He was fighting for his life and felt he did not need another burden.

People who suffer are often told that they are strong and that they must carry on even though they are not able to do so. Further, if individuals respond to suffering in perhaps a culturally unique manner, they may experience criticism from those upon whom they depend for support. Knowledge of cultural, religious, and secular beliefs as well as the impact of personality on these issues is critical to accurate diagnosis and effective assessment. These matters must be part of the continuing medical education of all health care professionals. While medical science searches for the "truth," suffering requires an understanding of that which is perceived. Unlike past homogeneous societies, clinical decision making in contemporary multicultural societies is complex and challenging.

Clinical Decision Making and Suffering: Contemporary Challenges

Contemporary clinical decision making in suffering requires knowledge and understanding of the patient as an individual as well as knowing the "origins" of the person's suffering (16). Treatment interventions demand careful attention to the story the patient relates and involve demonstrating and sharing with the patient an understanding of the concerns expressed. This approach is different from the discursive methods currently employed in medicine, in which the listener has a preconceived "script" against which the patient's complaints are compared for diagnostic purposes. In this latter method, the clinician listens for information relating to a specific disease or illness. There is usually no sharing of experience, and only disease-specific information is valued. The diagnosis of suffering, however, demands knowledge of the patient as an individual, knowledge that encompasses understanding the impact of culture, personality, and societal values on the person's beliefs about suffering. These skills are sometimes referred to as "empathetic listening" and "nondiscursive thinking," skills not currently emphasized in medical education (2, 17–19).

Another challenge to the diagnosis of suffering is to understand that suffering is not restricted to terminal illness and palliative care. Previous research shows that some individuals with epilepsy, arthritis, migraine, and spinal cord injuries may experience suffering and provides evidence that suffering is an entity separate from the construct of pain (10). Prevailing medical attitudes that consider suffering to be the secondary component of pain must be re-examined. Current research confirms the belief that to meet the objectives of client-centred and cost-effective care, suffering must be assessed as an entity separate from pain (20–22).

Some health care providers, who do not understand suffering as a perception of threat to idea of self and personhood, believe that the assessment of suffering is captured in measures of quality of life. This belief is fallacious because suffering scales measure perceptions of threat to the integrity of the self, while quality-of-life measures assess the impact of an illness on an individual's abilities and opportunities. While it is important to assess quality of life in those who suffer to further delineate the reactions to personhood, such measures do not identify those who suffer or describe the nature of individual suffering. In summary, the major challenge to incorporating measures of suffering into general clinical practice is the recognition that clinical decision making is not confined solely to the identification of disease. Consequently, when considering the construct of suffering, contemporary clinical decision making requires a clear understanding of the differences and specific purposes of assessment and diagnosis.

Diagnosing and Assessing Suffering

Diagnosis is the art of distinguishing one disease from another. Clinical diagnosis is based on signs, symptoms, and laboratory findings during life. Differential diagnosis involves the determination of which of one, two, or more diseases or conditions a patient suffers from by systematically comparing and contrasting their clinical findings. The diagnosis of suffering has long been avoided because suffering has been thought of as a totally subjective experience. In the area of suffering, the role of diagnosis is to ascertain underlying factors that may be perceived as threats to self and personhood. The cluster of signs and symptoms of suffering, which involve perceptions of threat to idea of self and personhood, loss of central purpose, and self-conflict, are usually not part of the diagnosis or assessment of patients' complaints.

Assessment, unlike diagnosis, is the determination of the status or value of a problem and requires both objective and subjective analyses. In the assessment of suffering, the value is simply whether a person suffers or not. Value judgments of severity are of limited clinical value. The real challenge is to determine the nature and extent of the perception of threat to the individual's life. The management of those who suffer is often the mandate of family members, nurses, therapists, chaplains, and social workers. Assessment tools that objectively delineate key characteristics of suffering are critical to effective treatment planning.

Helping People Who Are Suffering: Key Issues

Determinations of suffering require information about what the current illness/ injury means to the patient's felt experience. These questions are framed within the context of worry or concern individuals have that their illness will have a significant negative effect on their idea of self and personhood. Issues such as personal relationships, job performance, and community acceptance and involvement are measured. These concerns differ from impact-of-illness scales in which the main focus is on abilities and opportunities. For example, a suffering question might be: How much worry or concern do you have that you will never be the person you once were? The patient's worry and concern, for example, might focus on feelings of humiliation because of loss of independence, of not being seen as competent to make personal decisions, or of being a coward. A corresponding impact-of-illness question might be: Does your illness/injury prevent you from getting to work on time? Patient responses might focus on the fact that because of their present impairment or disability, they cannot drive a car and public transportation may not be available.

Further, suffering questions relate to negative beliefs about threats to the self and personhood in the future due to aging, loneliness, and sorrow. How has the individual managed adversity in the past? Does the patient believe the illness or injury will resolve in a manner compatible with his/her perceptions of body image, and/or emotional and spiritual stability? What does resolution mean to the patient? Sometimes a clinician's anticipation of resolution is different from the patient's perceptions.

The above example questions focus on the characteristic of suffering relating to personhood and loss of central purpose. Determining whether people are experiencing suffering also requires inquiring what patients think will happen to them during the resolution of their illness/injury. Do they fear that they will not manage pain, impairment, or disability in a manner that is acceptable to them? Are they worried about how they will cope emotionally in terms of autonomy of decision making? Are there feelings of guilt or shame? How much effort does the patient believe will be involved in the resolution of the problems, and do they want to expend the effort? Do they believe that they will be able to cope with their problems within the context of the person they believe themselves to be now and will be in the future? Do they believe that because of their illness or injury they are no longer acceptable members of the community at large? These questions must be addressed by health care providers with their patients if optimal treatment interventions for the resolution of suffering and/or any underlying pathology are to be achieved.

Responses to the above queries relate to "idea of self" and self-conflict and are best heard within the context of diagnosing and assessing suffering rather than within the context of psychological pathology. Some persons who suffer may be clinically depressed, but others may simply be expressing sorrow. Suffering is not an illness, and the impact of psychological distress can be determined once the nature of the individual's suffering is revealed. It is also important to clearly differentiate between the diagnosis and the assessment of suffering and the treatment of suffering. Treatments will usually focus on an individual's personal interpretation and expression of the experience. Cultural, religious, and societal attitudes may have considerable influences on outcomes.

Treatment Planning: Development of Strategies

The first challenge is to overcome professional reluctance. The roles of healer, scientist, and educator are common to clinical practice. Health care professionals are committed to trying to fix that which is "broken." Contemporary medicine is used to being the authority figure. Often this relationship negates the felt experience of the patient and, in fact, may increase suffering. The management of suffering demands an equalization of the power differential between patient and health care clinician. Expectations of "cure" and/or "care" must include and value strategies that provide comfort.

The first goal is to determine if the patient's expectations match the clinician's knowledge of probability. If expectations and probability are incompatible, the health care professional must also determine whether he/she is sufficiently skilled in the interventions needed to assist patients as they attempt to reach their goals. This approach may involve abandoning the authority role and joining the patient in their experience of uncertainty. We do not all have the professional knowledge and/or skills to deal with uncertainty in an empathetic way. It is the clinician's responsibility to evaluate his/her skill set.

Prolonged sorrow, for example, may be very distressing to the clinician who does not have the personal skills to deal with his/her own feelings about death or possible catastrophic life events. If inappropriate referrals for psychological counseling are made because of professional skill set inadequacy, the patient may feel abandoned. Not only is the patient harmed but other clinicians may inadvertently presume that the person has been referred because of mental illness.

The end result is that patients feel betrayed by those in whom they put their trust. Management of suffering does not require heroism on the part of patients or their clinicians. It does demand an empathetic approach to problem solving.

Further, some health care professionals are not able to accept a sense of ceremony in their clinical practice, particularly when the person who suffers must repeatedly tell the story of his/her suffering. Such clinicians argue that the treatments of suffering are subjective, time consuming, and costly. However, the diagnosis and assessment of suffering requires the same amount of time as other medical evaluations and does not require expensive technological confirmations. Moreover, failing to engage with patients' experiences causes them to continue seeking assistance to no avail. The end result of not addressing suffering is exceedingly costly, both economically and in human terms (12).

In addition, the question must be asked whether ethical practice permits the suspension of the patient's symbols, actions, and sensibilities because of the health professional's inaccurate interpretations of the person's suffering. Even if clinicians cannot directly address suffering, they can still help patients by acknowledging their own limitations to the patient. Appropriate referrals can then be made and the patient's experience of suffering validated and respected.

SUMMARY

There are many challenges in managing suffering in contemporary health care practice. The construct of suffering as a phenomenon separate from pain is proposed for consideration based on research studies (20–22) that report evidence that pain and suffering are separate entities that are only sometimes related. Perceptions of threat to idea of self, loss of central purpose, and self-conflict are measurable characteristics that identify the process of suffering. Differences between diagnosing suffering, which requires empathetic listening skills and assessing suffering to determine perceptions of threat, are delineated. The treatment of those who suffer requires slight shifts in approaches to clinical practice towards a less authoritative stance and an awareness of how individuals are able to change their idea of self. The identification of suffering is the responsibility of all health care providers. Referrals to colleagues in psychology and/or psychiatry are made when the clinician's skill set is not optimal and/or when patients request psychological counseling. The management of suffering requires the enhancement of clinical skills by practitioners in all divisions of medicine, such as nurses, social workers, chaplains, physicians, and therapists.

This chapter has focused on the theoretical hypotheses obtained from clinical observations and experience. The following chapter provides objective evidence to support the theory that suffering and pain are separate entities that are only sometimes related.

CHAPTER 1 QUESTIONS

1. Define suffering as a phenomenon separate from pain. How does this definition differ from traditional definitions of the past?
2. What are the universal characteristics of suffering?
3. What is meant by "idea of self"? How is idea of self different from identity?
4. What factors contribute to "personhood"?
5. Give some examples of the "central purpose" of an individual's life.
6. What is the difference between the type of question that describes the impact of illness as opposed to questions that delineate suffering?
7. What is the difference between assessment and diagnosis?
8. Why are some health care providers reluctant to address suffering in clinical settings?
9. Critically analyze the story of "Mr. Whitehead." What characteristics and factors indicate suffering?
10. Review the story of "Marlene." What factors differentiate between the universal characteristics of suffering and the personal expressions of suffering?

2 Suffering Is Not Pain

THE EVIDENCE

Science promised answers to all the mysteries of life, and postmodern society is the recipient of many of the wonders revealed and described by science. Unfortunately, contemporary society seems to have forgotten the revelations achieved through art and intuition. Consequently, in the attempt to conquer disease, many in medicine have forgotten that often it is not the disease that is the patient's real problem but rather the experience of illness. Suffering is not a disease, but it may well be the prime cause of the patient's experience of illness. Academic pundits may argue about the definitions of physical pain, psychic pain, and emotional pain, and these arguments have value because they stimulate creative thought, but in everyday life, those who suffer because of chronic illness or disability may require a more pragmatic approach.

Clinically, it is critical to understand the nature and origins of individuals' beliefs about the nature of suffering. It is not useful to combine suffering and pain as one entity. We know that some individuals who suffer experience little pain, and others who experience considerable pain report little suffering. The most useful understanding of suffering in medical practice is to acknowledge that suffering is a perception of threat to an individual's idea of self and personhood. Pain, whether physical, emotional, or psychic, is simply only one of many factors that may contribute to the experience of suffering.

The purpose of this chapter is to provide research evidence that shows that suffering, as defined above, and pain are separate and only sometimes related entities. The focus is on the relationship between (a) suffering and pain intensity in various diseases; (b) total suffering scores and pain intensity obtained from patients assessed using a self-administered, valid, and reliable questionnaire (MASQ); and (c) pain intensity and total pain scores in a group of patients with chronic illnesses such as arthritis, epilepsy, migraine headache, and spinal cord injury. Analyses of these data will show that some people who experience considerable suffering have low pain scores, while others with high pain scores have low suffering scores. These findings support the argument that if pain is eliminated, suffering does not always abate. The chapter concludes with a discussion that focuses on the significance of incorporating these research findings on suffering into clinical practice. The example given explores the relationship between suffering and monetary compensation in chronic illness or injuries. Emphasis is on cases of litigation involving tort law.

Research Evidence

Background

Considerable controversy exists about the ability to objectively identify those patients who experience suffering. Proponents of the argument for objective measures argue that universal characteristics of suffering such as a threat to idea of self and personhood, loss of central purpose, self-conflict, and impaired interpersonal relationships can be identified (1–3). Those against objective assessment argue that the experience is idiosyncratic and cannot be objectively evaluated (4–6). Our research team adopts the view that the characteristics of suffering are universal and measurable and it is only the expression of the experience that is idiosyncratic. Based on this theory, a self-administered questionnaire, the Measurement and Assessment of Suffering Questionnaire (MASQ), was designed and validated. Details of the items evaluated and results of statistical analyses relating to the validity and reliability of the questionnaire are reported in more detail in chapter 8. The hypothesis that suffering and pain are separate entities that are only sometimes related was tested on 381 patients who had chronic illnesses and who were attending either a hospital outpatient day program or were attending outpatient clinics.

Seventy-nine patients had migraine headache, 113 people had epilepsy, 23 had spinal cord injuries and 166 persons with arthritis were assessed. There were 66 females and 12 males in the migraine headache group with a mean age of 42.77 ± 12.22 years. Illness duration was 20.51 ± 11.98 years. The epilepsy group consisted of 58 females and 55 males with a mean age of 41.56 ± 11.42 years and the illness duration was 22.88 ± 12.96 years. The spinal cord injury group was considerably younger, with a mean age of 46.21 ± 8.54 years and an illness duration of 10.95 ± 11.91 years. There were 9 females in the group. The arthritis group consisted of 127 females and 39 males with a mean age of 60.31 ± 14.23 years. Illness duration was 10.95 ± 11.91 years (see table 2.1).

Of the 166 persons with arthritis, each subject was assessed at intake to a hospital outpatient day clinic and after approximately three weeks of treatment. All other subjects were assessed at intake only. Of the 113 persons with epilepsy, 13 people were part of the pilot study and data were collected and reported on another 100 people. Further, 38 of the 113 people with epilepsy had pain at the time of assessment and 2 of the 79 individuals with migraine headache had an aura only and were excluded from the analyses.

Measures of pain consisted of pain intensity, ability to endure the current level of pain, ability to endure more pain, anticipation of pain, ability to cope with more pain and belief of restoration of self if pain were removed. Suffering items focused on how much concern the patient had that their illness or injury would have a

TABLE 2.1 · Demographic Data of Participants (N = 381)

Disease category	Mean age	Gender	Duration of illness
Arthritis (N = 166)	60.31 ± 14.23 yrs	127 females	10.83 ± 11.16 yrs
Epilepsy (N = 113)	41.56 ± 11.42 yrs	58 females	22.88 ± 12.96 yrs
Migraine (N = 79)	42.77 ± 12.22 yrs	66 females	20.51 ± 11.98 yrs
Spinal cord (N = 23)	46.21 ± 8.54 yrs	7 females	10.95 ± 11.91 yrs

TABLE 2.2 · Relationship between Total Suffering and Pain Intensity, and between Total Suffering and Total Pain in Various Diseases

	Pearson correlation coefficients	
Disease category	Pain intensity	Total pain
Arthritis (N = 166)	0.343 (p = 0.000)	0.462 (p = 0.000)
Epilepsy (N = 100)	0.500 (p = 0.000)	0.428 (p = 0.000)
Migraine (N = 77)	0.210 (p = 0.060)	0.241 (p = 0.200)
Spinal cord (N = 23)	0.576 (p = 0.004)	0.648 (p = 0.001)

Note: p = the statistical probability that a phenomenon occurred by chance alone. The lower the p value the less likely it is that the finding occurred by chance. *Correlation coefficient* is a statistical measure of the interdependence of two or more random variables. Ranges in value are from −1 to +1. A value of −1 indicates a perfect negative correlation, 0 indicates an absence of correlations and +1 indicates a positive correlation.

negative impact on various aspects of self and personhood. Suffering item details are presented in chapter 8.

Mean scores, Pearson Correlation Coefficients, and Z score values were obtained for all groups and subgroups to determine the relationship between total suffering and pain intensity and total pain scores. Z scores are calculated to determine the exact location of a score in a distribution. The Z score indicates the number of standard deviations above or below a given mean.

Data analyses show that the relationship between suffering and pain is not strong (see table 2.2). The relationship between pain intensity and total suffering scores is: Pearson Correlation Coefficient $r = 0.343$, $p = 0.000$ for the arthritis group; $r = 0.500$, $p = 0.000$ for the epilepsy group; $r = 0.210$, $p = 0.06$ for migraine headache subjects; and $r = 0.576$, $p = 0.004$ for the spinal cord injury group. If pain and suffering were the same entity, correlation coefficients would be $r = 1.0$. These data show that factors other than pain contribute to suffering. Data also show that the probability of results obtained being due to chance is also slight (1 chance in 1,000, for a p value of 0.000).

TABLE 2.3 · Mean Differences within Disease Categories between Pain Intensity and Total Suffering Scores

Disease category	Pain intensity	Total suffering
Arthritis (N = 166)	02.99 ± 0.83 SD	03.27 ± 0.65 SD
Epilepsy (N = 100)	01.97 ± 1.37 SD	02.31 ± 0.83 SD
Migraine (N = 77)	01.69 ± 0.98 SD	02.69 ± 0.71 SD
Spinal cord (N = 23)	02.70 ± 1.66 SD	02.55 ± 0.74 SD

Note: Standard Deviation (SD) = a statistical measure that indicates the amount of variability in a group of scores.

TABLE 2.4 · Correlation between Total Suffering and Pain Intensity for Pain Subgroups

Disease category	Pearson correlation coefficients
Epilepsy (N = 38)	0.363 (p = 0.02)
Migraine (N = 30)	−0.03 (p = 0.86)
Spinal cord (N = 18)	0.538 (p = 0.02)

Note: See table 2.2 for definitions of p and correlation coefficient.

The relationship between total pain scores and total suffering scores is also weak (see table 2.2). With Pearson Correlation Coefficients of $r = 0.462$, $p = 0.000$ for arthritic patients; $r = 0.428$, $p = 0.000$ for the epilepsy group; $r = 0.241$, $p = 0.20$ for individuals with migraine headache; and $r = 0.648$, $p = 0.001$ for patients who have had a spinal cord injury.

Mean scores for pain intensity ranged from "a little pain" to "a lot." The scale ranged a score from 0 to 5 ("no pain" to "a great deal" of pain) (see table 2.3). We then looked at the subgroup of patients who had pain while taking the test. Again, Pearson Correlation Coefficients were not strong (see table 2.4). The relationship for the epilepsy patients was $r = 0.363$, $p = 0.02$, and a value of $r = 0.538$, $p = 0.02$ was found for the spinal cord injury group. In the migraine headache group there was a very inverse relationship($r = -0.03$, $p = 0.86$). When pain decreased, suffering increased, and when suffering decreased, pain increased. The $p = 0.86$ value indicates a high probability that this finding was due to chance.

Figures 2.1 and 2.2 illustrate the fact that pain and suffering are separate entities that are only sometimes related. If the relationship were strong, one would see the data points all clustered on the line of fit. This finding does not occur in any of the groups tested. Some of the data points do fall on the line of fit, which indicates that in some individuals pain and suffering, while not the same entity, are closely related.

Figure 2.1

The Relationship Between Total Suffering and Total Pain

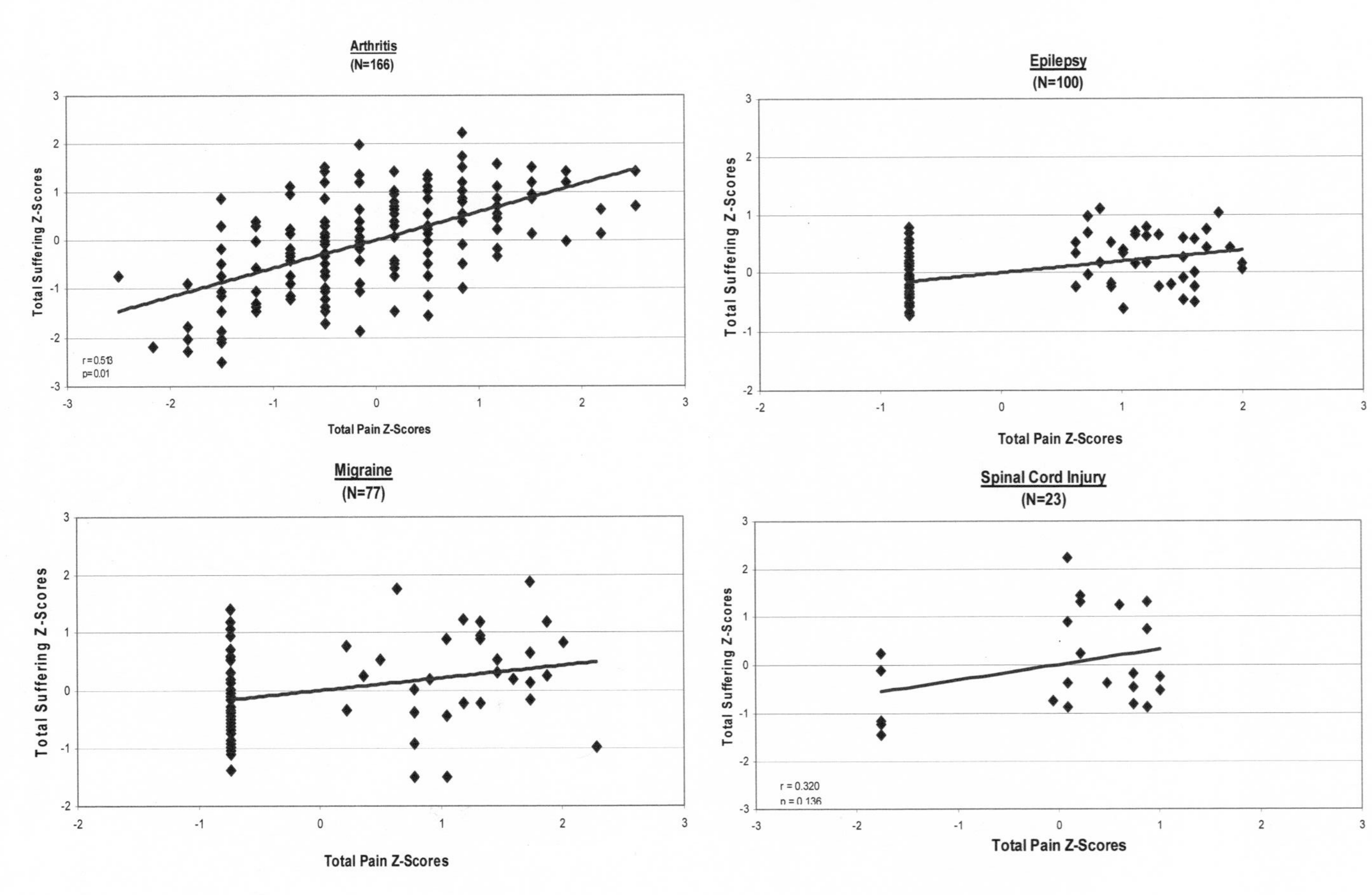

Figure 2.2
The Relationship Between Pain Intensity and Total Suffering

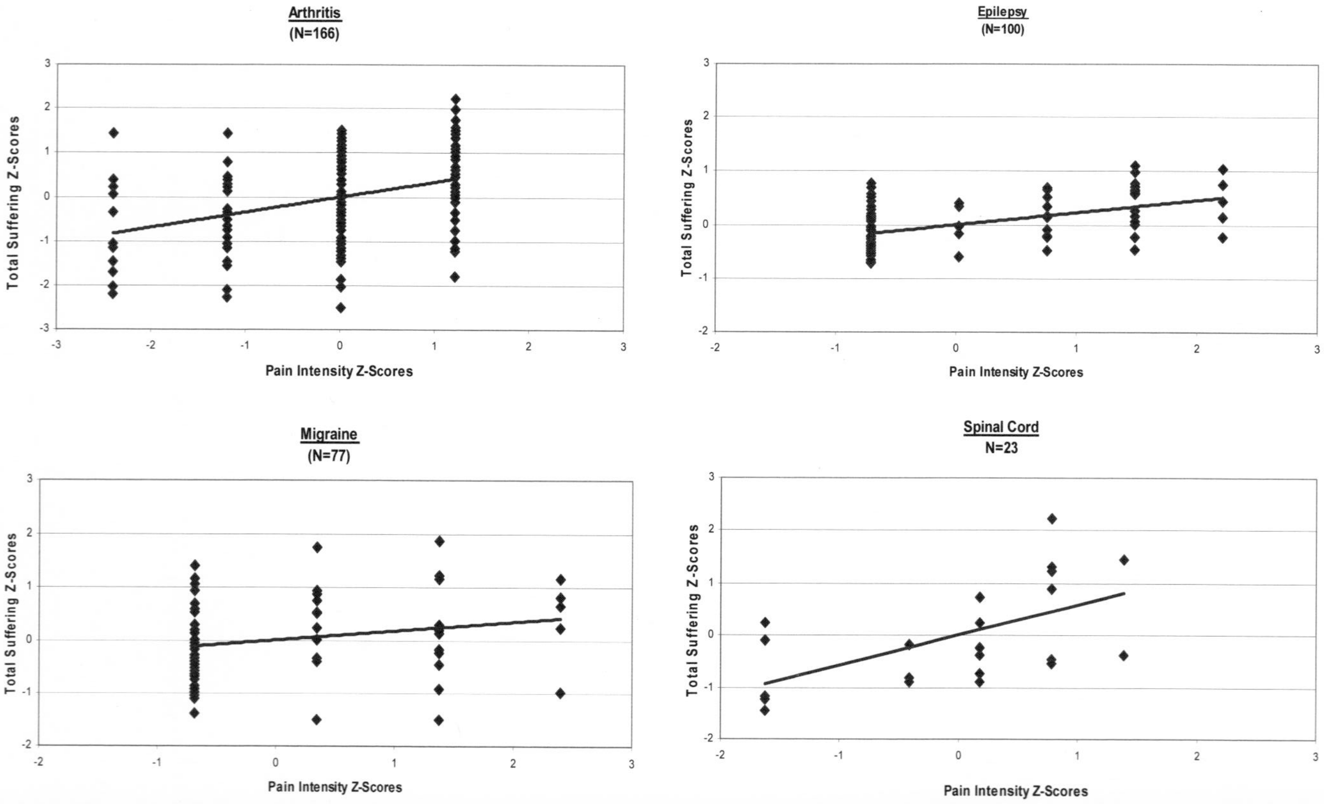

Arthritis
(N=166)

Total Suffering Z-Scores
3
2
1
0
-1
-2
-3
-3 -2 -1 0 1 2 3
Pain Intensity Z-Scores

Epilepsy
(N=100)

Total Suffering Z-Scores
3
2
1
0
-1
-2
-2 -1 0 1 2 3
Pain Intensity Z-Scores

Migraine
(N=77)

Total Suffering Z-Scores
3
2
1
0
-1
-2
-2 -1 0 1 2 3
Pain Intensity Z-Scores

Spinal Cord
N=23

Total Suffering Z-Scores
3
2
1
0
-1
-2
-2 -1 0 1 2 3
Pain Intensity Z-Scores

These objective research results provide evidence to support the hypothesis that suffering and pain are separate entities that are only sometimes related.

Traditionally, treatment objectives are to apply interventions that decrease pain with the anticipation that there will be a corresponding decrease in suffering. Sometimes this assumption is correct, but in many instances, particularly those in which there are multiple injuries or progressive disease, it is not. In chronic illness, failure to recognize suffering as a separate entity can lead to chronic disability and an escalation of health care costs. To illustrate this point further, we will consider an example of patient Neal, who had severe shoulder and neck pain due to a whiplash injury sustained in an automobile accident.

THE STORY OF NEAL

Neal has been referred to physiotherapy for treatment of a whiplash injury. He is a bright young advertising executive who spends a great deal of time in front of his computer. His job also involves considerable travel by car, and he is expected to play golf and tennis with business clients. Neal is married with two young children who are used to rough play with their father and who look forward to their time together.

When patients are referred to physiotherapy, the most common current model of practice usually involves an initial assessment to identify patient problems by the physiotherapist (figure 2.3). Problems are identified and treatment interventions begin. Most assessments involve determining the nature of the patient's complaints. Areas of focus are pain and swelling, pain location, type of pain (dull, sharp, or burning pain) and duration and intensity of the pain. Examinations also involve observation of the anatomy of the affected part, condition of the skin, palpitation of the muscle, determination of joint range of motion, and evaluation of muscle strength. Rarely are patients asked what impact the injury has on the patient's everyday life or what fears the patient may have about the injury or recovery.

Patients are often anxious to know whether the physiotherapist thinks full recovery will occur. At this point the physiotherapist knows the natural history of the disorder but does not know for certain what degree of recovery will occur. If the patient believes that the probable outcome of treatment is negative or even uncertain, then the injuries may be perceived by the individual as a threat to him in his roles as successful businessman and father. His idea of self may be perceived as threatened, and suffering occurs. If at some point in the treatment process, the patient is able to develop a new idea of self, even if he cannot do his job in exactly the same way or be the same father he once was, suffering ceases. If the patient cannot form a new idea of self or imagine his life evolving in a new acceptable way, then suffering persists. In such situations patients do not achieve maximal

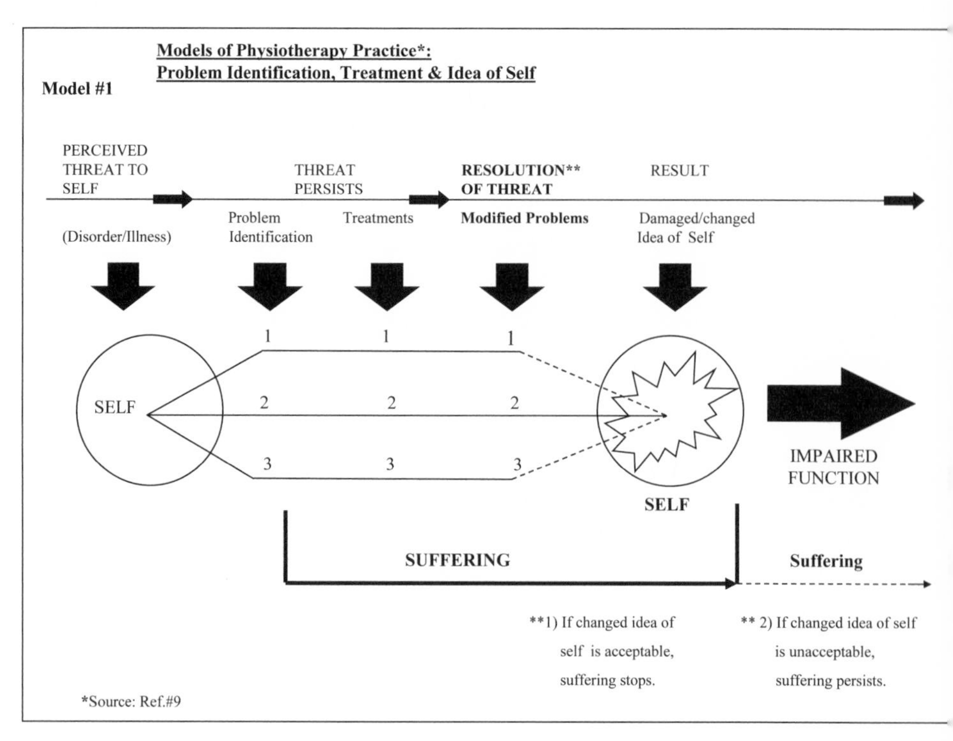

Figure 2.3

functional return, do not manage their everyday life optimally, and may seek repeated treatments for nonspecific complaints. The end result is an escalation of health care costs. Further, the physiotherapist may be left with the impression that the treatments were not effective or that the person was not putting his maximal effort into getting better. In Neal's case, which involves a motor vehicle accident, such opinions on the part of the medical personnel may have serious financial implications if insurance claims are being pursued. If Neal is seen to be not participating fully in his treatments, he may be labeled as malingering and his claims for fiscal compensation may be inappropriately assessed or denied.

Using the same scenario in which Neal has sustained a whiplash injury with severe shoulder pain and limitation of movement, there is another common set of events seen not only in physiotherapy clinics but also observed in the doctor's office. If the patient experiences suffering and the issue is not identified and addressed, the patient may try to tell the health care professional about the suffering using the language of pain. The physician may respond with a prescription for more or different medications, and the physiotherapist will likely reassess the patient. Because medicine is an inexact science that relies largely on qualitative evidence and patient complaints, the physiotherapist will probably identify more

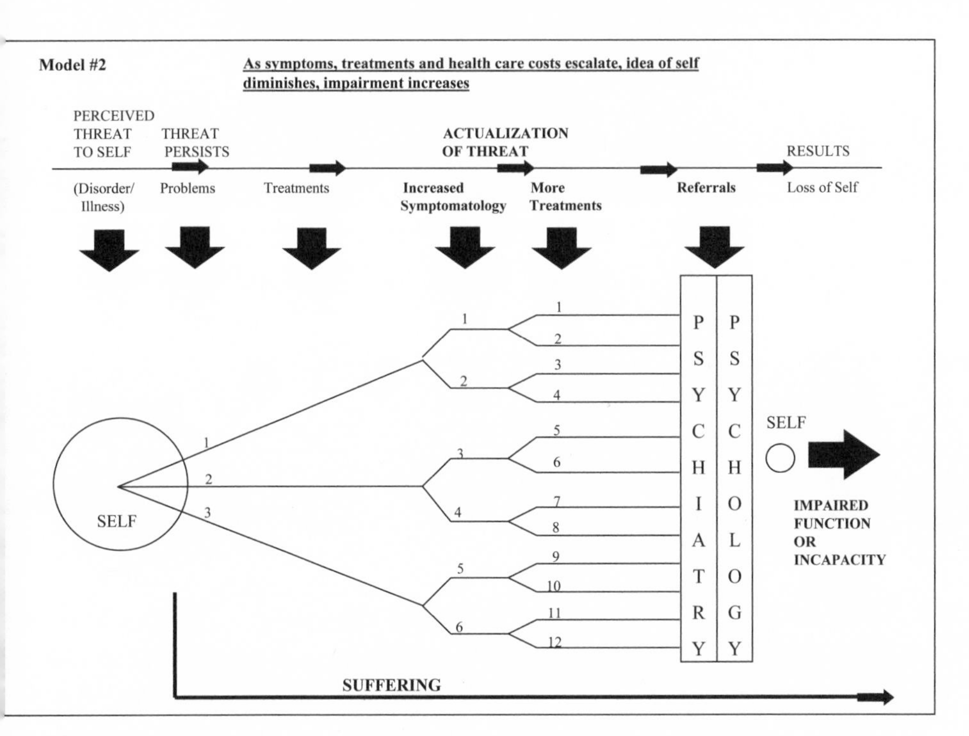

Figure 2.4

problems based on these new patient complaints and then try more interventions. The end result will still be unsatisfactory, and the patient, who originally sought treatment for perhaps three problems, now complains of several more (see figure 2.4). Usually, the physiotherapist will try to determine the relationship between the symptoms and known pathophysiology. If little or no correlation between the symptoms and known pathology is found, the health care provider may come to the conclusion that either the pain has become chronic, the patient has some other unexplained pathology, or the patient is not truthful. The patient may then be referred to myriad other health care professionals where complaints may continue to escalate. This process is detrimental to both the patient's idea of self and personhood and to the containment of health care expenditures. Studies of this process occurring with physicians are also documented (10–12).

Watkins et al. (11) report that patients who are treated for chronic pain make an average of 8.6 ambulatory visits to their doctor per year, and those who do not tell their doctor about pain (one in five patients with chronic pain) make an average of 5.2 return visits. Further, the authors report that the impact of pain on lifestyle is comparable between groups. Treatments in the study were traditional pharmacological interventions and modalities such as acupuncture, massage,

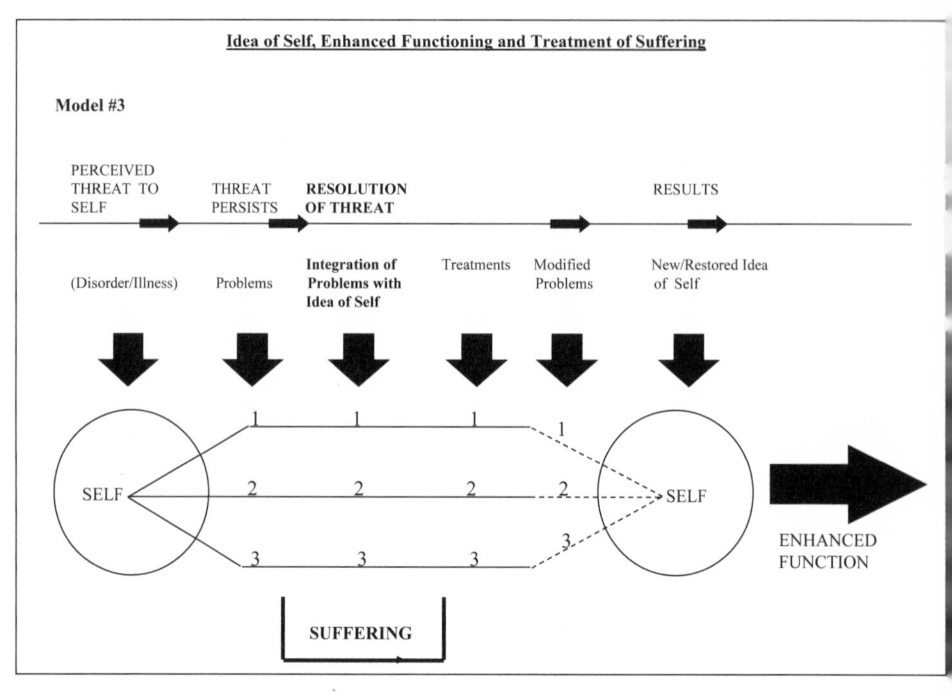

Figure 2.5

and chiropractic interventions. More research is needed to determine if physician visits decrease further when suffering strategies are part of the treatment regimens.

In a previously published paper (9) we have shown that the identification of suffering as an entity separate from pain as soon as the patient is assessed for physical complaints and the application of suffering specific treatment strategies prevents an escalation of symptomatology, a resolution of suffering, a preservation of an individual's idea of self and personhood, and improvement in physical function and a decrease in health care delivery costs.

The above examples are applicable to all types of disorders and are independent of the severity of the experience. The main question is to determine whether the patient can imagine a self that is acceptable for his life.

The impact of the failure to acknowledge suffering as an entity separate from pain in clinical practice is illustrated with an example of practice models from physiotherapy. An enhanced model for care (see figure 2.5) that incorporates identifying and implementing suffering-specific strategies shows the benefits to individuals with chronic illnesses as well as to cost containment concerns relevant to efficacious, client-centred health care delivery systems.

In summary, figure 2.6 compares treatment models in which suffering is or is

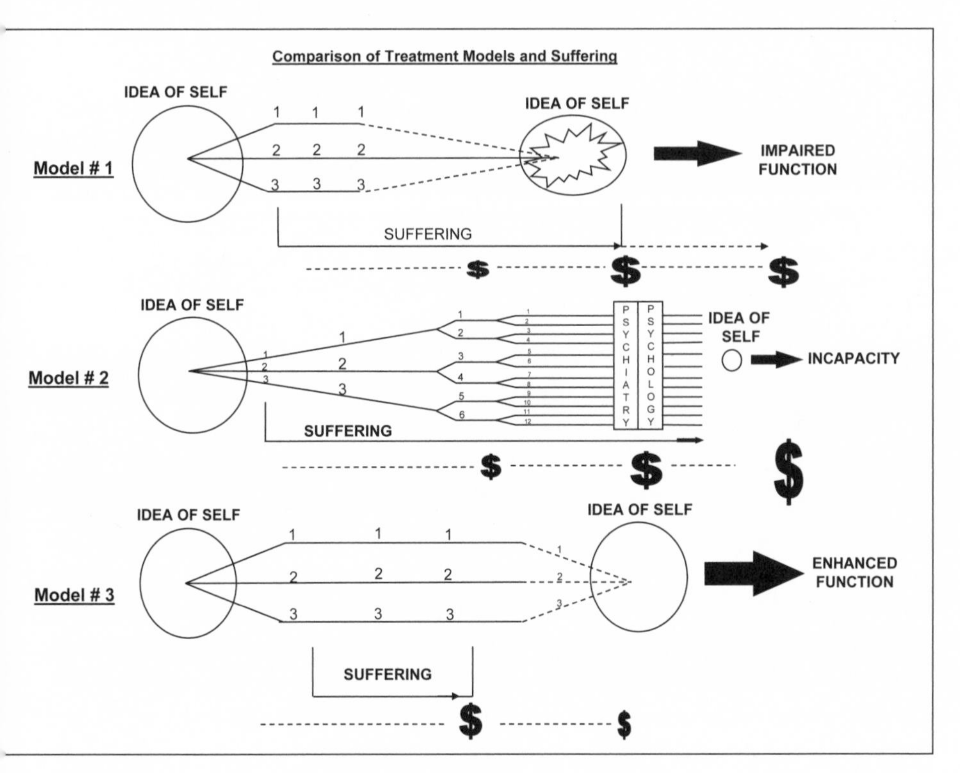

Figure 2.6

not addressed. The impact of suffering on idea of self and on fiscal expenditures and abilities to participate in everyday life are illustrated.

Significance of Research Findings: Clinical Challenges

Research evidence (1–3) shows that suffering and pain are separate and only sometimes related phenomena. To adhere to the principle of medical ethics in which all clinicians are committed to "doing no harm," the issue of monetary compensation for the effects of injury may negatively intrude. Currently, tort law, both in North America and Europe, is a legal mechanism for compensating people for pain, suffering, and loss of enjoyment in life. A study by Wissler et al. (4) showed that in the United States monetary awards allotted to individuals are greatly influenced by the characteristics and consequences of the injuries and are only marginally affected by the cause of the injury and the patient's responsibility in the accident. The more severe the injury, the higher the pain and suffering compensation. Further, disability, rather than degree of impairment, made the greatest contribution to the allotment of monies, followed by mental suffering, visibility of the disability, and lastly the degree and duration of pain. The ability of health care professionals to objectively assess suffering is of critical importance if ethical practice is to be maintained.

Without a valid and reliable tool to assess suffering, the veracity of patient complaints may be challenged. Coupled with the fact that in North America the amounts of monetary awards are extremely variable, the veracity of the patient's story is often questioned. Is the patient telling the truth about suffering, or is the individual a fraud? The challenge for health care professionals is to avoid becoming engaged in this adversarial argument. Ethically, objective evidence based on facts must be the goal of all health care assessments.

In the North American tort system, there is considerable unfair variability of plaintiff awards. The greatest source of differences in the monies awarded is the calculation of noneconomic damages and the calculation of punitive damages to the defendant. Economic damages are the easiest to calculate because they relate to medical bills and lost wages. In the United States, noneconomic damages estimated in 2001 made up 50% of all monies awarded, for a cost of $40 billion. Punitive damages are designed to punish the defendant for highly culpable behaviours. Less than 4% of all lawsuits involved punitive damages. In the United States, 60% of all pain and suffering awards are allocated on a purely random basis. Lawyers, judges, and juries all have idiosyncratic understandings of suffering in medicine. Because of the nature of the randomness of allocating awards and the fact that lawyers fees are closely associated with the amount of monies granted, some lawyers do not want to be able to objectively determine the cost of pain and suffering. Further, such determinations are objectively difficult to ascertain because lawyers are forbidden, on the rules of evidence, to make comparisons between cases (11). Consequently, one person may be given $1,000 for twenty minutes of pain, and another individual may receive $100,000 for the same event. Without a valid and reliable assessment tool, determinations of suffering are even more difficult.

Health care providers, often inadvertently, influence the outcomes of awards to patients for pain and suffering by providing opinions and not facts based on science. In the following chapters, this issue will be explored in more detail and an objective, reliable, assessment tool (MASQ) is presented to show that suffering can be objectively identified, separate from pain.

In multicultural societies such as Canada and the United States, health care professionals must realize that both individuals and health care professionals trained outside these countries may have different understandings of tort law and its impact on health. In Europe, attitudes towards fiscal compensation are vastly different from those in North America. For example, in Germany few patients engage in litigation, possibly because of the availability and nature of insurance coverage in that country. Lawyers earn less than one-third of the contingency fees paid in the United States and receive compensation whether or not cases are won. There are no awards for punitive damages. All damages awards allocated in every trial court in Germany are recorded in a book called the *Tabellen*. This book is published and used to estimate damages in new cases.

These differences between the German and American systems show the need for clinicians to provide precise objective assessments of suffering. In North America, personal liberty is of utmost importance to the personhood of all individuals. Only with objective evidence will health care professionals continue to provide ethical care to those who succumb to chronic illness or injury. In countries such as Germany, where the theory is that everyone owes duty to everyone else, the ethics of medical practice are based on the tenets of fair play substantiated by the *Tabellen*. Legal systems worldwide are constantly being revised, as is evidenced by publications on the need for the European Union to advance the unification of the legal systems of the various members of the union (12). It is clear that ethical health care practice is best advanced through a comprehensive understanding of suffering as an entity separate and only sometimes related to pain.

In chapter 7, entitled "The Disclosure of Suffering: Medical and Legal Discourse," the importance of understanding the tenets upon which the law is based and their impact on ethical health care delivery will be explored in more detail. All clinicians and their patients benefit from a clear understanding of the purpose of the various laws of their respective countries. A failure to comprehend these laws can result in a violation of medical ethics and facilitate an escalation of patients' health care complaints with a corresponding escalation of health care costs.

SUMMARY

This chapter has provided the results of Correlation Coefficients that provide evidence to support the hypothesis that suffering and pain are separate and only sometimes related entities. To review: Suffering, defined as a perception of threat to the individual's idea of self and personhood, is an entity separate and only sometimes related to pain intensity, pain beliefs, and pain coping. Addressing suffering as separate from pain may also facilitate the reduction of pain. Other scientific studies show that the risk of suicide in pain patients is double that of controls (12). This finding supports the need for further investigation of the relationship between suffering and pain.

The objective evidence shows that suffering as an entity separate from pain is important also to the component of personhood that involves fiscal compensation for debilitating illnesses or injuries. Differences between tort law in North America and Germany show that health care professionals must fully understand suffering as a unique entity if the medical ethic of "doing no harm" is to be upheld.

To be of clinical assistance to individuals with chronic illness who experience suffering and pain, clinicians must have at least a basic understanding of factors that may impact on idea of self and personhood. The next chapter will explore the power of traditional spiritual and religious beliefs on individuals who suffer.

CHAPTER 2 QUESTIONS

1. What is the relationship between suffering and pain intensity in patients with arthritis, epilepsy, migraine headache, and spinal cord injuries?
2. What is the significance of the relationship between pain intensity and total suffering in patients with migraine headache?
3. What factors constitute "total pain" in the MASQ?
4. Describe a practice model based on the goals of your own profession. What is the impact of suffering on idea of self and health outcome measures?
5. Using the same model, what health outcomes can be improved if suffering is identified and treated from intake to discharge?
6. What are the fiscal expenditure and health status outcomes if suffering is considered to be the secondary component of pain?
7. In the American tort system what percentages of pain and suffering awards are allocated on a purely random basis?
8. Why is it important to understand the difference between suffering and pain and issues of personhood?

3 The Power of Religious and Spiritual Beliefs

Postmodern medicine has, to a large extent, abandoned its passionate commitment to the whole person to embrace the cold, distant anonymity of the technological age. We have forgotten the wisdom of the words of the poets of the past. The British poet William Wordsworth lamented that "The world is too much with us" and that "we have given our hearts away" (1). In the poignant words inspired by Persian poet Hafiz, "Now is the time to know that all you do is sacred." Many others are lost to antiquity (2). In medicine, such losses come at great cost to those who are ill and suffer and to those whose job it is to heal and cure. As seen in the previous chapter, failure to understand suffering results in a loss of human potential and an increase in health care expenditures. To fully understand the experience of suffering in medicine, it is critical to understand the power of an individual's spiritual and religious beliefs, past and present.

The purpose of this chapter is (a) to briefly outline key aspects of personal suffering in several major world traditions, including the Judeo-Christian tradition, Hinduism, Buddhism, Confucianism, humanism, Islam, and North American and African aboriginal worldviews, and (b) to show how these belief systems may impact on clinical practice. Because extensive examination of these issues is beyond the scope of this text, a comprehensive reference list is provided for those desiring more intensive study.

Perspectives on Suffering

The challenge to modern health care practitioners is, first, to understand the origins of patients' cultural, religious, and spiritual worldviews about health and suffering and, second, to determine the influence of these belief systems in contemporary life.

A Western Worldview: Judeo-Christian Perspectives

Historically, the Western world view embraces the idea of a perfectly ordered universe in which there is an infinitely good, omnipotent God (3). Suffering occurs when there is a failure on the part of an individual or his soul to assume its proper position in the harmony of this ideal order. No suffering is senseless but rather is deserved or redemptive. In the most simplistic terms this worldview acknowledges that God is good, God is powerful, and evil exists. Because this perspective embraces the notion of original sin, the main task of the individual/soul, both in health and wellness, is to try to restore the natural order. Sources of suffering are imbalances in the body, distorted interpersonal relationships, difficulties with an individual's powers of self-possession, self-control, as well as influences from the external world. Self-possession in this latter sense is often referred to as "the will" (4, 5). In Judaism, Rosh Hashanah is a two-day holiday in which individuals assess their actions, existence, and choices in life. It is a time for personal restoration and is followed by ten days of penitence leading to the holy holiday of Yom Kippur (6). In the Christian tradition the confession of sins is also a practice of appraisal and renewal of the self. The Lenten holidays and Easter vigilance are further examples of Christian self-renewal. Great value is placed on the power of the will and individual choice. Some believe that humans choose and even create evil, as is depicted in stories of the fall from grace in the Garden of Eden.

There are many theories concerning the nature of evil. Some argue that there are natural evils such as earthquakes, physical pain, and death, and there are moral evils that are due to actions or omissions attributed to perversion of the will, knowledge, or love. Suffering is seen to be the consequence of evil in some form, and as humans we must experience suffering to help us grow in wisdom and grace. God does not cause or remove evil, but God does walk with those who suffer. Ancient teachings of privation theories (7) state that God created a wholly good but hierarchical universe. "Higher beings" have more good in them than "lesser beings," and evil is said to be an absence of God. Others believe that suffering cannot be explained but is part of the mystery of God and all individuals can do is enter into an encounter with the mysterious presence of God, who is always with us even in our suffering (8). People cannot escape suffering, but they can transcend it. Past teachings described a synthesis between suffering and pain, and early Christian narratives depicted suffering as powerful and redemptive. These narratives provided a mechanism to transcend the strictures of Roman ideology. Death was viewed as the ultimate victory for Christian martyrs. The martyr literature brought into social consciousness the view of the body in pain and the suffering body. Many aspects of these ancient texts persist in modern thought.

The effect of illness on the body results in suffering because in illness the body becomes an obstacle to the person, who can no longer shape the world in a way that is personally acceptable. Because of the limitations imposed by disease and/or illness, the patient's world becomes smaller, with an increased dependency on others. There is a loss of personal power (self-possession) and autonomy (will). In Judeo-Christian traditions, people often exert the power of the will through devotion and/or work. Limitations to work due to illness may result in perceptions of a lack of self-control or willpower. Further, the recollection of how one has dealt with past adversity and the belief that these methods are no longer viable, result in suffering. Individuals suffer if they violate their own principles of behaviour for whatever reason (9–17).

In Western thought, individuals strive to maintain an idea of self that is in harmony with a whole universe, consisting of God, history, the mind, a community of others, and an ultimate purpose. Consequently, in Judeo-Christian traditions, suffering has a purpose. Suffering is not senseless, because individuals are expected to learn from adversity and subsequently contribute to the restoration of the perfect order of the universe. The infinite goodness of God is omnipotent. Suffering is a way humankind enters into a divine relationship with God. For example, in the past, physicians were thought to have a divine relationship with God because they attended the sick (18, 19).

In summary, the key reasons humans suffer are that there is: (a) a failure on the part of people to be free from the restrictions of the body due to illness, (b) a perversion of the will, (c) a failure to submit to the will of God, and (d) a loss of central purpose that is sometimes interpreted in Christian traditions as failing to follow the teachings of Jesus and in Judaic law, the commandments given to Moses. Even people in our postmodern age, who often profess to have no belief in Judeo-Christian principals, may find themselves internally subjected to the demands of these past familial/societal traditions in times of severe adversity. Clinicians, to be effective, must have at least a cursory understanding of this worldview if effective, patient-centred care is to be provided.

As a result of these belief systems, Western contemporary health care delivery and research focus on the disharmony of the natural order of the body afflicted by disease. The above depictions of suffering in Judeo-Christian theology are very brief and are presented merely to provide a glimpse of how these beliefs can impact on health. They are presented to encourage health care providers to commit themselves to the necessity of lifelong learning about the beliefs of those entrusted to their care. Just as complex as Judeo-Christian teachings are those arising from an Eastern worldview.

Eastern Worldview

Hinduism · In early Hindu traditions, the universe is depicted in a series of ever-widening circles extending into eternity (20, 22). At the centre of these circles is a private self that is influenced by disturbances in these circles. Due to the complexity of society, the circles are not in fixed orbits and the goal of life is to maintain a balance between the influences of these circles and the centre (self). Good health depends on the person's ability to maintain a state of equilibrium. Health seeking is a religious obligation. Pain and suffering are not considered to be natural conditions, and nothing is to be gained by suffering.

According to traditional Hindu beliefs, the occurrence of suffering is thought to be due to several factors, such as wrongful thinking and disharmony between the cosmic order (dharma) and the laws of causality (karma). In cases of illness, the will must be preserved at all costs, particularly in a dying person. A poor prognosis must not be spoken to the patient for fear of hastening death. In Hinduism, the relationship between suffering and the self is seen through the perspective that all of life is part of the same community of religious thought, mythology, and legal practices. Reality consists of a non-decaying spirit (self, consciousness) and a decaying materiality.

Hindu traditions embrace the concept of two "selves." The true self (Atman) is transcendental, observing, and unable to unite the body. Only the false self (Ahamkara), which is phenomenal, has the capability to unite the body parts. Illness occurs because the unity of the body parts is precarious. It is not possible to rely on the transcendental self, and the phenomenal self is too fragile. Some evidence of the existence of self is breathing, blinking, biological functions, moving to another land in a dream, ability to shift from one sense organ to another, and concentration. In early Hindu thought the breath was associated with the notion of soul and self. It was the life force. Later, the concept of the self evolved as a true witness to the events of life freed from worldly connection. This freed self is not touched by death and is considered to be the absolute reality. The true self becomes part of the divine.

The body is considered to be capable of both malevolence and benevolence. It consists of wind, bile, and phlegm. The common belief is that all things are connected to the earth. Water is the essence of earth; plants depend on water to produce flowers, fruit, and seeds; and all is connected to humankind. This belief then evolved to five humors: earth, wind, fire, water, and ether or space. Body parts are associated with cosmic elements. For example, some believe the back is associated with heaven, the stars with bones, and the sun with eyes. Medieval views linked the body with gods and goddesses, and parts of the body with other spirits. Some yoga practices followed these beliefs. When the body is no longer viable the soul transmigrates. In addition, there is a hierarchy of body parts. Speech is the highest because it is the instrument of social interaction. The power of the mantra is thought to be the way one could communicate with the gods.

There are six schools of Hindu philosophy; one of the oldest is the Samkhya philosophy in which there is a belief that there are three unifying principles that form the natural world. They are called Sattva, Rajas, and Tamas. These principles are called *gunas*, and each one is intrinsically bound with the other. Rajas guna is responsible for action, energy, and preservation, while Tamas is the quality of laziness, darkness, and inactivity. Sattva is the quality of calmness and purity. Individuals may be defined as having too much of one or the other of these qualities; the ultimate goal of human life is to achieve a balance between them. The practice of medicine is derived primarily from the Ayurvedic school of thought.

In the Ayurvedic (*ayur*: life, *veda*: sacred) school of medical thought there are three mind/body principles that create specific mental and physical characteristics. Physicians practice medicine from a holistic perspective in which the mind, the self, and the body form the basis of living. These mind/body principles are called doshas. There are three doshas: Vata, Pitta, and Kapha. Vata is a force that is conceived as consisting of the element of ether (space) and air. Pitta is viewed as fire and water, forces that affect life transformations and are critical to the life process per se. Kapha is seen as the equilibrium between water and earth. It is concerned both with body structure and lubrication. Kapha maintains body resistance to illness and is responsible for biological strength and the immune system.

Ayurvedic medicine teaches the importance of eating proper foods, establishing good sleep habits, exercise, and stress management techniques to maintain health and facilitate healing. The patient can move from inertia to serenity or from an undesirable to a desirable state. People are subject to the same laws of the universe as the elements because they are made up of the same components. Therefore, all human contact has the potential to affect moral and physical well-being.

Health requires a suppression of negative mental impulses. Old age and congenital disorders are seen as natural conditions of life. Common social practice was to "shop around" for a suitable doctor, a practice not valued in contemporary medical thought.

Attitudes towards illness are that the laws governing a specific element are attributed to a specific bodily function. For example, fire and fever are related. Treatments also focus on the removal of poison, opening of channels, oiling of passages, and loosening of body parts. Language is very powerful, and great care is taken with the spoken word.

Buddhism · Buddhism does not recognize an individuated ultimate reality and does not incorporate the idea of a unique self. Suffering occurs because individuals believe in the power of the self. Belief in an individuated self is illusionary. The goal of Buddhism is to rid the world of suffering, and the way to achieve this goal is to get rid of a belief in this individuated self. It is believed that as reality constantly changes so does the mental and physical self. Everything is impermanent. The only thing that one may possibly control is the rate of change (23–28).

Several types of suffering occur in Buddhist thought. Ordinary suffering occurs with everyday events. Suffering occurs when there is awareness that all is decaying. Suffering also occurs because the nature of existence is conditioned or constructed. To achieve salvation, it is necessary to deconstruct the self. Spirituality is the awareness of the contrast between what life is and what it should be like when considering the body and suffering. In Buddhism, this awareness is true suffering. The body is seen as an entrapment for the soul.

Patients who follow this tradition may spend considerable effort in trying to understand the meaning of the adversity that afflicts them and what deficit in consciousness may have contributed to their illness. They believe an enlightened consciousness contributes to wellness and subscribe to a philosophy of trust and patience. Health care clinicians who wish to assist persons who adhere to Buddhist traditions must be prepared to address issues from the perspective of consciousness and patience. Failure to do so may lead to diagnostically incorrect interpretations of psychological denial and pathological passivity, with subsequent clinical outcomes of poor compliance and ineffective treatments. Patients are often willing to tolerate considerable pain because of the belief that pain and suffering are a natural part of life and the discomfort associated with these phenomena will pass.

Buddhist patients may have spiritual teachers who may be of assistance to health care professionals in understanding the relationship between mind and spirit. Contemporary health care team meetings may expand to include personal spiritual advisors.

Confucian Belief · This tradition focuses on the ideas that it is possible to perfect human nature and that learning to be human is a lifelong commitment. The self is constantly evaluating and transforming itself. Followers of this belief system have faith that humankind is good and can become what it once was before the "fall." Human uniqueness is not only a responsibility but also a privilege (29, 30).

In Confucianism, suffering is deserved and is endured because people make mistakes. Life is viewed as a burden caused by self-consciousness. Through mental and physical discipline, people can transcend the self. Humanity cannot bear the suffering of others. A valued response is to sacrifice oneself (altruism). Everyone has the capability to regard heaven and earth as one. There is nothing that is not oneself. Once a person cannot feel pain or understand suffering, that person has lost his/her humanity.

Buddhist and Confucian beliefs may seem, at first, to be incompatible with definitions of suffering in which suffering is seen as the perception of a threat to a person's idea of self. Further exploration, however, shows that these viewpoints are not in conflict, for while Buddhist and Confucian thought do not value adherence to the demands of the self, they do not deny the existence of the self and the human struggle for coherence. Postmodern medicine neither accepts nor rejects the self as an inherent cosmic value, but rather sees the self as one of the components of human beings.

Islam · In this tradition, God is the basis of life. The Holy Spirit is the essence of all life and arises from the world of divine commands (31–34). Health, illness, and death are preordained by God. The body is the vehicle by which the Holy Spirit manifests and functions in this world. The spirit within a person is a conscious, changing force which evolves as the body develops. The spirit determines each individual's unique personhood through the person's commitment to learning, reflection, beliefs, and worship. Individuals consist of a union between body and soul and health in the context of well-being. Wholeness is granted from God.

Suffering and illness are indicators that the originally intended wholeness has been disturbed. Suffering appears to exist within the context of wholeness and occurs so that one may learn a lesson from wrong doing or because humans must directly experience the consequences of human sins. Medicine and theology are closely linked. The prayers of the sick have the highest priority with God, and those who are ill are encouraged in their devotions.

Medical knowledge and practice is seen to be directed by God. This view may, in some instances, be in conflict with contemporary medical practice, which adopts a secular perspective, as it serves a multicultural society. The challenge for medicine is similar to that of individual health care practitioners who may have to find methods of dealing with systemic differences that occur between their own personal religious convictions (e.g., abortion, end-of-life controversies) and that of the health care organizations (scientific evidence). Modern medicine strives to develop methods of integrating the cultural beliefs of individuals within the larger framework of optimal health care delivery strategies.

In Islam, medical practice is a religious necessity for the society at large and should always be practiced in a climate of respect and awareness of the presence of God. The patient's feelings, privacy, and body are treated with the utmost dignity. The goal of medicine is to help people who are under stress and not exploit their need. The doctor is the servant of the patient because the patient is in the sanctuary of his illness.

Three major tenets of spirituality and their relationship to health in Islam are: (a) faith (to be safe and at peace), (b) wholeness (integral, not disintegrating), and (c) piety (conscious of God, protected). The mind is the rational aspect of the soul, the spirit is the intellect, and the body is the material faculty. The mind and spirit can work together to overcome the limitations of the body. There is a strong belief that the choices made by the body, spirit, and mind throughout a lifetime have consequences extending into eternity. Health is viewed as a blessing. Sickness is a test and may occur to indicate death is at hand.

If one body system fails, then the spirit becomes disconnected from the body. If illness causes a disconnection of the whole body with the spirit, the body dies. Both the body and the soul may have illnesses. Sickness of the soul may involve forgetfulness of the divine presence. Examples are jealousy and avarice. The valued response to illness is endurance. The sleep of the ill person is sometimes viewed as a form of worship, and the cries of patients are a litany in praise of God. No disease is sent without a corresponding treatment. It is a person's obligation to maintain health, to seek treatments, and to observe religious traditions. Further, it is considered a blessing and privilege as well as an obligation to visit the ill. To do so is to be in the presence of God. Incorporation or reaffirmation of these principles in clinical practice has the potential to enhance the practice of client-centred care.

Aboriginal Traditions

North American · There is a strong connection between health and the power of the supernatural world in North American aboriginal traditions (35–37). Healing occurs through persons whose inspiration and training have enabled them to become mediators between human beings and the supernatural world. In ancient times, healing was thought to be the result of a supernatural blessing. Human beings, the supernaturals, and the world form a unified whole. Human beings contribute to this universal harmony through rituals. Health is totally dependent on one's relationship with the supernatural. Suffering is accepted as inevitable, and individuals strive to find ways to restore the relationship with the supernatural in a positive way. Great value is placed on the ability to withstand hardship, cold, and physical pain.

In North American aboriginal traditions, suffering is not related to pain. Past reports from various tribal groups on suffering focus on the fear and stress that occurs when individuals believe that their way of life is threatened (floods, drought, forest fires, etc.). Death is viewed as a way to prevent overpopulation and was devised by the creator and a trickster companion.

Disease is believed to be a gradual dying. In dying, the soul moves towards the realm of the dead and when it reaches its destination the person is dead. Health is a supernatural gift or a consequence of having good relations with cosmic powers. Not all injuries have a supernatural origin. Examples include fractures, muscular strains, and cuts and bruises. Such disorders may be healed by senior members of the community who are experienced herbalists. Medicine men, who are thought to be supernatural beings, use supernatural means such as inspirational visions. Healings may occur either when the medicine man is lucid or semiconscious. Shamans are doctors working in a deep trance and with the aid of a guardian spirit. The shaman may enter a deep trance and send his soul or one of his souls for assistance. Shamans are medicine men but are not always doctors.

Diagnoses made by shamans may take two major forms, object and/or spirit intrusion or loss of the soul. In the case of object intrusion, a damaging spiritual being of minor dimensions or an object may enter a person's body, causing pain, swelling, or wounds. When a spirit acts to cause illness, it is believed that the spirit has been enraged because the individual has broken a taboo or ritual rule.

Patients who believe their illness is due not only to a disease (viruses, bacteria) but also a spirit force may seek care from both a shaman and a medical practitioner.

Failure to be aware of these worldviews may result in incomplete treatments and poor outcomes.

In cases of soul loss, the belief is that human beings have two different soul complexes. One soul complex sustains the individual during consciousness and one soul, known as the free soul, is active during unconsciousness (sleep, trance). The two souls interact with each other. A soul may leave the body unexpectedly due to a shock or injury and go to the realm of the dead. As long as someone's soul remains with the individual, the person's life is not in danger. Only in exceptional cases is the shaman able to rescue the free soul and restore the person's life.

Health and life are a supernatural gift. Human beings exist in the supernatural world before they are born. When one is called to be born, the supreme creator gives the body the life soul and free soul. Death is set aside and secluded from the worlds of humans, spirits, and gods. Death holds no fear. In general, the realm of death is not articulated and beliefs focus on living well and in harmony with the physical and spiritual worlds.

African · There are approximately 3,000 African tribes and each has its own religious system (38–42). In general, African worldviews contend that there is no separation between the sacred and secular. Religion is part of all aspects of life and is often thought to begin before birth and extend after death. Religion is not specifically for the individual, because the belief is that to be human is to be part of a community. The concept of time is unique and defines an individual. For example, actual time is what is present and what is past. There is no concept relating to a future. A person's identity is established partly in his own life and partly through generations to a time before his birth. In some of the African societies a person is not considered fully born until he/she has undergone the process of physical birth, naming ceremonies, puberty, initiation rites, and marriage/procreation. After death the person returns to the original pre-birth state and is present on earth through those who remember his name. Consequently, it is important to have children who will remember your name. People may be remembered for several generations. While remembered, an individual is in a place called the living dead. Incorporating the value of community and health for persons who subscribe to these views may be a challenge for health care administrators who are not able to merge a sense of ceremony involving patient, family, and community with fiscal restraint.

African religions are older than Christianity and Islam and there are no sacred scriptures, missionaries, or conversions in this tradition. Religious participation begins before birth and persists after death. The names of people have religious meanings. Suffering occurs when the individual experiences hardship, is the victim of evil spirits, or is punished for contravening customs or traditions. Suffering is not the providence of God. God is holy, wise, and creative. God's will determines everything. God heals the sick even when medicines are used. African aboriginal teachings hold that God is the originator and sustainer of the universe. All spirits, people, animals, and plants are of God, and to destroy or remove the mystical relationship is an affront to God. As in North American aboriginal traditions, sickness is a religious experience, and people go to both traditional doctors and medicine men.

Humanism

Humanism is defined as a rationalistic system of thought attaching prime importance to human rather than divine or supernatural matters. It is a Renaissance cultural movement that turned away from medieval scholasticism and revived interest in ancient Greek and Roman thought (40–42). Contemporary understandings of humanism vary. Some argue that humanism is a religion, others that it is a nontheistic belief system, and still others maintain that it is an educational method. Adherents of humanism philosophies divide humanism into three categories: (a) nontheistic nonreligious humanism, (b) nontheistic religious humanism, and (c) theistic religious humanism.

A basic understanding of the tenets of humanism is important because medicine is based on humanist principles. Terms commonly used to describe humanistic thought are secular or scientific humanism. Understanding humanism is important because it encompasses the educational methods under which all health care providers are trained. Humanism subscribes to the idea of perfect health for all and is concerned with solving problems through rational thought.

Secular humanism states that all dogmas or traditions need to be tested using reason, evidence, and the scientific method. All individuals must strive for personal fulfillment, growth, and creativity. There is a constant desire to seek truth and to seek meaning in life both personally and historically. Adversity may present many challenges to patients who adhere to humanist principles, because the process of suffering per se does not have an intrinsic value. It does not necessarily provide meaning or absolute truth; it is simply a process in which there is a perception of threat to an individual's idea of self and personhood. Surviving suffering may result in new life meanings and "truths" for some individuals, but the experience per se does not have redemptive power. Suffering from the perspective of humanism is neither bad nor good. In humanism, viable social and political principles pertaining to ethical conduct are essential to society. Each individual must strive to greet the ideas of others with goodwill, tolerance, and reason for the advancement and well-being of the world. Understanding the spiritual and religious beliefs of patients is a basic tenet of humanistic thought.

The challenge of addressing suffering and humanism in medicine is twofold. The clinician must understand humanism as a spiritual tradition and as an educational system. In general, postmodern medical organizational systems usually subscribe to secular humanism, which is devoid of religious traditions. Private hospitals with religious origins are also challenged by the need to care for patients who follow humanist philosophies. Public system health care workers may find considerable organizational resistance to any type of ceremony. The successful management of suffering involves the ability to integrate evidence-based methodologies with a degree of ceremony, which is an integral part of the management of those who experience the process of suffering. Early identification and treatment of those who suffer is critical if the goals of ethical practice and cost containment are to be achieved.

SUMMARY

The world traditions described in this chapter touch only on the very basic tenets of a select group of belief systems. There are many other traditions and subcomponents of the above groups, but the issue of idea of self and its relationship to various aspects of human life and the cosmos is evident in all traditions. Further, while many in contemporary society hold views based on philosophical humanist perspectives, it must be remembered that ideas of self and personhood are key issues. Awareness of cultural/spiritual teachings are important, not to profile individuals, but rather to form a basis for therapeutic dialogue leading to comprehensive, effective care of the patient.

In addition, issues of culture, ethnicity, and nationality are components of individuals' idea of self and personhood in pluralistic multicultural societies. Effective health care delivery occurs when clinicians fully understand the tenets of assimilation, acculturation, customs, and rights and practices from a framework of cultural sensitivity and competency. These issues are examined in chapter 4.

Past mythology may persist, in part, in modern medicine. It is most important that health care providers have at least a basic knowledge of a person's cultural heritage. The value of this knowledge is not to make assumptions about an individual but rather to have the skills required to be sensitive to potential patient concerns based on past/present cultural teachings. In contemporary medicine, the efficacy of treatment interventions may be enhanced if the diverse belief systems of patients and the various ways individuals pray are recognized. Failure to do so may result in patients feeling isolated and/or abandoned, factors not conducive to achieving optimal treatment outcomes.

An additional challenge to contemporary medical practice is that in North American society, many persons subscribing to Buddhist beliefs have been educated in other traditions (Catholicism, Judaism, etc.) in their formative years. The management of suffering may be complicated by these different perspectives.

Again, the unity of theology and medicine in many of these worldviews requires understanding and a creative ability on the part of the health care provider if client-centred care is to be accurately assessed and provided.

CHAPTER 3 QUESTIONS

1. How is suffering viewed in Judeo-Christian traditions?
2. How do Hindu beliefs about "self" impact on health?
3. In Buddhism, how does the illusionary self relate to the secular "ideas of self" in contemporary society?
4. What types of suffering occur based on Buddhist thought?
5. What are the Islamic beliefs about suffering and illness?
6. What is the process of healing in North American aboriginal traditions?
7. How is the self understood in African aboriginal belief systems?
8. What is humanism?
9. How does contemporary medicine view human suffering?

4 Suffering and Culture

Cultural traditions have a profound effect not only on individuals' idea of self but also on the identity of families and the community at large. Cultural traditions may augment not only the experience of suffering but also its expression. Insensitivity to transcultural issues can result in ineffective health care treatment outcomes, increased suffering of individuals, and an escalation of health care delivery costs.

The purpose of this chapter is to: (a) review common definitions of culture, ethnicity, and nationality in contemporary society; (b) illustrate the difference between a patient's idea of self and self-identity; (c) explore the dynamics of cultural identity and idea of self; (d) discuss the impact of cultural traditions on health; and (e) provide a case study in which cultural sensitivity and competency were important components of successful treatment outcomes.

Culture, Ethnicity, Nationality

Culture

Culture has many definitions. It has been defined as a patterned behavioural response that develops over time. Giger et al. state that culture can be defined as the end product of an imprinting on the mind of patterned responses that occur through social, religious, intellectual, and artistic experiences and that it is also the result of acquired psychological mechanisms that are affected by internal and external stimuli (1). Values, beliefs, norms, and practices that are held in common among members of a group are what shape a culture. Culture guides an individual's thinking and doing and becomes a stereotypical expression of the person. Culture guides an individual's actions and decision making while fostering ideas of self-worth and self-esteem.

Others (2) define culture as a socially transmitted behaviour pattern that is based on the acceptance of beliefs, attitudes, language, and practices that are typical of a community at a give time. These authors argue that geographical, economic, and social segregation of any ethnic or racial group reinforces the culturally influenced behaviour pattern. When considering suffering in such groups, these points are of considerable importance. In health care, changes in usual patterns of behaviour may be regarded as evidence of pathology when, in fact, the person is simply retreating to a time and place of emotional safety because threats to his/her personal idea of self are perceived.

In the arena of health, individuals may be forced into a culture of chronic illness or disability. People with asthma, for example, may become part of a culture in which members advocate for clean air, the abolishment of smoking in public places, or a fragrance-free society. Others with physical disabilities may lobby governments for wheelchair-accessible buildings and subsidized public transportation. Other individuals may find themselves in an illness culture when lifesaving drugs are not subsidized by public resources. In many such examples, an individual may belong to several cultural groups. One may be based on illness, another on disability, and the third on ethnicity. The most useful definition, in clinical practice, is that culture is the sum of the beliefs, practices, habits, likes, customs, norms, and rituals that individuals learn from their families during their years of socialization (3).

Culture is the mainstay of personhood; that is, it is how people live in society. Adherence to cultural traditions is a conscious experience and functions as a device for creating as well as limiting human choices. Cultural traditions not only determine the nature of personal identity but also can mold individuals' ideas of self. When considering suffering as a perception of threat to ideas of self and personhood, it is important to acknowledge that in some cases, cultural traditions are not always compatible with an individual's idea of self.

Self-conflict and impaired interpersonal relationships, two characteristics of suffering, may be magnified when the patient is confronted with conflicting ideas of self. Conflicts may arise when the person's idea of self based on past cultural teachings is incompatible with aspects of the self that are influenced by factors in contemporary life. While idea of self is determined by internal psychological stimuli, it is not always influenced by external cultural norms. Idea of self is an internal perception that reassures an individual of his or her uniqueness in the world. Culture is the external influence of others that shapes one's identity in society. Factors such as ethnicity and nationality define cultural habits.

Ethnicity and Nationality

Ethnicity · Ethnicity often refers to a common and distinctive racial, national, religious, linguistic, or cultural tradition. People of a specific ethnic background usually have a common geographic origin, migratory status, race, language, and dialect. They have many ties that transcend the boundaries of kinship, neighborhood, and community. People of like ethnicity share traditions, symbols, values, literature, folklore, music, and food. Their settlement patterns and employment patterns are similar, and individuals belonging to the group have both an internal and external sense of distinctiveness. When suffering is experienced, this sense of distinctiveness may be exacerbated by increasing feelings of isolation from the community at large, whose cultural demands are beyond those of the individual's own cultural group (4).

In contemporary society, however, ethnicity also refers to non-Western cultural traditions. For example, in North America, food that is not derived from Anglo-Saxon traditions is labeled as "ethnic." Individuals whose first language is not English are referred to as "ethnics" even though each person may belong to a different cultural group. In medicine, ethnicity usually refers to an individual's origins by birth rather than present nationality.

Nationality · Some scholars (5) argue that nationality and culture are symbiotic. For health care professionals who have an ethical commitment to care, nationality is simply the status of belonging to a particular nation. Nationality also can refer to an ethnic group that forms one or more political nations. When considering the relationship between culture and nationality, culture is seen to provide meaning to a life because people share a language, memories, geographic territory, and common practices. In some instances, people choose to become part of another minority culture rather than be identified with a less favourable minority due to immigration or political policies. An example is that of immigrants from the Caribbean who choose not to identify with African Americans. The ethos of the Caribbean culture is perceived by Caribbean immigrants to be different from that of African Americans.

Ethos, Ethnocentrism, Xenophobia

It is critical to understand the ethos or characteristic spirit of a culture or community if respect and validation of others is to be truly achieved. Health care professionals who are committed to the preservation and enhancement of the health of all members of society must guard against ethnocentrism, or the belief in the superiority of one's own ethnic group. An example of ethnocentrism in medicine occurs when health care professionals assume that attitudes based on religious traditions in which suffering is seen as a punishment for a life poorly lived are considered to be "primitive" in the eyes of scientific medicine. Many cultures do not subscribe to the views of medicine.

In health care, as well as in society at large, ethnocentrism may also occur because of xenophobia, the undue fear or contempt for strangers or foreigners usually because of inaccurate perceptions of political or cultural practices. It is important to realize that lack of understanding of the ethos of a culture, ethnocentrism, and xenophobia occur equally in minority cultural groups as well as in dominant cultures. Consequently, patients may believe that the cultural customs of the dominant society are inferior to those of their own cultural inheritance. Because of such misunderstandings suffering may escalate in individuals with chronic illnesses. Failing to understand the ethos of a community or to understand the nature of ethnocentrism and xenophobia may cause health care providers to fail to hear and validate the story with the patient. Sometimes individuals voluntarily change their nationality and cultural practices. This change usually evolves through either assimilation or acculturation.

Assimilation and Acculturation

When individuals assimilate, they become more like the dominant culture. Assimilation may be cultural or due to intermarriage. Some persons totally abandon their cultural background, and others absorb parts of the dominant culture while maintaining part of their original culture. Assimilation is usually a matter of choice, while acculturation usually occurs over three generations. Acculturation occurs when people are forced to learn the ways of a new culture for reasons of survival. Individuals who experience acculturation may be living between two cultures. Immigrants to North America and the aboriginal peoples often live in two different cultures due to the demands of acculturation. They live both their own aboriginal or immigrant traditions as well as the customs of the dominant Anglo-Saxon society. When such individuals experience suffering, self-conflict may be very intense because patients may emotionally move from one belief system to another. In such instances the experience of suffering may be prolonged. Further, the situation may be even more complex if those same individuals become physically disabled. They then must embrace the culture of disability.

Because organized heath care delivery is a social institution, governance is determined by popular politics. Health care providers in North America and throughout most of the world believe that they have a duty to administer, without prejudice, to all who are ill, but they are bound, in part, by the rules and regulations of their health care organization and the political norms of the dominant culture. The end result of trying to meet the sometimes divergent objectives is that individual health care providers can also experience considerable self-conflict.

Cultural Sensitivity

Customs vs. Rights

The clinician who effectively manages suffering with cultural sensitivity has a basic knowledge of the patients' cultural customs. A constructive approach towards patients' attitudes and practices, particularly if those beliefs are different from those of the dominant cultures, is advanced through an awareness of both social customs and human rights policies. Knowledge of cultural beliefs, language, and practices can help clinicians determine the nature of the patient's world view.

Knowledge of the nature and customs of minority groups is critical to effective health care delivery. Few health care professionals realize that members of a minority group have the "right" to protect their culture if their identification with it has been voluntary. However, some argue that only those born in the country of origin have established legal rights (6–8). In health care it is important to realize that some members of minorities who were born and raised in their social cultures did not choose minority status but may find themselves in a minority group because of circumstance or chronic illness. The relationship between the social isolation of minority status and the existential loneliness of those who suffer is a critical factor in understanding the nature of suffering in medicine.

In North American society, individuals and families belong to several cultural groups. They may belong to particular groups based on the primary characteristics of culture or race, skin colour, gender, age, or religious affiliation. Cultural identity is also determined by geographic location. Some individuals live in urban areas and others in rural settings. Marital status, physical characteristics, migration history, and immigration status are all factors upon which cultural customs are constituted (9). The purpose of group membership is that individuals have the need to live in familiar, safe environments. Those who suffer often express the feeling that they now live in a world others do not know. They become immigrants in their own lives.

Other group memberships are due to the secondary characteristics of culture such as educational status, socioeconomic status, occupation, military experience, and political beliefs. Membership in these groups is due to economic reasons and is entrenched in human rights and freedoms. Some individuals choose their collective identity for economic and/or political gain. Shared race, language, or practices are not requirements of this type of membership. The dynamics of group functioning are usually based on the formal laws of the group and can form an individual's social identity. Further, other individuals subscribe to a symbolic ethnicity. For example, through intermarriage some people may choose to follow the ethnic customs of their partner rather than their own customs or blend more than one tradition into their family identity. There are no real benefits or costs to the individual's choice in these instances. For health care professionals, whose task it is to help those who suffer to reintegrate into their respective societies, it is critical to understand the nature of the group to which the patient once belonged (12, 13).

Attitudinal Shifts

Cultural groups change slowly over time, even in stable societies. To be useful to patients who suffer, effective clinicians understand their own cultural backgrounds and are aware of how their attitudes, beliefs, and practices could negatively influence care. For example, if the health care provider's culture focuses on independence of the individual, difficulties may arise in cases where the patient is from a culture that does not specifically value the individual but rather involves the family or the subgroup within the larger group in decision making. In such situations, the health professional's task shifts from that of being an authoritative expert providing scientific information to functioning from a more holistic perspective that includes synthesizing the tenets of personal respect; caring; being present; and offering protection, reassurance, and compassion as well as scientific information (14). Such changes involve reassessment of one's own value system and the desire to objectively consider the views of others.

Another challenge facing clinicians is the need to be culturally appropriate. Naive, superficial knowledge about other cultural traditions can be harmful and unproductive in the management of suffering. To provide the best possible care, health care providers must have a solid knowledge base about cultural diversity. Awareness that visible minorities have considerable internal diversity and that subgroups may have cultural traits or social customs that are vastly different from the main cultural group helps the clinician avoid stereotyping patients on the basis of ethnicity and/or presumed cultural practices. Clinicians can avoid making incorrect assumptions about any particular individual or group by seeking information directly from the patient. Questions relating to cultural sensitivity should be part of every health professional's initial clinical assessment. Focusing on the fact that all cultures share similarities and that suffering is a life experience with universal characteristics leads to the effective care of those who suffer. It is important to recognize that it is the expression of suffering, not the experience per se, that is idiosyncratic and culturally bound.

Many health care providers show considerable cultural sensitivity, but sometimes these individuals may lack cultural competency in the administration of health care planning and delivery (9, 10). To be culturally competent when dealing with suffering, it is critical to remember that suffering, in medicine, does not refer solely to pain or a plethora of unpleasant events. Suffering is a perception of threat to an individual's idea of self and personhood.

Cultural Competency

Purnell's model and Lenninger's Sunrise model for cultural competence and transcultural nursing practice provides a useful framework upon which to examine the challenges of cultural competency faced by those who are managing suffering in medicine (11, 14). Examination of definitions of culture in health care delivery indicates that cultural customs significantly contribute to the development of identity and often ideas of self. When considering suffering as a perception of threat to idea of self and personhood, understanding the ethos of minority cultures, ethnocentrism, and the relationship of idea of self to identity is critical to cultural competency.

Self

Self is often defined as a person's particular nature or personality, the essential being that distinguishes the person from others. Idea of self is an internal perception, a dream or wish that a person holds in which the behaviours and action that are honorable and acceptable to the person are seen as his/her own. Sometimes idea of self is culturally bound, and sometimes it is not. Idea of self is personal and determined by the individual. A person's idea of self is sometimes totally incompatible with how the person is perceived by others. For example, a woman may perceive herself as being risk taking and having a contemporary worldview. She may see her past and present ways of managing life's challenges as daring and bold. Family and friends however may see her as being sensible, reliable, extremely competent, and subscribing to their culture's worldview. These differing perceptions of the individual and family separate the individual from other family members and give the individual a unique place within the family constellation.

When faced with overwhelming adversity, illness, or disability, an individual may be forced to re-examine his/her idea of self. If the expectations the individual has about his/her behaviour do not match family cultural expectations, the sudden revelation of these differences may result in interpersonal conflict. Some people can readily change their internal beliefs about how they must now behave to maintain personal integrity. Other patients may have considerable difficulty changing their idea of self and require help from health care providers. Changes in idea of self in conjunction with changes in physical and/or emotional performance may also cause considerable upset within the family complex. Clinicians in these instances must also address family concerns. If clinical assumptions and expectations of patients are based on stereotypical cultural attitudes, the management of those who suffer is compromised.

Identity

Identity, on the other hand, is an accumulation of factors such as culture, ethnicity, and nationality that determine the social characteristics of an individual. Identity is also based on external factors determined by others. Cultural identity is important to individuals because it is a collective identity that does not require an essential self. Cultural identity provides individuals with guidelines for a successful life. While most people are socialized into a collective identity from birth, anyone can also choose to adopt a new one. Cultural identities are important for individuals because they determine the values and cognitive symbols for everyday life. For example, belonging to a cultural identity automatically gives meanings to marriage, religion, moral behaviour, and language. Cultural identity also gives individuals social and political power.

Idea of Self and Self Identity

The relationship between idea of self and identity can be said to be symbiotic. One may incorporate the cultural teachings of childhood into his/her idea of self or not. When incorporation occurs, a culturally based idea of self and identity may be the gold standard to which all future behaviour is compared. Those who choose cultural groups other than the one inherited at birth may find themselves in considerable personal conflict as they try to synthesize past and present identities into a cohesive idea of self. The challenge to health care providers is twofold. It is imperative not only to acknowledge and validate the individual's personal idea of self but also to understand the origin, nature, and demands of their cultural identity and how these factors contribute to their everyday life or personhood.

Personhood and Heritage

To understand the many manifestations of perception of threat to an individual, it is useful to have some knowledge not only of the person's dream of self but also of his/her heritage. Factors such as country of origin, current residence, economics, political experience, reasons for immigration, educational status, and current occupation are key factors that may have significant impact on health status, illness prevention, and coping with illness or injury.

When considering the construct of culture and idea of self and identity within the family unit, determinations of gender roles and power structures are important. For example, who is the head of the family? What is the role of the elderly? How are members of the extended family viewed? What are the priorities within the family structure? Factors such as family attitudes towards single parenting, sexual orientation, child-rearing practices, childless marriage, and divorce are powerful contributors to idea of self. An individual's idea of self may be incompatible with family expectations and this may only become apparent to the patient and family in situations of stress and adversity. This familial incongruence may be the source of a great deal of additional suffering. Suffering in chronic illness, when considering culture, identity, ideas of self, and personhood, has an additional set of challenges. Conflict between health care providers and patients and their families about patient autonomy, acculturation, assimilation, ethnic communication styles, individualism, and the desire of families to incorporate customs of health care practices from their countries of origin with Western methods may all enhance patient suffering. These factors are all components of personhood, that is, the tasks of everyday life, which may be seen by individuals to be threatened by the onset of chronic illness and/or disability and by insensitive transcultural medical practice. When personal autonomy is overruled by the authority of health care practitioners, idea of self and self-image are damaged. The patient may feel a loss of power over his/her own life. In cultures where individualism is not valued, adherence to strict codes of personal autonomy in health care organizations may be experienced by patients as abandonment. Further, struggles of second-generation immigrant children can escalate because of the demands of managing chronic illness from the perspective of immigrant family members who are accustomed to methods that are different and sometimes not appreciated by current scientific practice.

Sensitive transcultural care of individuals who suffer involves helping patients preserve not only their idea of self and personhood but also their cultural identity. All these factors constitute the construct of personhood. Clearly, cultural competency depends on knowledge, empathetic listening skills, and effective communication. In addition to ethno-history, the impact of the patient's dominant language and how that language is usually expressed must be known. For example, some individuals who have recently emigrated from Russia may speak more loudly when confronting authority figures because of traumatic incidences that occurred while in their native country. Those behaviours may be misinterpreted as being abusive or ill-informed. Others, such as people from India, may speak more loudly because of ancient religious beliefs relating to the power of the voice and respect given to God.

Knowledge of illness beliefs is useful. Some groups of Asian background may avoid eye contact because of ancient beliefs that looking at someone directly may invoke evil and cause illness. Many traditions adhere to beliefs in the "evil eye" in a variety of formats. Facial expressions, the use of touch, and body language are all culturally driven and have a variety of meanings. In health care, spatial distancing, the meaning of time, the use of names and acceptable greetings can all impact on the establishment of trust, compliance, and effectiveness of treatment interventions. Once again, the health care professional becomes the non-knower and the power differential again shifts from expert (the patient) to novice (the clinician). Such shifts may be very threatening to clinicians who not only believe that their cultural traditions are superior but also that their traditions must take precedence. In such situations, patients quickly determine those behaviours that are deemed threatening and either withdraw from care or only give the clinician the information the patient believes the clinician seeks. In both cases the end result may be an increase in suffering, ineffective treatment interventions, and an escalation of health care costs.

Effective management requires the ability to accommodate and negotiate cultural differences, and restructure individuals' idea of self and personhood when necessary. It is critical to know patients' past patterns and practices of health, particularly in the fields of rehabilitation medicine. Respectful expressions of care along with knowledge of the importance of the environment to the individual and the language and ethno-history of the patient are essential components of ethical, efficacious, cost-effective health care delivery. Clearly, culture has a considerable impact on personhood for the individual as well as the family and social group.

The Power of Cultural Customs on Suffering: A Case Study

The power of cultural customs on suffering is best understood through explorations of ritual, privacy and, spiritual beliefs. The following is a case study that demonstrates the need for all health care practitioners to address suffering in their respective fields. The story of Marron takes place in a physiotherapy rehabilitation facility.

MARRON'S STORY

It was my second day at work in a rehabilitation unit when I received a requisition to treat Marron, a young woman of aboriginal descent who was complaining of muscle weakness in both legs and an inability to walk after experiencing a traumatic event. Apparently, after wild partying, the woman had slipped and fallen and was injured. While such events may make some smile wryly, in health care, it was just another story. I entered Marron's room, and my greeting was met with silence. She did not meet my gaze as I introduced myself and explained the reason for my visit. Questions began to surface in my mind. What did the silence mean? Was Marron's silence a function of her personality or was it a cultural response? Perhaps it was both. In some cultural traditions silence is an indication of respect and in others a sign of fear and distress. Had I been more experienced I would have asked the patient. Time would tell me what silence meant to this young woman. I had learned from past experience to be slow in making judgments about the meaning of behaviour. Many thoughts flicked through my mind as I stood at her bedside. I remembered reading that in the Navajo tradition, personal privacy was very important and revelations of mating practices or sexual information was not readily given and often withheld from health care providers. I did not know if this was an issue for Marron and perhaps a reason for her silence, given the circumstances of her accident. I knew that it is important not to make assumptions about a patient's cultural heritage or to think that traditions were constant across groups and subgroups. I resolved to ask Marron to explain her belief systems about personal space, touching, and privacy needs within the context of assessments and treatments offered through physiotherapy. As I glanced around the room I noticed that there were no visitors in the room. The nurses later informed me that they had not seen anyone visit during the week. I took mental note of this observation because my past experience with people of North American aboriginal decent, who lived in isolated environments, was that family and community were usually very present when a member of the group was ill. Of more concern to me was the fact that some of the hospital staff seemed to be interpreting Marron's silence as an indication of hostility and noncompliance. Further, because there was little scientific evidence that any severe damage to Marron's spinal cord had occurred during the accident, it seemed some of the medical staff were beginning to have suspicions that perhaps Marron was experiencing hysteria.

On physical examination, Marron complained of severe pain in her low back and on the front of one leg. I began treating her in her room on the ward. Marron always spoke with a very quiet voice. She seldom smiled. One day, she told me that she felt that the staff did not like her because she was an aboriginal person and that they thought she was a liar. Being an experienced and perhaps overly protective therapist, I felt the need to shield my patient from the power of labels and scientific controversy. I switched our sessions from the ward to the gymnasium in an attempt to legitimize her impairments in the eyes of some of the medical staff. Several days later, Marron was discharged from the hospital as an outpatient. She was to see me the following week at 1 P.M.. On the day of her appointment Marron did not arrive until 3 P.M., much to the exasperation of our receptionist. Fortunately, I was free to see Marron at that time. As she entered the gym, I noticed that she no longer used the gray metal cane that I had given her but rather was using a carved wooden stick with a beautiful hand grip into which was inserted a series of bells. I made no comment. We began the stretching and exercises and, after a while, Marron began to speak. She told me that she had been cursed by the grandmother of her boyfriend who believed Marron had caused them disgrace. I listened and said nothing. Marron went on to say that a medicine man she knew in another village gave her the wooden cane because it had magic that would heal her. She showed me the cane and I admired its beauty. She said nothing else and I asked no questions because I did not know what questions would be helpful and which would not. We continued to work. Later, Marron and I talked about the routines that determined her life, and I explained the obligations that governed mine. It became clear that Marron believed that I would be able to help her get better and that she also had great faith in the traditional healing practices of her culture. She was only a few minutes late for the rest of her appointments. I never told anyone about the spell, and I argued on her behalf at team meetings so that she could continue to have treatments as long as she showed improvement. One day, Marron came in to the gym without the cane, and after she left, I never saw her again. To me, this was not an unusual experience because I had some slight understanding of aboriginal traditions and belief systems. From my perspective this was appropriate and acceptable behaviour.

Some of my colleagues had considerable difficulty accepting this approach to treatment because, from their perspective, Marron was abusing health care resources and I was not advancing the cause of science. I believed that part of my job was not only to offer Marron my technological skill but also to support her idea of self and personhood. Marron had told me that she believed that she had behaved dishonorably prior to her accident and that she had disgraced herself and grandparents with whom she lived. Marron did not know what she was going to do because she felt shunned by her community and by the medical staff, who, she believed, thought she was "faking" her illness. She was afraid that she would be disabled for the rest of her life as punishment for her poor behaviour. She was very angry, with herself, her family, some of her community members, and sometimes with me. I interpreted Marron's behaviours as indicators of suffering. I believed she perceived her idea of self and personhood as being threatened. Marron's treatment regime involved not only the exercises I was showing her to improve her muscle strength and mobility but also a restoration of her idea of self and personhood. Restoration of Marron's idea of self now involved atonement and forgiveness for her behaviour. She believed she was receiving help from the medicine man in her village. The nature of her personhood, that is, how she had dealt with adversity in the past and believed she would manage in the future, was expressed, in part, through her belief in spirits and spells and by attending her village healing circle. Usually, I prefer not to treat patients who are simultaneously being treated by other health care practitioners because it makes it more difficult for me to determine the efficacy of my interventions. Further, there is always the danger of negative interactions between treatment modalities.

In Marron's case, no drug therapies were involved, and she believed that traditional medicine would also help her. I believed that it was important to validate the nature of Marron's personhood and that she have the freedom to combine folk methods with Western medicine techniques. In this particular case, I believed that the art of medicine (both folk and Western) took precedence over the science. Further, I believed that part of my therapeutic responsibility was to avoid contributing to her suffering.

After her discharge, Marron did not return for repeated visits complaining of pain, as is often the case with patients who have had similar problems and in which suffering is not addressed. While Marron may still have some physical impairments she was not disabled.

In retrospect, I believe that Marron and I worked together successfully. I did my job, and she did hers. At the time, I believed that my job was to objectively identify the health care problem, discuss with Marron the interventions that I believed would be effective, and be aware of the cultural factors that could influence treatment outcomes. Marron's job was to accept my help and to tell me about what would constitute a successful health outcome for help. Our relationship was not an easy one because I was not sure that I was addressing all of Marron's concerns from the perspectives of cultural sensitivity and competency. My approach was based mostly on past experience and instinct because my professional training did not include courses in transcultural care.

I learned a lot from Marron. I learned that when providing culturally sensitive care, it is very important to be clear in my own mind about my obligations both to the art and science of medicine and to the cultural needs of my patients. It is important to know about the routines and rituals of the patient and the family as well as the community at large. The role of the family and how illness impacts on family routines and rituals as well as the power structure within the family are particularly important when addressing suffering. Who makes the decisions in the family unit? What is the attitude towards individualism? What are the beliefs about personal space, modesty and touch, and communication methods? It is critical to know the patient's place in the family structure, the expectations of the family subgroup, and the rules and regulations of the larger community group. These factors must be considered for all patients, but there are other vital factors to be explored when evaluating the impact of cultural traditions and suffering within minority groups.

Questions of acculturation and assimilation are pertinent when addressing suffering with patients from minority groups. From the perspective of health outcomes, the involuntary transfer of people from one minority group to another may escalate the process of suffering. For example, had Marron become disabled, she would have belonged to two minority groups: one group determined by ethnicity and nationality and the other by health status. How do aboriginal groups view those who are handicapped or disabled? What would be the challenge to Marron from the perspective of rehabilitation? Were her parents born in the country in which they lived? Determinations of when people have immigrated may also play a significant part in suffering. The expectations of self of first-generation immigrants are often vastly different from those of their parents, as are religious and spiritual practices, the use of herbs, and other complementary health care techniques. Cultural traditions have a significant impact on ideas of self and personhood in those who suffer. Cultural sensitivity and cultural competency may well be critical factors that prevent the development of both physical and emotional disability.

I have told the story of Marron to my students over the years as I've tried to instill in them the importance of cultural sensitivity and cultural competence. I believe that had my undergraduate training involved courses in cross-cultural sensitivity and competency, I may have been even more helpful to my patients.

SUMMARY

This chapter has explored the relationship between cultural traditions and suffering. It is clear that a full understanding of the concepts of culture, ethnicity, nationality, and heritage and their relationship to the experience of suffering must be thoroughly understood. Further, health care professionals must also know that suffering, defined as a perception of threat to idea of self, personhood, and identity, occurs not only with individual patients but also with their families and the many subgroups to which individuals belong. We have explored also the power of subgroup beliefs on the experience of suffering and have seen how cultural sensitivity and competency enhances everyday clinical practice. Another critical factor in understanding the nature of suffering in contemporary health care delivery is that not only do individuals experience suffering because of threats to their idea of self that are related to physical and emotional illnesses and/or injuries but also because critical life-stage tasks are also perceived to be threatened. The following chapter will explore suffering from the perspective of developmental life-stage tasks.

CHAPTER 4 QUESTIONS

1. Define Culture.
2. Differentiate between ethnicity and nationality.
3. How does xenophobia impact on health care delivery?
4. Give examples of ethnocentrism in medicine and describe how ethnocentrism may negatively affect those who suffer.
5. How does acculturation impact on the health care delivery of individual patients?
6. Describe the critical components of cultural sensitivity.
7. What are the characteristics of culturally competent health care providers?
8. What is the relationship between idea of self and self-identity in patients who suffer?
9. How does an individual's heritage impact on the construct of suffering?
10. Analyze the story of "Marron" from the perspective of cultural sensitivity and cultural competency.

5 Crises of Suffering across the Life Span

Personhood is defined as those responsibilities and activities of individuals that constitute a life. When considering the experience of suffering, personhood has a further meaning. Personhood, within the context of suffering, also involves an individual's perception of threat to those developmental psychosocial tasks and behaviours that must be addressed throughout the life span. Failure to understand the nature of these tasks and behaviours, and the impact of the variety of family roles and cultural traditions on an individual's life tasks, can result in increased suffering and failed clinical interventions.

The purpose of this chapter will be to: (a) briefly outline some theories of human psychosocial development across the life span, (b) show how various understandings of what constitutes a family impacts on the achievement of these life tasks, (c) demonstrate how health care organizational policies may be in conflict with the life tasks of patients who have chronic illnesses, and finally (d) delineate the challenges to effective health care of those who suffer. For clarification, examples will be drawn primarily from the perspective of Western cultural traditions.

The Life Cycle: Developmental Tasks, Behaviours, and Challenges

Developmental Tasks

The clinical management of the experience of suffering has long been relegated to the fields of palliative care and mental illness. Treatment has been the domain of psychologists, psychiatrists, chaplains, and social workers. To the rest of the medical team, suffering per se was considered to be outside their scope of clinical practice because suffering is often considered to be the secondary component of pain. Many still believe that without pain there is no suffering. Currently, few regulated health care professions include the alleviation of suffering in their formal statements of practice goals and objectives. Yet suffering, defined as a perception of threat to self and personhood, is encountered by all health care practitioners in the course of their everyday work. Physiotherapists encounter suffering when they treat patients whose impairments become disabilities or when families must suddenly cope with a child who has birth defects or is developmentally impaired. In such cases treatments may be required throughout the various stages of the life cycle of both child and parents. Nurses, who have the most contact with patients, encounter suffering when patients have surgical procedures that may be life threatening or when individuals await news of the fate of loved ones after health emergencies. Social workers, chaplains, and many other health care personnel help those who suffer not only in the field of palliative care but also whenever there are patient perceptions that life-changing events may be unmanageable. Psychologists and psychiatrists have advanced skills to treat those individuals who are unable to restructure or adapt to a new idea of self and personhood. Awareness of the behavioural life cycle tasks and behaviours enhances effective patient-centred health care delivery.

As previously discussed, suffering does not necessarily correlate with pain, but occurs when there is a perception of threat to an individual's beliefs and ideas of self and personhood. Most of the previous chapters have focused on idea of self. It is important also to explore more fully the construct of personhood from the perspective of the psychosocial development of individuals across the life span. There are many psychoanalytical theories but we will begin first by demonstrating the need for clinicians to be aware of the many internal demands placed on patients who suffer using the classical theories of Erik Erikson (1). These theories were developed from the pragmatic study of people of various ages and abilities.

People face many psychological developmental challenges throughout life. I became aware of the power of these tasks early in my career when I was working in a school for physically challenged children. At the time, children with disabilities were not automatically integrated into the public school system but attended special schools. These special schools had the mandate to provide education, rehabilitation, and eventual integration into the regular school system. The school in which I worked was fully staffed with teachers, physiotherapists, occupational therapists, speech therapists, and social workers. The professional health care team was well integrated with education objectives. Unfortunately, in contemporary health care many children do not have these resources readily available in public schools.

THE STORY OF ROBBIE

One day, Robbie, a skinny little seven-year-old boy came to school with his hair dyed green. His teenage mother had dyed his hair in an attempt to make him appear more normal and less handicapped. Needless to say, the other children had a great deal of fun at Robbie's expense. It is difficult to be "cool" and independent when you need others to wheel your wheelchair and help you go to the toilette. Having green hair in those days did not help Robbie socialize.

Robbie was born with cerebral palsy, a medical condition in which his arms and legs were usually spastic and at times flayed about in twisted athetoid contortions. Robbie was the product of a sexual encounter between his mother and her high school boyfriend. Upon finding out about Robbie's conception, his father quickly abandoned Robbie and his mother, as did both the mother's parents. Robbie and his mother faced a life of hardship and poverty. It was a life filled with a series of "uncles" and unconventional parenting practices. Professional meetings with Robbie's mother were filled with anger and frustration, but Robbie was a remarkably happy little guy who did very well in school.

Several days after the hair-dying incident, the occupational therapist asked Robbie to draw a picture of himself, and he drew a picture of a traditional little boy with arms and legs intact and sitting in a wheelchair. The child Robbie drew had brown hair (the natural colour of Robbie's hair), blue eyes, and a big smile. "That's me" Robbie said proudly with a big smile on his face. In spite of his many disabilities Robbie had an intact self-image. But what about his idea of self? Robbie had many conversations with both the occupational therapist and the physiotherapist about what he wanted to do when he grew up and how he saw his future life. He was very clear about differentiating between impossible dreams and reality.

How did a child with a severe physical disability; an impoverished family life; and a poor, depressed, emotionally fragile mother maintain such a healthy idea of self? What was the nature of the family unit and its everyday functioning? If the clinical staff had so much personal information about Robbie's conception, why was there not a clearer understanding of the family unit?

There is a prevailing belief that families are to be examined to determine the extent to which they contribute to health problems. Opinions of staff are based on health care organizational attitudes of right and wrong. Rarely are developmental life cycle tasks taken into consideration when assessing family dynamics. For example, what were the life tasks of Robbie's mother, who was fourteen years old when he was born? Were there internal conflicts between the developmental life cycle tasks of the mother and those of Robbie? Many health care professionals at the time were advising very young mothers to not place their children for adoption. Little regard was given to the fact that the mother's developmental tasks might not be achievable or compatible with those of an infant or young child.

Knowledge of the crises that can occur when life cycle tasks are not addressed is very important to health because the psychosocial tasks of each stage of life are integrated with each other. For example, in infancy the challenge to the infant is the dichotomy between basic trust and basic mistrust. Babies test their environments and the people in them to determine issues of safety and survival. The resolution of this dichotomy lays the foundations of the human strength of hope. In early childhood the challenge revolves around autonomy and personal shame. Parents of very young children are very aware of how proud young children feel when they are able to toilet independently and how ashamed the child feels when mistakes occur. The third stage of childhood developmental tasks involves the tension between initiative and guilt. Successful resolution results in establishing the foundations upon which children begin to develop a personal purpose in life. School-age children, usually six years old and up in Western societies, have the much larger world of the neighborhood to operate in, and their challenge is to reconcile the crises that can occur between feeling industrious and successful and feeling inferior. Foundations for feelings of personal competency are being formed at this stage of the life cycle (2).

In puberty, there is considerable confusion about identity and the desire for an identity separate from others, particularly family members. At this stage, the foundations of leadership and fidelity are established (3). In young adulthood the struggle is around intimacy needs and feelings of isolation. Young adults struggle to develop an ideological worldview. They begin to explore intimate love relationships, and struggles between competition, compassion, and friendship arise. Adulthood is a time in which individuals are divided between cultural traditions and creativity. Issues of authority involving generational differences are at the fore. The main tasks involve care of self and others.

After age fifty-five, the tasks involved require maintaining integrity and avoiding despair. Mastery of the psychological tasks involved in resolving this dichotomy results in achieving wisdom (1).

The above very brief summary of the psychological and sociological tasks, based on Erikson's comprehensive theory, outlines key issues that may underlie the experience of suffering. The emerging human strengths required to resolve development challenges in this theory show that individuals are subject to vulnerabilities that may, even in ordinary circumstances, require healing. If patients feel that they will not be able to meet the life challenges because of illness or injury, suffering may be profound and prolonged.

Clinical Challenges

Assessment and treatment interventions must consider the relationship between perceptions of suffering and developmental psychosocial crises.

In clinical practice, health care professionals are more effective if they consider the age and gender of the individual, the age-specific life crises to be resolved, and the impact of illness or disease on achieving these obligations. Further, incomplete or distorted performance of life cycle tasks, due to chronic illness, can negatively impact on future stages of psychosocial development because all these psychosocial stages are inter-related.

Erikson's model of psychosocial development, discussed above, is an endogenous model of human development based on the principles of rationalism (1). The importance of understanding psychosocial developmental tasks and the impact of suffering on an individual's ability to successfully complete these tasks is only one factor to be considered in helping people resolve suffering. Those who suffer may also be helped by therapists who use therapeutic interventions based on exogenous models of development (4). In this latter model, all ideas derive from sense impressions of the external world and sense impressions coming from an individual's internal state.

Simple ideas become complex through association with other simple ideas. In suffering there is considerable internal self-conflict, and individuals try to meet the challenges of a changed external world. Understanding these theories in relation to suffering, defined as a perception of threat to an individual's idea of self and personhood, provide yet another way to help patients. Still other models of human development, known as structural models of human development, focus on the relationships between the id (instincts), ego (the internal mediator between the id and external reality), and the superego, which dominates the ego (5). Once again, these theories provide methods to help individuals restore an impaired or changed idea of self.

There are also many other theories that address, moral and ethical developmental stages, cognitive learning processes, as well as cultural and gender-based developmental methodologies (6, 7). While it does not seem reasonable to expect every health care provider to be expert in all these approaches to care, medical education can include these subjects in undergraduate curricula so that all clinicians will have a better understanding of the nature of suffering and how patients may best be helped.

When suffering is understood in medicine as a perception of threat to ideas of self and personhood, it becomes clear that there are many health care professionals who can assist the patient to restore or change ideas of self. The idea that coping and adjusting to adversity demands patients to be quiet and carry on with their life even though they are also experiencing suffering is the result of incomplete problem identification and incomplete application of appropriate suffering-specific treatment interventions.

In the field of family systems therapy, some (8) argue for an ecosystem approach to care. Effective family therapy using this approach involves obtaining pertinent information about family dynamics. Information about what constitutes a family from the patient's perspective is critical. What are the family's values and social boundaries? What constitutes a harmonious life? How does the family understand suffering? Is suffering synonymous with hardship? Is there a value in suffering? What is the family's worldview? Is all of life suffering? How does the family manage suffering? What are the family and community attitudes towards those who suffer? How do individuals manage internal conflict? Many individuals do not have families; single senior individuals and homeless people are often without family. Idealistic attitudes about the composition and/or dynamics of "healthy" families should be avoided.

Other ecological theories focus on differentiating between the general population and the individual (9, 10). The main thrust is on enculturation and socialization. The physical environment of the individual and the social environment are key concepts in these theories. Customs about child-rearing practices, parental and cultural beliefs, social representations, and caretaker psychology are also key components (11, 12). The main thrust of ecological theories is that the cultural organization of human beings is so important that it affects all biological skills, even those such as eating. These theories advocate linking the individual to the physical environment in which life is lived as well as the social constructs and dynamics of the interpersonal relationships in the family and immediate community.

Regardless of the model of care chosen to address suffering, it is important to have a comprehensive understanding of patients' family structures and their dynamics.

Family Dynamics and Suffering: The Challenges

The Family as a System

The family paradigm is often described as a unit in which members function within a broad social network that evolves over the life cycle (13, 14). Family systems theory argues that changes in one part of the system are followed by compensatory changes in another part. If one member of the family is unable to meet the developmental age-appropriate challenges required because of illness, disability, and perceived threats to self and personhood (suffering), then other members may not be able to actualize their own developmental tasks. For example, young children who have established an embryonic trust in life as a domain of safety may find this fragile belief system shattered by the premature death of a parent or the onset of chronic disability. Further, other senior family members may feel emotionally shattered as their life cycle task of managing the dichotomy between wisdom and personal integrity appears to be thwarted because of poor health of their children (15).

Perceptions of the family differ between therapists who follow an ecosystem approach to care and therapists who adhere to a family systems approach. The ecosystem theory of family dynamics consists of four principles. The first is that individuals are not viewed from the perspective of pathology. Difficulties within the family unit are the result of interrupted growth and development. The second principle is that a variety of interventions may be applied to the various subsystems that make up the family unit. These various interventions may all produce the same effect or outcome. The third principle is that the family is a natural helping system, and health care providers are most effective if treatment strategies make use of natural systems and life experiences of various family members. The last principle, which is compatible with family systems theory, is that only one part of the family system needs to change to produce overall change in the whole system. The role that the family plays in the resolution of an individual's suffering is significant, and clinicians are challenged to fully understand family dynamics if effective treatment interventions are to be achieved.

For example, if knowledge of the family as a systems unit is incomplete and clinicians erroneously emphasize a factor such as loyalty obligations, a value that may not be held by the family, suffering may escalate. Issues of role rigidity, adequacy of problem-solving capabilities, clarity of power boundaries, and effective communication skills are key issues influencing the effective resolution of suffering. Often patients react more strongly to how the family as a whole responds to the illness or disability than the actual threat to self presented by the illness. Some individuals will sacrifice themselves to protect the family. A high level of engagement of family members with the chronically ill patient may sometimes interfere with the needs and perceptions of individual family members. When one member suffers, so does the rest of the family. Each family member's perception of threat will be related to their own specific idea of self and how they perceive the threat to the personhood of the family unit. When assisting those who suffer, it is critical to recognize not only the nature of the patient's idea of self and personhood but also that of individual family members and the family as a unit (16).

Challenges for Care

Family relationships are constantly changing. Children leave home to go to school and eventually leave the parental home to form other family units. After the first has left the family unit, the second child may suddenly find himself or herself in the role of the first child. Roles reverse again when the first returns home for family celebrations or in times of crisis. Illness or disability may also produce shifts in social roles within the family. These role changes can have adverse effects on the highly personal expressions of an individual's achievements, age-specific psychological and social developmental objectives, and behaviours. To solve family problems, families use coping strategies that may sometimes seem inappropriate to others.

When considering suffering, the family unit presents many challenges for the health care provider. For example, patients with a Japanese cultural background may have strong beliefs about the value of filial piety, and the necessity of living a harmonious life (17). Factors that determine a harmonious life in the Japanese tradition are compassion, respect for life, moderation in behaviour, self-discipline, patience, modesty, humble expectations, and a hesitation to intrude on another's time or energy. Such belief systems may impact on how health care providers can be useful to those who suffer. If effective care depends on gathering pertinent information from the patient and family, families who hesitate to take up too much time during a visit may not provide a complete picture of the problems to be addressed. Clinicians who have knowledge of the beliefs of others may have a greater understanding of the nature of their patients' perceptions of threat to idea of self and personhood. A major cross-cultural challenge to the role of the health care provider is to try to understand and relate these family belief systems to those of the health organizations, whose values are usually grounded in middle-class, secular perspectives (13–18). One strategy is to begin by working with a family member who is most acculturated to the social values of the health care professional or the health care organization.

Problem-solving styles are different for every family. Some individuals who suffer from chronic illness may sacrifice themselves for the sake of the family. They may refuse treatments that are costly in order to spare the family financial hardship. Individuals may refuse treatments in which outcomes are uncertain so that they avoid family conflict over the feasibility of trying such interventions. Consequently, key issues of suffering such as a loss of central purpose, impaired interpersonal relationships, and considerable self-conflict may not be addressed. In such instances, the severity of the illness may then escalate. A study that explored the problem-solving skills of families of patients who had end-stage renal disease who were treated with dialysis over a thirty-six-month period found that the family's emphasis on a strong sense of unity was negatively correlated with the early death of the patient. Other patients may choose to suffer silently within the family structure. The study showed that behaviours associated with silent suffering, such as withdrawal from family life and profound sorrow, affect all family members (17).

In clinical practice, health care providers cannot assume that all persons have or all cultures subscribe to the model of the nuclear family. For example, African families often comprise many extended family members. Issues such as child-rearing practices relating to dependence and obedience, autonomy and self-reliance, and permissiveness versus authority may be very intricate. An individual's development of self-identity and idea of self may be very convoluted and fragile in such cases. When illness or disability occurs, decision making may often be the province of people other than those of the traditional nuclear family. Health care organizations face many challenges around social issues of confidentiality with extended family members. These issues can be addressed as matters of routine information gathering on admission to care or at the time of initial physical assessments. If family members are regarded as a nuisance by hospital staff and the family, suffering may escalate. These factors are particularly relevant when the issue of the role of minor children with severe illness is considered.

From ecological perspectives of family dynamics there is no family culture outside an environment context. Ecological theories have explored the relationships between hunting and gathering societies and the role of the father, as well as the value various societies place on the child (12–18). Some parents value children solely for economic reasons. In North America, past practices of having many children were based not only on religious beliefs but also on the need to have workers who could help sustain the family unit financially. Particularly in developing countries, children may be the only aspect of human life that presents family members with any joy and hope. These attitudes may prevail to varying degrees in contemporary society. The role of the child and decisions made about children in modern family units is very important from the viewpoint of suffering. Understanding the dynamics of family structures encompasses knowledge both of the ecological context and of the sociopolitical demands, particularly in cultures where adults determine the nature and worth of the child (19, 20).

Some aboriginal and African societies do not consider a child to be a full person until weaned. Some groups value children based on gender. In some African cultures, the life cycle involves a passage from one life at death to another world where an individual is born and comes back as an ancestor. The role of the adults for these reborn children is not to mold them or condition them but rather to provide an environment that will fulfill the child's needs. Unfortunately, such beliefs may be viewed by some health care providers as primitive and incompatible with contemporary science. If clinicians embrace the tenets of medicine as both an art and a science, then unfamiliar beliefs are respected and suffering is more likely to be addressed.

In contemporary litigious societies, secular beliefs may dominate. In one of my classes at the university, a graduate student brought a hypothetical clinical problem to class. The case involved the relationship between a father and his very ill young adult female child. The student was to role-play the problem case and arrive at a care plan.

THE STORY OF MR. CJENCHUCK

Mr. Cjenchuck spent every day with his daughter, taking time away from his place of business and other children in the family. Because the nature of the patient's illness was not life threatening but rather chronic in nature, hospital staff found the father's behaviour excessive, and questions about the appropriateness of the relationship between father and daughter were starting to arise. My student was worried because some colleagues might be suggesting that the relationship was improper.

In class, our discussion focused on the importance of clearly identifying the problem. What were the tasks of the patient? How was her inability to reconcile the need to be independent with a desire not to be isolated being perceived? Did the patient have a perception of threat to these tasks? What were the dynamics of personhood for this young woman? What was her idea of self? What were the cultural expectations of father and daughter? What evidence was there of any impropriety? Staff concerns were found to be speculative and unsupported.

It became evident that the father's presence was an inconvenience and disruption in the staff's normal routines. We talked further about the father's age and his probable life cycle tasks. What were the expectations of the rest of the family? Did they believe that their father, as protector of the family, should be with the patient? Did the family trust authority figures? Our discussions were lively, and the student was challenged to seek further answers.

On her return to class, the student was enthusiastic and energized. As part of her hypothetical role with this family, the student told us that "she spent" considerable time both with father and daughter. She discovered that the daughter was a first-generation North American child but the father had been born in an Eastern European country. The father and his wife believed that the father's job was to care for his family. He was the final decision maker, although issues were discussed with his wife and other family members before any formal decisions were made. The family history was one of persecution in Europe, and therefore, the senior family members did not trust authority figures. The patient felt comforted and safe with the father's presence. His attention and caring dispelled her fears of isolation, which she believed would become a permanent condition of her life in the future. In the role-play scenario the issue of idea of self was gently explored with the "patient," and the student expressed confidence that not only did she believe that the patient benefited from the student's new insight about the power of life cycle tasks and suffering but the rest of the staff had learned about the dangers of accepting popular contemporary attitudes about sexual abuse without objective evidence.

Consequently, the student said that the care plan would involve instituting in-service teaching sessions to discuss suffering as a threat to an individual's sense of self and personhood and the impact of life cycle tasks and behaviours on patient health outcomes. She told us that the father would now start being seen as a member of the health care team. Needless to say, the rest of the students were impressed by our colleague's approach to problem solving. We asked about how she thought it would be possible to facilitate so much change, and she said simply, "It's the job for which I was trained but I am just beginning to fully understand the nature and dynamics of personal suffering and health."

Family units are determined and influenced by beliefs, values, environments, and religious and cultural systems. Health care providers are well equipped professionally to deal with the challenges presented by those who suffer once (a) suffering is seen as an entity separate and only sometimes related to pain, (b) suffering is understood as a life experience that is characterized by a perception of threat to idea of self and personhood, and (c) suffering is recognized as involving a loss of central purpose in life and impaired interpersonal relationships and results in considerable self-conflict.

SUMMARY

This chapter presented the argument that knowledge of life cycle developmental, psychosocial tasks is critical to effective management of those who suffer. The resolution of suffering is influenced not only by highly individualized perceptions of self and the nature of an individual's personhood but also by the fact that people may suffer because they are not able to accomplish life cycle psychosocial developmental tasks. To provide effective care to patients who suffer, clinicians must be aware of the types of tasks the patient may need to accomplish at various ages and how illness or injury can thwart the successful accomplishment of these tasks. In addition, the basic tenets of family systems theory and ecosystems theories of families and how the family is affected by the suffering of one of its members were outlined. In health care delivery, human behaviour must be viewed from the sociocultural context in which it occurs. Explorations of the age-specific stages of development life cycle tasks show that each stage is integrated with another and that illness may follow interruptions in the completion of any one of these life cycle tasks. In-depth study of family systems theory and ecosystems theories demand attention if effective care of those who suffer is to be achieved.

The resolution of suffering from the perspective of individuals, the family, and the health care organization requires not only the ability to understand and implement theoretical approaches to care but also a new approach to patient communication in which individuals' personal autonomy is acknowledged and respected. The next chapter will explore the language of suffering and its relevance to personal power and autonomy.

CHAPTER 5 QUESTIONS

1. According to the tenets of Erikson's theories of human psychosocial development across the life span, what are the key concepts?
2. Choose three psychological milestones. What are the respective psychological tasks that may be affected when suffering occurs?
3. What are some of the conflicts that may occur between patients who suffer and their families?
4. How may potential conflicts arise between hospital staff, patients, and families when patients and families are unable to accomplish their psychosocial developmental tasks?
5. What is an ecosystem therapeutic approach to the care of those who suffer?
6. What is a family systems approach to care?

7 How do perceptions of families differ between an ecosystem and family systems therapeutic approach to care?
8 What type of care plan could have avoided the conflicts described between Mr. Cjenchuck's daughter and family and the hospital staff?

6 *The Language of Suffering*

Beneficence, that is, doing good, is the primary goal of all health care providers. The challenge in clinical practice is to do what is considered to be morally good as opposed to performing self-serving acts that one determines are for the "good" of the patient but are really attempts to derive personal prestige and reward. The moral obligations imposed on medical acts of beneficence are to respect the autonomy of the patient, to do no harm (non-malfeasance), and to ensure justice prevails (1). Regulated health care providers have a fiduciary relationship with the patient as determined by their respective professional colleges, which set the scope of practice and quality of care. Health care professionals have the trust and confidence of the patient and the responsibility to act solely for the benefit of the patient. When considering the relationship between health clinician and patients who suffer, the patient's primary goal is to restore his or her idea of self, to resolve issues of self-conflict, and to pursue the central purpose of his/her life in the face of adversity.

To meet the objective of beneficence with those individuals who suffer, one must have a clear understanding not only of the language of suffering but also of the concept of autonomy and its relationship to personal power and personal responsibility. The preservation of personal autonomy in individuals who have chronic illnesses and who experience suffering is particularly challenging in culturally pluralistic contemporary societies.

This chapter will explore: (a) some aspects of the language of suffering and its value when there is a loss of autonomy and personal power, (b) the historical roots of autonomy and its social ramifications, (c) the problem of patient autonomy in medicine, (d) the dimensions of personal power and health, and (e) the dimensions of power and the need to hear the patient's voice.

The Loss of Power and Autonomy: The Language of Suffering

. . . And then
From reasonableness to the village idiot
Always aware of the fool,
Stumbling here, stumbling there
How long before the idiot succumbs
To the cold winds of winter
A frozen corpse, no telling of past passions

No fire of love, all stiff and awkward
Not even the peace of decomposition
A restlessness, fear, pain
Drained . . . blood . . . spirit . . . personality
All depleted.
And still the frozen zombie gets up and walks
Searching with sightless eyes, a mindless creature
Searching for a soul.

This poem, along with several others, was given to me as a gift from one of my patients who, on discharge from the hospital, told me that I could use it for teaching purposes as long as I kept the authorship anonymous.

LAURA'S STORY

I first met Laura (not her real name) many years ago when I was working in a rural rehabilitation unit. I was doing a twelve-month locum in orthopedics and Laura was a patient of mine who was the sole survivor of a terrible car crash. Her entire family perished in the tragic accident. Laura sustained multiple fractures of both her legs, pelvis, and right arm. Fortunately, she did not have a head injury.

Laura's rehabilitation process was long and often physically very challenging. She seemed to be a quiet, well-groomed, reserved woman. She smiled only occasionally, but her attendance in the clinic was punctual and she worked hard.

Prior to her accident, Laura was working on a doctorate of philosophy in art history and continued with her studies while in hospital. Other patients whispered to the staff that they thought she was a hero, given the circumstances of her accident. Laura told me she hated the label because all she felt was an all-encompassing fatigue and profound sorrow.

One day, after the resident on the ward had made a referral for Laura to Psychology, she broke down and tearfully told me about how badly she felt because she believed that the staff thought she was "crazy." I tried to explain that seeking psychological help after a traumatic event was a brave and courageous act and referrals were not made because she was "crazy" but rather to help. I felt uneasy and more than a bit guilty saying this to her because although I believed that no one thought Laura was "crazy," I was not sure that she had not been diagnosed and subsequently labeled with clinical depression, a psychological illness. The dual messages that Laura was receiving were that she was either a hero or mentally ill. Because of my limited skills at that time, I did not understand the language Laura used to describe the extent of her fear that maybe she really was mentally ill.

Because the health care team did not understand the language of suffering, we did not hear or understand the power of her suffering. Perhaps that was why Laura became quieter and more withdrawn. Later on I realized that Laura was trying to tell us about her felt experience. She was trying to tell us about her loss of self and personhood, which we misheard and labeled as possible mental illness. Suffering is not a mental illness but simply a life experience. Fortunately, the psychiatrist who treated Laura quickly discerned the true nature of Laura's experience. Unfortunately, the rest of the team seemed to adopt the attitude that Laura's suffering was outside the boundaries of their respective scope of practice. It may be that Laura felt that she no longer could trust the medical personnel and her only way of validating her experience was to write poetry.

In the above poem, Laura talks about becoming "the village idiot" and "always the fool." I now realize that suffering involves a loss of the individual's old self and suddenly being confronted with a life that seems the same but is not. It is a new life, one in which there are few or no internal supports. Some patients feel that they can no longer trust themselves. It was only after Laura's discharge and after reading some of her other works that I became aware of the many concerns she had for her mental health and the power of the almost existential loneliness that formed the basis of her life.

While in hospital, Laura sometimes spoke of her frustration as being unbearable, particularly after family/patient meetings. She said staff made decisions for her. She would complain that no one asked her what she wanted. She did not want people coming into her house to feed her. She told me quite emphatically that she was not a child. When I asked her, as gently as I could, how she planned to cook with only one arm and from a reclined position in her wheelchair she began to cry. She told me that it was not that she did not want help but that she was upset because decisions were made not with her but about her. After a while, we talked about developing a plan and I asked her if she would feel comfortable if I asked the occupational therapist to join us. She agreed, and the three of us worked out a strategy that Laura then presented to her doctor and the rest of the team. Fortunately, the team agreed to follow Laura's lead. Often this is not the case, and such attempts can be misinterpreted; patients can be labeled as being controlling and uncooperative.

There were other such incidents during Laura's hospital stay involving various members of the health care team, but we still failed to hear the language of suffering, and each of Laura's concerns had to reach a crisis state before resolution occurred. The process of trying to communicate these feelings to staff required a lot of energy on Laura's part, energy that might have been spent on enhancing her recovery process. In retrospect, I still have the uneasy feeling that we missed hearing many of Laura's concerns and as a result abandoned her to further suffering.

On discharge, Laura presented me with a gift of a notebook filled with poems and thoughts that she had written down during her stay in the rehabilitation unit. I used to read these poems at night before I fell asleep. It occurred to me that in many ways we had failed Laura because we were so focused on her pain and physical limitations that we did not hear the language of suffering. Because we did not hear the language of suffering we did not acknowledge the importance of her autonomy. We did not realize that our actions may have robbed Laura of her dignity and need for personal power.

Rereading the first line of Laura's poem, "from reasonableness to the village idiot, always aware of the fool," it's clear that Laura was writing about the fact that she believed she was now living in a world that had lost all sense of reason. She speaks of her loss of central purpose because she was always "stumbling here, and stumbling there." She spoke of living in a place were there was no light, no way out of her terrible situation. She described herself as a "frozen corpse," all "stiff and awkward." There was no place in her emotional and/or physical world where she could find peace or comfort. Her great angst was that while the passion of her soul had died, there was still an energy inside her that persisted. She speaks of searching, of being mindless, and of looking for her lost self and personhood. Clearly, this poem speaks to a loss of idea of self and central purpose and feelings of self-conflict, the universal characteristics of suffering.

Other writings spoke to the need to be silent, to seem to be managing so that staff and friends would be pleased. She once told me that she felt alone, that she was living in a different world from the rest of us. Many of her poems passionately addressed her fear that perhaps she was going mad and that there was no way out of the dark world in which she now lived. Many of the writings expressed a profound existential loneliness. She kept asking the reader to look at her and see if they could see a person, because she had lost herself. In other poems there were images of suicide, yet this issue was never mentioned to the staff, nor did any of us address the subject. Did Laura try to tell us and we did not hear? Other images were descriptive of emotionally hiding away from friends and family while still participating in normal daily tasks. There were expressions of rage and profound sorrow. The most significant observation was that the rage expressed seemed to be directed at her belief that the rest of the people she knew would not let her back into the world of the living. I decided to share Laura's poems with the health care team.

Laura's poems were disturbing to our staff because they were all dated and we realized that as Laura became more skilled at pleasing us, her suffering escalated. Even when her physical health had shown significant recovery, expressions of suffering were still very high. We recognized in Laura's behaviour elements of many of our other patients. We then began to explore issues of language and assessment and diagnosis and we discussed the concepts of autonomy and personal power as it relates to health care delivery. We examined the history of autonomy and compared our findings to contemporary life and then spent considerable effort examining autonomy and its relationship to personal power and human dignity in clinical practice. The relationship between suffering and autonomy is a prime factor in effective health care delivery. There is a critical need for courses in moral philosophy to be included in the basic education of all health care clinicians. Our team meetings began exploring the issue of autonomy and its relevance to the care of those who suffer.

Autonomy and Power

Historical Perspectives

Moral philosophy arose after great political change in Europe. The power of the monarchies declined, as did the influence of religious authority (2). Egalitarian rights expanded and individuals began to view autonomy in terms of personal responsibility. Diverse views could only be accommodated in pluralistic societies if mutual respect was considered to be the moral imperative. Autonomy and personal responsibility became factors for health care professionals, who needed to obtain permissions from patients. The problem with viewing autonomy as permission is that individuals no longer make their own decisions in health care and in other social arenas; rather, they are asked to either agree or disagree with the decisions made by others. A health care example is the agreement concerning when and if further treatments are to be stopped. Individuals either agree or disagree that treatment should cease when certain parameters, determined by others, are reached. Autonomy has become a form of collective bargaining.

Tauber argues that, because there is no overall societal moral imperative in modern society, we have become social pragmatists and tend to live without moral and ethical guidelines (3). Other scholars argue further that without a moral ethic there is really no such thing as freedom or autonomy (4–8). In democratic institutions, there is a prevailing belief that freedom and personal autonomy are key components that must be part of obtaining patient consent. Patients must be free to agree or disagree to treatments offered without prejudice or fear of future reprisal (9–11).

Such differing views are a challenge to health care providers, and hospitals now have ethics committees to advise staff when conflicts arise. Ethical modern health care delivery must be aware of the social perspectives of autonomy. Modern health care delivery must encompass the diversity of needs of people from all walks of life.

The Social Origins of Autonomy

Past understandings of autonomy in North American society are based on the works of Kant, in which autonomy is the equivalent of self governance, freedom of action, independence, and liberty. Current views are that autonomy is based on contracts and agreements (2). These current perspectives have evolved because societies are now very diverse and there is no overall moral imperative to which all persons subscribe. Further, not all cultures place the same emphasis on the value of the individual in decision making. For example, Korean-American and Mexican-American patients often prefer to have decisions made by families (4, 5).

Many persons who subscribe to the spiritual teachings of Taoism, Buddhism, or Confucianism, traditions that emphasize the power of the community over that of the individual, may not embrace the construct of individual autonomy. Harmonious relationships in concert with others are of prime importance to these patients. Personal autonomy may be interpreted by these groups as an unnecessary burden on the patient who is trying to get well. Some research studies add support to these points of view and results show that while many people may practice personal autonomy in everyday life, they may not want to make direct decisions when they are ill (6). Consequently, postmodern definitions of autonomy embrace both the individual and a variety of views based on cultural diversity. Confidentiality becomes a critical factor in the ethics of autonomy based on contractual agreements (7).

Contemporary understandings of the nature of autonomy in medicine and the need of those who suffer to be autonomous are germane to ethical, patient-centred care. Loss of autonomy is manifested through the loss of idea of self and personhood. The objective of medicine, then, is to help the patient maintain or restore his or her idea of self.

Autonomy in Medicine

In health care decision making, the definition of personhood is more confined than that presented in earlier chapters. From the perspective of suffering, personhood refers to all aspects of an individual's life. The definition of personhood encompasses ways people have lived their lives in the past, how they live now in the present, and their anticipations for life in the future. In medicine, personhood is often viewed from strictly pragmatic terms involving people's ability to feed themselves, toilet, bathe, dress, and ambulate independently. Work and recreational objectives and competences are of secondary importance, and issues such as ambitions and dreams are rarely considered to be within the realm of health care delivery (8–10).

Autonomy, in medicine, when it refers to permissions, is defined as moral competence (11). In current medical decision making, patients are deemed morally competent if they can conceive of rules and actions for themselves, exhibit rational thinking, provide evidence of a moral sensibility, and demonstrate that they think of themselves as being free to make decisions.

The difficulty with this approach is that patients are often unable to conceive of rules and actions for themselves when they are ill because they are frightened or are in psychological and/or physical distress. In addition, patients are unskilled in medical practice, and while the Internet provides a great deal of information, it does not provide knowledge or skills. Because of the prevailing injury or illness, individuals are often not able to see themselves as free agents. They must then appoint health care providers to make decisions for them. Health care professionals have the obligation to make decisions on behalf of their patients based on rules of beneficence, competency, and justice. Autonomy becomes the province of the law and lawyers, and moral competency becomes a question of adequacy. Autonomy in clinical practice is no longer the sole responsibility of the patient but rather a shared responsibility between patient and health care provider. Often this relationship does not exist, and personal autonomy becomes an act of professional paternalism. When patients are able to make decisions for themselves, they become personally responsible for their actions.

Autonomy becomes self-rule when there is a deep agreement between an individual's moral self and the rules this self imposes on itself. In such instances, patients are able to understand, evaluate, and determine what is at stake and the consequences of their decisions on the self and on others. The patient is morally responsible for his/her decision if a moral choice is involved. Moral choices are those decisions based on a principle or a moral belief, such as those arising from religious or philosophical teachings or an appeal made to one's own true self (7–10).

Not all autonomous views are considered valid in medicine. For example, euthanasia and selling of human organs are usually not acceptable social constructs and can be a source of conflict within the clinical setting, particularly in situations involving terminal illness.

In medicine, autonomy not only involves the tenets of morality but also demands accountability, both of patients and health care decision making (7). Manipulation of information, failure to provide information, the perception of threat or evoking fears of retaliation, and coercion limit a patient's individual autonomy. Those who are ill or suffering may be afraid that staff will become angered and not treat them well if they do not agree with the professional's advice or decisions. Patients may also be afraid to disagree with the doctors because they fear that they will find themselves without the medical expertise they need to get well. In these circumstances the patient does not have an active voice. He/she either gives permission or keeps silent. Silence is often a strategy used by individuals who suffer as a method of maintaining personal power.

The issue of personal power in medical practice is paramount to achieving autonomy (9, 10). Patients and families must be accountable for their decisions. Individuals who fail to follow medical advice, or who seek several advisors simultaneously and then sue individuals at random for poor advice, must also be held accountable. However, when considering those who suffer, such activities on the part of patients are rarely encountered. In suffering, the health care dynamics usually revolve around the power differentials that exist between clinicians and patients.

The Goals of Health Care Delivery

Aspects of Power and Responsibility

Power is commonly understood as the ability to act in a particular way. It is the capacity to influence other people or to affect the course of events. Power involves political authority, control, and physical or emotional strength. Responsibility involves being morally accountable for one's behaviour. It is an obligation to do something.

There are many types of powerful people. For example, people with extraordinary skills and knowledge who are willing to take responsibility for their actions have "real" power. In health care, physicians have "real" power because they assume full responsibility for their patients. Political leaders may have "real" power as well when they make policy decisions that affect the health and welfare of citizens. Chief officers of organizations may appear to have power, but in fact, decisions and actions are determined by politicians, board members, union representatives, and others. Health care administrators have apparent power when obtaining health care fiscal resources and real power in the distribution of these monies. Charisma is another form of power in which individuals appear "larger than life" to others. Charismatic people are able to exert considerable influence over others and events but they usually do not assume responsibility for their actions. They do not participate in the actualization of their ideas. In health care, charismatic people may be professional fund raisers who raise money for various causes but do not become involved in accountability of the funds raised or whether the monies are actually used for the purposes proposed by the fundraising event.

In families, there are those who have real power, apparent power, and may even have charismatic power. As in the community at large, power differentials among people shift depending on circumstances. Individuals have absolute power when they exert full control over situations or others.

When objectively considering the issue of suffering in contemporary society, it is the individual who suffers who should have the real power because he/she is the only person who knows the felt experience and is the only person accountable for the behaviours that arise in response to the experience. The responsibility of the individual is: (a) to maintain the present perception of self by incorporating new demands on the self caused by the current adversity or (b) to develop a new sense of self that the individual deems acceptable. In reality, the patient feels powerless because suffering involves a perception of threat to his/her idea of self.

The personal management of suffering, particularly in chronic illness, often seems to be a daunting task for patients. Some individuals can embrace this task alone and others cannot. Clinical practice shows that people with social support systems manage better than those without. The successful restoration of the self requires a shared experience of power, autonomy, and social responsibility between health care providers and patient. This objective remains challenging to achieve, particularly if the health care organization's power structure is hierarchical in design.

Power and the Health Care Professional

In current clinical practice, the health care clinician is usually regarded as most powerful and is awarded the respect associated with the knowledge and responsibility assumed. The physician is often the member of the health care team with absolute power in hierarchical organizational structures (9, 10). The patient may be the least powerful, as is illustrated by the fact that others determine the veracity of the patient's story of suffering as well as the appropriateness of the sufferer's response to the experience of suffering.

In fact, the health professional knows medicine but does not know the patient's felt experience. Consequently, because of the present power differential between the clinician and patient, the health professional has considerable ability to influence the patient and family as well as the society at large. In cases of suffering, the power of the health care provider can negatively impact patient autonomy if the construct of suffering as an entity separate from pain is not understood and if the patient's voice is not heard.

In the case of Laura discussed above, the patient believed that telling the story of her suffering would result in her being labeled with a mental illness. She was convinced that if she did not follow the wishes of her care givers, her care would be compromised. She sometimes asked why her therapists were trying to "reframe" her experience. She kept saying that the suffering that she experienced was not the story that was being retold by others. Her response to these events was to become silent. She felt that she was powerless. From a therapeutic perspective, silence can be very powerful because it creates a distance between the individual and the clinician.

In medicine, clinicians often speak of empowering patients, which is a contradiction in terms. One person cannot empower another. Power is attained by the efforts of individuals. Opportunities such as those suggested above may be provided so that a person may develop the skills required to be independent and subsequently powerful, but the process is personal and determined by the individual. For example, rehabilitation medicine is one aspect of health care in which the therapeutic goal is to assist individuals to become physically and emotionally independent. The impact of an individual's real power on motivation is remarkable, particularly in cases where the physical rehabilitation outcome far exceeds scientific probabilities.

Autonomy and Suffering

Managing suffering involves resolving the perception of threat to an individual's idea of self, eliminating self-conflict, and developing a new central purpose in life. The importance of autonomy and personal power is critical to the restoration of health.

To successfully help those who suffer, clinicians must be willing to sometimes take the risk of reversing the current power dichotomy. Because autonomy involves permissions and agreements determined by health care providers, the responsibility for shifting the power relationship is that of the clinician. When pragmatic power shifts are made, the potential professional risks are that the clinician is now at the service of the individual and has less absolute power, but he/she still has the legal and moral responsibilities for the patient's care. This approach to the patient-clinician relationship can be very threatening to some health care providers. Such fears are unfounded because the management of suffering is an integral, though often undocumented, component of all professionals' scope of practice.

In the case of the management of suffering, a shift in the real power differential must occur if health care providers are to be able to provide the patient with relevant suffering treatment interventions. At times, the patient will have real power because the health care provider has agreed to accept the patient's authority about the impact and nature of the suffering. The health professional agrees with the individual's determination of the factors that constitute a resolution of suffering. In return, the patient agrees to assume responsibility for the outcome of such decisions when there are differences between clinician and patient. The exceptions are when there is potential harm to the individual and/or others that is unacknowledged by the patient. In these situations, clinicians who understand suffering as an entity separate from pain still have real power, but not absolute power. Clinicians determine the scientific medical care of the patient and have the specialized skills to manage both the illness and its effects.

The issue of risk is common in medical practice. Health professionals constantly face the potential risks of personal error, accidents, and unexplained or unknown scientific factors. Risks are taken every day in medicine as health care professionals try to help those in need. Compared to these real risks, the potential risks in shifting power differentials in suffering are minimal.

The issue of power differentials is more important to some health care providers than to others. Studies have shown that physiotherapists, for example, value power for themselves far less than they value beneficence to their patients (12, 13). Results show that physical therapists highly prize values that give benefit to others and view their own professional success in terms of beneficence (14). In physiotherapy, treatment of suffering separate from pain does not require a significant shift in the power differential between therapist and patient. Efficacious care in physiotherapy demands the skill to recognize suffering as separate from pain and the ability to implement suffering-specific strategies into assessment and treatment.

All professions have expectations of their members. In professions such as nursing, social work, and chaplaincy, beneficence is the prime moral value, but in nursing, the prime objective is to care for the patient during illness and help the patient not only to understand the nature of the illness but also to obtain the care needed to restore health. In physiotherapy, the prime goal is to facilitate motivation to overcome the effects of illness. In professions such as chaplaincy and social work, the objectives are often to help people redeem the inner self after the onslaught of illness or injury and help them find a sense of meaning in their lives. Once again, the power shift in these professions requires acknowledging and validating the voice of the patient in the management of suffering.

Physicians, on the other hand, have a primary commitment to "curing" a disease. Caring, in the sense of comfort and consolation is often a secondary component. The ultimate legal and moral responsibility for the patient is that of the physician. Consequently, issues of authority, power, justice, and malfeasance can be more complex and more challenging for physicians, but not more important than those facing other health care providers. Extrapolation of scientific evidence into clinical practice is very difficult, particularly in litigious societies. Physicians are faced with resolving the demands of absolute power and moral responsibility with those caused by the shifting dynamics between real and apparent power in health care delivery.

Patients also have expectations of health care providers that impact on their autonomy, dignity, and personal power. A study involving occupational therapists (15) showed that patients' expectations of occupational therapists were for therapists to show concern, direction, fellowship, and guidance. Patients did not want to experience the effects of political coalitions between health care professionals and they did not want to be rejected or treated in a detached manner if they did not agree with the advice of the therapist.

Patient expectations are of considerable importance in the management of suffering. If health care providers have not successfully addressed suffering in their own lives and are emotionally stressed by evidence of suffering in others, they may react to patients in a detached manner in an attempt to self-protect. Detachment is not helpful to patients who suffer. The management of suffering involves empathetic engagement in the patient's experience rather than an instructional approach where the health care clinician is the ultimate authority.

SUMMARY

This chapter has explored the importance of recognizing the language of suffering in clinical practice using a patient's poem as a reference point. Analysis of the poem revealed the importance of autonomy and personal power when managing suffering as separate from pain. The historical origins and social manifestations of autonomy and its relevance in health care practice were discussed. The need for a shift in the current power differential in which the health care professional is the ultimate authority to one where the patient and his/her felt experience dominate was examined. The importance of understanding the language of suffering and its relationship to the goals of health care delivery were emphasized.

The management of suffering involves not only an understanding of the language of suffering but also a willingness to engage in power shifts between health care professionals and patients and to recognize the importance of the sufferer's voice, personal autonomy, and social responsibility.

We have seen in previous chapters how culture and religious and spiritual traditions impact on the experience of suffering. In this chapter we have made reference to the litigious component of secular society. It is now important to explore the impact of legal and medical discourse on those who suffer due to chronic illness and/or injury.

CHAPTER 6 QUESTIONS

1. What are some of the key themes expressed using the language of suffering?
2. What constitutes beneficence in health care delivery to those who suffer?
3. What are the main tenets of the historical evolution of autonomy?
4. What are the social origins of autonomy?
5. What is the nature of autonomy in contemporary medicine?
6. How does the lack of personal autonomy affect health care outcomes?
7. Define the various types of personal power. What are their respective impacts on the health of those who suffer?
8. What is the relationship between power and professional responsibility?
9. What is meant by personal responsibility?
10. What is the nature of the power differential between health care professionals and those who suffer?

7 Medical-Legal Disclosure of Suffering

The issue of suffering in contemporary medical practice is of considerable concern. Legally, the law regards pain and suffering as one and the same entity, and proof of suffering is found in the realm of psychological illness. Some clinicians fear that acknowledging suffering as separate from pain will result in insurance adjusters denying legitimate claims for fiscal compensation to those individuals who require considerable assistance after traumatic injuries. Against this argument is the definition of suffering as a perception of threat to idea of self and personhood. Accepting this definition does not negate the results of impairment or disabilities as determined by quantitative and qualitative measures of abilities and opportunities (quality-of-life scales) or impact-of-illness measures. Acknowledging suffering, as defined above, simply takes the experience out of the realm and stigma of psychological illness and places it within the context of cause and effect. In medical legal cases, the patient may be entitled to fiscal compensation because idea of self and personhood are adversely affected due to traumatic events. Further, suffering, as defined above, would most likely not have occurred if the impairments had not led to disability or chronic illness.

Many health professionals and their patients do not realize that the prime concern of insurance companies is to be sure that monies are awarded in accordance with rules and regulations determined by formal legal agreements and the duty of the law is to uphold these rules when disputes occur. Often patients and clinicians believe that the purpose of the law in personal injury disputes is to determine the rightness or wrongness of an event or the goodness or badness of the people involved. Consequently, ignorance of the purpose of the law may result in failure to understand the impact of health care providers' careless or inappropriate note taking and inappropriate and incomplete problem identification in determining the degree of assistance required by patients. Failure of health care providers to understand the basic tenets of the law in relationship to suffering may result in poor treatment outcomes and an increase in patient suffering.

The purpose of this chapter is to present a brief introduction to the history of the law and a description of how rules and regulations are made. The focus of this chapter also raises questions about: (a) the difference between medical and legal definitions of suffering, (b) similarities between medical and legal discourse and suffering and the loss of personal autonomy, (c) the justification for loss of personal power in legal and medical discourse, (d) ethical considerations in medical and legal discourse, and (e) cultural implications in pluralistic multicultural societies and the impact on suffering.

In this section it is argued that it is the ethical responsibility of all health care practitioners to be familiar with basic tenets of the law as it relates to patient suffering. Issues relating to law and professional misconduct are beyond the scope of this discussion. For purposes of clarification, examples of legal discourse are taken from the British, U.S., and Canadian legal systems because both the U.S. and Canadian systems have evolved from the British system. The need for health care providers to understand the basic principles of the legal systems of their own countries is a global medical responsibility.

A Brief History of the Law and Its Impact on Contemporary Health Care Delivery

Sometimes, patients experience a great deal of distress when legal judgments appear to violate laws of natural reason and perceptions of justice. If health care providers can provide patients with brief explanations of how, throughout the centuries, there were many difficulties encountered in determining the relationship between the law and individuals, patients may be less likely to feel victimized and abandoned.

The law arises from the needs of society and may be based on religious or social customs (1–3). In ancient times (500 B.C.), Greek laws were such that claims were made against manufacturers, bank officials, or accountants. Crimes involved murder, robbery, and slander. Initially, murder was a crime against a family, but later became a crime against the state. Generally, the notion of justice is based on ideas of morality and fairness. Health care providers who are not aware of the history of the law may not realize that justice was originally based on ownership of property and possessions. In the language of modern society, justice and fairness relate to monetary gain. The needs of contemporary society are often more complex, but the underlying basis of justice is still very rooted in fiscal compensation. The component of morality in the construct of justice was not based on the personal autonomy of individuals but rather on a business ethic involving goods and property. The implication for health care providers whose responsibility is the health of their patients is that care must be taken to avoid contributing to the suffering of their patients by engaging in a process in which the patient and his/her illness become commodities in the marketplace.

In 621 B.C. the Athenians began to codify laws. Draco wrote the first code of laws, which were very severe (draconian) and the impact of these laws is still evident in modern society (1). A series of reforms were established in which jurors were paid for their time and sometimes thousands of people were involved in decision making. The process of secret ballots was soon corrupted by special interest groups. Judges had little training, and the procedures were very much like religious rituals. These practices are evidence of the beginnings of an adversarial system, once again based on a business model rather than on an ethic of compassion and care. Currently, health care providers must be aware of how modern adversarial legal processes may impact on the health of their patients. It is important also to acknowledge that lawyers who are employed to assist patients must work within the constructs of this adversarial system even at the cost of the patient's felt experience. Often patients are afraid of the legal process, afraid that they will not be believed. Consequently, they may not fully engage in rehabilitation programs for fear that should there be improvement in their physical condition, all their legal claims for compensation will be denied. For some patients, the refusal of a claim for compensation may cause considerable fiscal hardship. For example, the cost of necessary assistive devices and/or automobile/home adaptations critical for rehabilitation may be prohibitive for the patient if claims are denied.

The Athenians soon realized that some crimes were against society as a whole and should not be dealt with by the aggrieved individuals who sought vengeance. The Athenians developed a structure to deal with the predictability of various areas of potential conflict. The process of presenting arguments was determined. There were three main precepts. One, the speaker must obtain the good will of the audience; two, arguments must be presented; and three, there must be a summary of the arguments presented. These precepts became the basic tool of the courts and the basis of formal education. Trained orators began to represent clients in court and the foundations of the legal profession were established. Examples of the origins of this historic process in contemporary medicine are encountered by patients who must appear before "discovery" committees of lawyers. In cases where there is litigation against insurance companies patients can be subjected to interrogation by panels of lawyers from several insurance companies. The role of the legal personnel is to determine the veracity of the patient's complaints and to determine the monetary value of the case. The objective is to keep potential monetary compensation negligible or nonexistent. Participation in this process may be extremely threatening to patients, not only because of the psychological stress incurred but also because patients may feel their job will be in jeopardy if extra time is taken away from work to attend these proceedings. Settlement of such cases may take decades to resolve, with considerable harm to the patient. Patients may believe that if they show any improvements, such improvements may negate their legal claim. Lawyers sometimes fail to explain to patients the nature of the legal arguments being presented and assure patients that the legal issues do not prohibit improvements to health.

Health care providers must be scrupulously accurate in reporting the health status of patients and refrain from giving nonscientific opinions about those in their care. Clinicians who are aware of the law are better able to assist patients by advising them of the process, helping them manage stress, and modifying treatment regimes to account for such disturbances.

In the fifth century B.C., Roman class distinctions of people were based on birth and wealth. A code of laws known as the "Twelve Tables" was passed to create some equality of rights between the classes. The main tenets of the code focused on interest rates, property and personal rights, and some aspects of family relationships. At this time the purpose of the law began to slip away from religious and social custom to the notion of justice and fair play. Interpretation of the code by persons other than those who created it was considered to be treachery. Judges helped to draft the code and were deemed the appropriate people to be appointed to interpret it. This process formed the basis of modern judicial process whereby courts now interpret statutes without referring to legislative bodies. Today, informed health care practitioners who are supportive of patients' decisions to be involved in litigation can reassure patients that their experiences with the law are appropriate by explaining, in simple terms, how the court system works. By doing so, clinicians can refocus patients' attention back to improving health.

During Roman rule, difficulties arose because the same laws were applied over many thousands of miles and involved many cultures. Roman emperors created many new laws that were not uniformly applied. Judges and lawyers had no access to new laws made in Rome. The government at the time did not collect and store the thousands of edicts issued, and by the year A.D. 300 Roman law consisted of 3 million edicts. Private lawsuits took years to be resolved. While lawsuits are now settled more quickly, few health care practitioners realize that their patients may be struggling with the court system for decades, and as a result, accurate assessments of health care interventions may be severely compromised by such processes. It is important to ask patients if they are involved in litigation so that they may be reassured that the clinician will do all that is ethically and legally possible to be of assistance.

In A.D. 429, the Eastern empire established the Theodosian code, after Emperor Theodosius II, which codified all the edicts since the time of the Emperor Constantine. That same year the code was also adopted in Rome. About one hundred years later, the Justinian code was established by the Eastern empire. The first published version of the Code of Justinian was completed in A.D. 529 and forms the basis of modern European law; the law of Quebec, Canada; and the law of the state of Louisiana. The Code of Justinian also forms the basis for the Canadian Charter of Rights and Freedoms and the U.S. Constitution. The fifth century saw the fall of the Roman Empire and Europe reverted to religious and customary laws.

Later in England, under William the Conqueror (1066), the "Domesday Book" was the census of a new kingdom. The legal relationships that were established saw the crown as the head of the courts. Trials were based on religious and customary beliefs, and in the early stages, implementation disputes were settled by a series of physical ordeals endured by the accused. If the accused person's body healed after a prescribed time, the accused was declared innocent. In 1215, the Magna Carta was signed and these practices were discontinued. Disputes were settled by professional fighters. Justice was not an issue. This method forms the basis of our modern adversarial system in which lawyers are the patient's professional fighters. Patient recognition of lawyers as professional fighters can also be useful in managing feelings of loss of personal autonomy and perceptions of victimization, symptoms common to those who suffer.

In the sixteenth century, Henry VIII tried to reinstate the Justinian code of the Romans but failed. At the same time however, England broke away from the Roman church and established the Church of England with Parliament at the head. Large sections of religious doctrine became the source of law. The Renaissance in Italy in the fourteenth through sixteenth centuries saw the resurgence of interest in Greek and Roman literature and the re-establishment of the codified Roman system. In France, in the early nineteenth century, Napoleon Bonaparte codified French law and it became known as the Napoleonic code in 1805. Under this system of codes, the status of women diminished, minority rights were abolished, and tolerance of religious beliefs was retained. The code established principles of equality before the law, and all issues pertaining to the French Revolution of 1789 were included. Understanding these historical events will help clinicians address patients' perceptions of unfairness or injustice, factors that may contribute to the development of clinical depression. Simple explanations of the meaning of equality before the law may help patients avoid feelings of victimization.

Many social changes have evolved since the signing of the Magna Carta, but the influence of this document prevails in modern life. For example, in Canada, the conquest of Quebec led to the Quebec Act of 1774 in which the criminal laws of England and the civil law of France were instituted. Currently, Quebec law is based on the Napoleonic code. Many legal systems in countries throughout the world have been influenced by the these historical events, which have a powerful influence on the lives and health of those who seek redress through the courts. In the United States of America, British parliamentary rules and regulations were overridden by the U.S. Constitution, as the United States of America developed its tenets as a democratic republic.

While it is important to understand the historical basis of the law, if the relationship between suffering and the law is to be understood, the process of how rules and regulations are determined in modern life is also important. Historically, the legal system has been shown to be and continues to be an organic entity. To do no harm is the objective of all health care personnel. Professional organizations and educational institutions are beginning to offer programs to help their members understand legal rules and regulations. In law, such rules are called statutes. The value and power of statutes in contemporary society are outlined below, using the Canadian parliamentary system as an example.

Rules and Regulations: The Power of Statutes in Contemporary Society

A statute is a document that sets out legal rules that are usually passed by both Houses of Parliament in the form of a bill and agreed to by the crown. Exceptions are made in which some bills do not need approval from the Senate. Statutes are commonly known as Acts of Parliament and consist of personal, private, and public Acts. It is important for health care providers to know how specific rules and regulations established by the statutes affect the lives of their patients. Some statutes refer to professional practice issues of health care providers and some to the ethics of patient care.

Common Law

After the Norman conquest of 1066, the statutes developed by the English Royal courts were not changed. The common laws established by the Royal court applied to the whole country and not only to local regions. The main purpose of these rules was to preserve the Royal treasury through the establishment of a central administration. These rules were part of the court system for three centuries after the Norman Conquest. Common law is usually not written down or codified but is derived from centuries of judicial resolution of disputes. Sometimes, complex judgments involving health are decided according to the tenets of common law.

Case Law

A codification of a common law becomes a statute and is then known as case law. If a statute is used to contradict an existing common law, it must be presented in such a way that is it absolutely clear and unambiguous. Statutes are not open to interpretation. Past judgments or decisions of a court can be used as an authority for reaching the same decision in subsequent cases. Case law is often used in litigation involving insurance.

Civil Law

The law of any state is based on Roman law rather than English common law. Civil law consists of a body of rules and regulations that govern the rights and obligations among individuals, institutions, and corporations, and relates to contracts, property, family issues, marriage, divorce, tort, negligence, wills, inheritance, insurance, copyright, patents and trademarks, employment, and labour. It is a private law as opposed to a criminal law. Under civil law, individuals are under a duty not to cause harm to another. Persons are at fault if they fail in that duty by not acting according to the expected standard of care. If clinicians are to provide optimal ethical health care delivery, it is important for health care professional association regulatory boards to ensure that professional licensing of their members is based on a sound knowledge of jurisprudence.

Torts

Torts are civil wrongs committed by one person against another such as to cause injury or damage. Torts may be intentional or unintentional. An assault is usually an intentional tort while an unintentional tort would involve negligence. The law of tort is mainly concerned with obtaining compensation for personal injury and property damage caused by negligence. It also protects other interests such as reputation, title to property, commercial interests, and so on. In health care, intentional torts involve battery and assault and issues around consent. Unintentional torts involve negligence or factors contributing to negligence usually by health care professionals. Patients, like all citizens, may be involved in intentional or unintentional torts. Health care professionals who listen to patient narratives to determine those who suffer and to ascertain the nature of patient suffering must know at least the significance of these processes to patients and their health.

Criminal Law

Medicine is committed to helping all who suffer, and some patients may be perpetrators of crimes. Consequently, it is important to have at least a cursory knowledge of the experiences in which a patient may be involved and to be aware of the language used to describe these events. Knowledge of the definition of the criminal code, at least, is critical if care givers are to understand patients' "felt" experiences, a factor critical to complete problem identification.

The criminal code is a federal government statute concerned with relations between individuals and the state. It is concerned with matters in which there is a breach of fundamental values and rules resulting in a threat to peace, stability, order, and the well-being of all the citizens. In Canada, the provinces cannot make criminal law, but they can impose fines and short prison sentences for breach of provincial laws (highway traffic, municipal by-laws, environmental offences, and health laws). Categories of criminal offences are indictable offences (murder, manslaughter, attempted murder, criminal negligence causing death, robbery, theft of property having value over $10,000, treason, and conspiracy to commit an indictable offence) and summary conviction offences. Summary conviction offences involve causing a disturbance, discharging a firearm in a public place, loitering, trespassing at night, and vagrancy. Dual hybrid offences are offences that may be tried either against the crown or as an indictable offence. Until the crown attorney makes the choice, the offence is deemed indictable.

The above discussion was based on examples of Canadian law. There are many commonalities between medical and legal discourse both in Canada and the United States. For example, in the law, jurors are often instructed that while their role is to give the defendant every benefit of reasonable doubt, their real job is to find the "truth." Some legal experts (4) argue that such instructions violate the right of the accused to the presumption of innocence. It is sometimes further argued that a criminal trial is an evaluation of the evidence presented to determine if the state has proved each element of each alleged offence beyond a reasonable doubt. Misunderstandings of the "truth" are perverted by legal rules such as the use of "higher burdens of proof." Burden of proof relates to the duty of a party involved in litigation to prove a fact or facts, persuasive or legal burden of proof is the responsibility of the party who, as a matter of law, will lose the case if the facts of the issue at hand are not proved. "Essential burden" is the duty to show that there is sufficient evidence to raise an issue for the consideration of particular members of the court. Misunderstandings of truth also occur because of legal rules that limit the ability to introduce new evidence, even if it relates to innocence, as well as rules that permit the exclusion of evidence. The results that occur from using non-expert jurors also impacts significantly on obtaining the "truth." Patients who do not understand the machinations of the legal system may personalize issues that occur in legal processes and feel that they are not believed and are being labeled a "liar." While it is not feasible for health care providers to be experts in the law, it is their ethical responsibility, particularly in the fields of nursing and physiotherapy to at least be able to explain basic principles to patients. These latter professionals usually have the most direct, consistent, and intimate contact with patients, and they have considerable influence on patients' attitudes towards health recovery.

The Patient and Medical Legal Disputes

In clinical practice seeking the "truth" in medical legal cases often follows procedures similar to those described above. In medical discourse, such "truth seeking" occurs under the guise of scientific evidence. Research evidence is used to determine whether the patient's felt experience warrants enough evidence to support the legal rules even though research evidence is always obtained from highly controlled settings. Such evidence may then be incorrectly extrapolated to situations that are outside the boundaries established by the original experiments.

Consequently, patients' complaints may then be deemed false because they do not coincide with the extrapolated evidence. Unlike the law, medicine does not always follow the strict rules of evidence, and medical opinions may sometimes be unduly prejudicial. Further, medical discourse may cause harm because of the nature of "privileged information" between doctor and patient. Referral letters for second opinions are often written with subtle prejudice. For example, a letter may begin "Mrs. X has been a patient of mine for several years. She reports persistent pain in her lower back, which she says causes her considerable distress. In spite of numerous tests, we have been unable to find any pathophysiology that explains her complaints. I would be most grateful for a second opinion." Before the second doctor even examines the patient, the letter suggests to him that the patient visits the doctor frequently, is anxious, and since science can not explain the reports of pain the patient is, at best, most likely over exaggerating her symptoms.

Medical discourse may also negatively impact on patients' health and well being. A further example is the release of medical information to the courts in cases where the law must determine legal harm. Legally, confidential conversations between patient and physician cannot be excluded and may be taken out of context when determinations of "the truth" are being made. If patients do not allow the release of their medical information, there is little hope of a positive resolution to the patients' problems. Further, all records of what patients say or do are interpreted by third- and often fourth-party recollections.

An example of how medical information can be misconstrued occurred in our department when one of our colleagues was involved in a car accident and admitted to hospital. While the staff member was in hospital he was visited by the hospital chaplain, a personal friend with whom the patient usually played tennis. A nurse on the ward saw the chaplain enter the patient's room and, without consultation with either party, recorded in the patient's chart that the patient was having psychological problems that were being addressed by the chaplain. This unsubstantiated note became part of the patient's legal medical record and cast doubt on the patient's emotional stability. This incident had severe ramifications for the patient because the car accident resulted in legal litigation. Record keeping must be precise and accurate and relate solely to the health care practitioner's scope of practice. Health care practitioners must know the basic tenets of the law and the potential for harm that exists through ignorance of legal tenets and precepts.

This brief outline of the history of the law shows that the original purpose of the law focused on property rights. Issues relating to the individual stemmed from the belief that human life was also a commodity, and consequently, murder became a punishable crime. Human rights were also based on economic concerns involving tithes and taxes. There seems to be little to suggest that the felt experience of individuals was considered. In fact, the opposite seems to be evident in early historical reports of accused persons being subjected to physical trials, such as the ability to hold a red-hot iron, in order to determine innocence. The concept of suffering was based on ancient religious dogma that sometimes viewed suffering as a method of purging humankind of original sin. It is important to understand the historical evolution of our legal system because while contemporary social science recognizes the concept of suffering outside the framework of past religious dogma, current legal discourse follows past historical patterns. Contemporary legal practice indicates that the responsibility of legal discourse is that suffering should not be enhanced (2, 3). Consequently, it may be argued that health care professionals also have a social responsibility not only to be aware of the impact of legal discourse on suffering but also to understand the nature of very basic legal procedures that may impact the health of their patients. Failure to understand the basic tenets of the legal system may result in clinicians causing patients harm. This may occur by poor record keeping, the expression of subjective opinions rather than objective evidence, and by questionable ethical practices associated with conflict of interest matters that occur when clinicians receive monies for these opinions from special interest groups such as insurance companies or company employers (5–7). It is argued that health care practitioners are obliged to refrain from engaging in adversarial experiences involving patients. To meet these objectives, knowledge of differences between legal and medical definitions of suffering is useful.

Questions then arise concerning the motivations and processes of legal juridical discourse, which are a point of reference for further investigation into the phenomenon of suffering and the law. The term *juridical* describes legal proceedings and their preparation for judgment by a court of law or judge. Similarities in medical and legal discourse and professional power as well as possible ethical, cultural, and spiritual implications are presented for consideration. *Spiritual* refers to an individual's internal belief system, and while these beliefs may be influenced by religious teachings, spirituality and religious dogma are not synonymous.

Differences between Medical and Legal Definitions of Suffering

The nature of suffering in medicine has been previously discussed (chapters 1 and 2). In summary, suffering in medicine is thought to be a process that occurs when an individual perceives a threat to his/her idea of self and personhood. Idea of self may not be reality based but rather a dream of self and how that self behaves under duress. Personhood relates to all aspects of being human and involves the present, past, and hopes for the future. In medicine, suffering has no moral value. It is the expression of suffering not the process itself that is idiosyncratic and culturally bound. In addition to a perception of threat, the process of suffering also involves the person's loss of central purpose, impaired personal relationships, loss of personal control over events, self-conflict, and a profound sense of meaninglessness. Suffering is a distinct phenomenon separate but sometimes related to pain. Patients with severe pain may not suffer, while others with minimal pain may experience suffering.

Legal definitions, unlike those proposed for medicine, consider pain and suffering to be one phenomenon. The *Oxford Dictionary of Law* defines "pain and suffering" as the "psychological consequences of personal injuries, in terms of pain, shock, consciousness that one's life has been shortened and embarrassment caused by disfigurement. Damages are determined on the extent to which the plaintiff actually experiences these feelings" (8). The legal definition of suffering has potential difficulties for the health care provider. How does one accurately assess the felt experience of "consciousness that one's life has been shortened" or "the embarrassment caused by disfigurement"? How does anyone know the extent to which individuals actually experience these feelings? Attempts to measure these perceptions are often based on an adversarial approach in which lawyers and medical personnel try to show that the patient does not actually experience any of the above feelings. The legal system and the medical system may, unfortunately, find themselves engaged in a process of trying to prove the patient is a liar, a malingerer, or psychologically impaired.

Medical and Legal Discourse: Power and Authority Differentials

There are major similarities between the legal process and medicine that may, in fact, be in common with any social process in which there are those who know how a social system works and those who do not. For example, lawyers know the law and clients usually do not. The same disparity in power exists between patients and doctors and students and teachers. Usually, those who are powerful know the rules and procedures of the law and those who are powerless are either victims or perpetrators of crimes. In medicine, the power structure is an even more rigid continuum, with physicians at the top of the power spectrum, other health care providers at various points along the scale, and patients at the bottom (9, 10). The doctor is the ultimate authority, and others contribute to the maintenance of this power base. The end result of these mechanisms is that the patient/client often loses personal autonomy. Decisions are made by others, and the person can become "lost" in the pursuit of a medical "cure" or legal argument. Consequently, suffering may be enhanced in individuals who seek assistance from these groups.

Philosophers of law (2) argue that, currently, suffering and pain must be legitimized by a third-party authority figure such as parents, judges, police, social workers, and/or legislators. This authorization depends on the authority figure's interpretation of the individual's verbal, gestured, and/or written expression. Failure of those in authority to recognize and respond to the individual's experience has the potential to impact negatively on the person's body. In the course of the legal discourse, the individual's story slowly transforms into a narrative that no longer expresses the person's lived experience. The person suffers not only because of the threat to self and personhood due to a specific set of events (injury/illness) but also because of the legal translations of these events. The person becomes a symbol placed in the centre of the argument about the law as lawyers try to place the story into categories that can be accepted by a judge. Personal privacy may be forgotten or violated and meanings of trauma ignored. The expert is powerful and the client becomes powerless (10, 11).

Similar parallels can be seen in medicine when symptoms are fitted into diagnostic categories and the meaning of the illness or injury is ignored. The trauma of a perceived threat to the individual's idea of self because of an illness/injury may be incorrectly reframed to suit psychological classifications such as depression or an anxiety disorder. Often, it is the health care provider who verifies or negates the person's descriptions of the presence or severity of symptoms. This verification takes the form not only of matching the symptoms presented to known pathophysiology but also making judgments about the individual's credibility. This process is particularly evident when the person complains of chronic pain or when the complaints describe symptoms in which the pathophysiology of the illness is unknown to the health care provider. In such instances, people may be labeled as being psychologically impaired or malingering.

Consequently, there may be costly and inappropriate referrals to other health care professionals or, of even more concern, the patient may undergo a loss of personal power which he/she may perceive as another assault on idea of self and personhood (12). In such instances, individuals may once again experience suffering because they are not believed or are thought to be emotionally unstable. The person experiences suffering due to (a) the initial assault, (b) the process of collecting "facts" by officers of the law and medicine, (c) the verification of the person's story by third parties (doctors, lawyers, therapists), (d) classification of story components to form legal arguments and medical diagnosis, and finally (e) determinations of an individual's credibility about the impact of the assault on self and personhood by third-party authorities.

If suffering due to medical and legal discourse is to be eliminated, practitioners must ask the following questions:

1. How and why does the legal/medical discourse of a modern state/organization conceal the experienced meanings of those who do not know the system? It

can be argued that the legal/medical discourse protects the authority of the law and medicine by placing a value on it that is superior to that of ordinary discourse. Every profession strives to have a unique language and a scope of practice that differentiates itself from other professions. Currently, these practices are historically based and often not applicable in contemporary society. It is conceivable that with the plethora of technological resources, such as the Internet and specialized medical devices, available to average people, the face of professional power will shift to one in which the patients/clients are more powerful.

The survival needs of human beings have not evolved at the same rate as society's technological advances. Persons still have the need to care for and be cared for by others, and the human body remains susceptible to injury and illness. Individuals still thrive in community with others and the need to communicate and be heard is still a fundamental human need. It may be that future power differentials in medicine and law will be more strongly based on precepts rooted in humanitarian objectives rather than property contract resolution as is currently the case in law. It may be that a less monetary/opportunistic approach to health and the law will evolve in a modern society.

2. If a person becomes ill or is the victim of a crime, does the medical/legal discourse recognize the harm from the individual's perspective? Some believe that if professionals in health care and law were to engage in the felt experience of clients, it would be too distressing for the professional, given the number of times such engagements would occur. The caregivers would become ineffective. This argument seems somewhat fallacious because it ignores the ability of human beings to listen empathically to a person's felt experience and then determine the most reasonable strategies for resolution given the circumstances. One obstacle to such an approach is the belief in fairness, which has its roots in a barter system. Little is fair in medicine and law. Is it fair that children are affected with terminal illnesses? Is it fair that seniors are victims of assault and injury? Must compensation for injury always be monetary? These questions are challenges for postmodern society as it struggles to aid those in society that are vulnerable and at the same time control fiscal expenditures.

3. Does the harm experienced by the individual sometimes slip through the juridical/medical categorizations? Sometimes, lawyers and health care professionals become so focused on the process of medicine or law that the person is forgotten. While lawyers win arguments and clinicians defeat diseases, considerable neglect is experienced by clients/patients. Contemporary medicine strives to educate health care students in the need for evidence-based decision making, in which categorizations are necessary, but it must be remembered that medicine is both a science and an art (13–17). Students who are trained the art of ethical care usually advocate for and mentor patients and colleagues. Currently, more investigations

into qualitative research methods are providing clinicians and lawyers with data that can be useful in situations in which patient behaviours fall outside statistical norms.

4. If the harm/illness is recognized, is it re-represented through a vocabulary, grammar, and gestured style that is familiar to the expert but not to the person harmed or ill? Historically, clinical practitioners have been trained to listen only for language that falls into specific patterns that are subsequently translated into diagnoses of illness. The expert rarely listens to the whole story being recounted by the patient. Modern medicine demands that students are educated in a process known as empathic listening in which the clinician acknowledges the patient's felt experience and responds in kind rather than using scientific jargon. A reply of "I know what you mean, my father had the same worries" as opposed to "the anxiety response rate is 14 percent in subjects with organic manifestations of this disease" is more helpful to sufferers. The latter response can raise more concerns, particularly if the patient does not believe that he/she is anxious. Responses of this type may establish power differentials between clinician and patient in which the clinician has dominance over the patient. In legal situations, the process is similar but with an outcome that may cast aspersions on the client's truthfulness and/or mental competency.

5. Can the medical/legal discourse of a modern state/health organization even translate an experienced event in the language of the person harmed? If not, why not? While it may not be possible to fully understand the indigenously experienced event of another, the felt experience can be acknowledged and validated, and an effort can be made to translate professional jargon to the patient/client.

6. Does the legal/medical discourse prevent the use of the other languages? Is the language of the individual disregarded in favour of legal and/or medical definitions? It is important for professionals in medicine and the law to consider implementing a mechanism of care into discourse in which the felt experience is addressed. Patients may say that they always have pain when what they really mean is their pain is so severe that it seems to always be present. Words like "always," "never," have less rigid meanings in common language than they do in medicine or the law. In the disciplines of law and medicine, such words have special power, often with monetary implications. The language from both disciplines can be explained to ensure that common language usage and the power of professional language are understood by both victims and perpetrators. Both medicine and the law must adopt a neutral stance in addressing the problems of individuals. Medicine does not serve only the good, and law does not serve only the innocent.

Answers to these questions depend on the professional individual's awareness of professional jurisprudence, cultural sensitivity, knowledge of spiritual and religious traditions, and the common attitudes of the society at large. It is the responsibility of all clinicians to understand the basic mechanisms of the legal system. Failure to do so may result in considerable harm to patients. One example would be a therapist who may suggest to a patient who is a victim of rape by a sports star that legal assistance be sought from the sports club lawyers. The end result may be disastrous for the patient because the objective of such lawyers is to provide a legal argument that protects the player and/or sports club and not the person claiming to be harmed. In other cases patients who seek legal help may become unwittingly manipulated into becoming a spokesperson for a political cause. Health care professionals have the responsibility to be informed and current about any potential harm to their patient's health that may result if the patient pursues such a path. It is the obligation of health care practitioners to advise their patients of potential harm. Few clinicians are fully aware of the implications of these issues.

Justification for Loss of Power in Medical and Legal Discourse

Conklin argues that in law, the expert cannot understand what clients say because the meanings of their stories do not fit into the official legal discourse. Therefore whatever the outcome is to the client, it is considered to be acceptable. Because the client has simply become a factor in an argument, he/she can be "consumed, excluded or ultimately executed" (2). The person becomes separated from his/her body in the minds of the legal professionals. Lawyers, police, and others collect information about this "body" and analyze the "facts," not the client's felt experience. The analysis is done by finding categories that others will accept as legitimate. The client's behaviour then becomes evaluated by determining whether it falls under the specified categories. The client's experience becomes enclosed within these expert boundaries and may not bear any resemblance to the actual lived experience. Personal autonomy is not considered.

There are similar parallels in medical practice, particularly in the area of suffering. The patient's suffering may be disregarded as the focus shifts to fighting the disease. The patient's story is interpreted to fit disease categories, and only when it fits these categories is the story really "heard." He/she may then become a symbol of the disease. The patient becomes the Parkinson's patient, or the MS patient, or even the fractured knee in room 402. Judgments are then made as to whether the patient behaves well or badly according to preconceived notions of behaviour attributed to those diseases or illnesses. The impact of the illness on an individual's idea of self and personhood is usually not considered. In those instances when the issue of threat is addressed, patient reactions are often reframed to suit professional categories of acceptability/unacceptability. Personal autonomy is not considered.

In both legal and medical interactions, everyday language cannot be recognized because to do so would contradict the professional need to maintain authority. Individuals suffer initially because of the original assault (illness) and then repeatedly as experts begin to recognize the harm and start to translate the suffering into acceptable professional discourse.

This need for professional authority, which may have had its roots in a paternalism that is no longer relevant, requires a new approach in contemporary society. While current approaches in medicine favour a multidisciplinary approach, there is still the problem of professional boundaries and power. The problem that persists is one of professional authority enacted at the expense of the patient's autonomy. If the expectation is that patients and/or clients are totally responsible for their own well-being, then those who serve may have to face the challenge of accepting a reversal in the patient/client power differential. The patient/client then becomes the person who "knows" the true story and the lawyer/health care provider becomes the one who "serves."

Ethical Considerations and Suffering

If ethics are the moral principle or the branch of knowledge concerned with moral principles, and if moral principles refer to the rightness/wrongness and goodness and badness of human character, is the process of legal/medical discourse ethical when considering human suffering? Are these processes ethical simply because they are accepted standards of practice? Do these practices contradict other ethical principles such as doing no harm and/or protecting those in society who are not able to protect themselves? What ethical basis is used to determine such standards, and are they reasonable in contemporary society? Some argue that clients/patients are informed prior to treatments and legal interventions. What factors constitute informed consent? Medicine attempts to clarify this issue when it comes to the mechanics of care involving "extraordinary measures," but the issue of personal power and the power differential between the professional and patient is usually not addressed. Legal mechanisms are sometimes clarified, but the issue of autonomy is often ignored. Is the right of legal discourse ethical only within the prescribed professional boundaries but not in human terms? What is the impact of an individual's cultural or spiritual beliefs? Is it possible to legislate behaviour? Is professional behaviour a belief system based on a clearly defined ethic? What contribution does medicine make to suffering when it engages in the process of legal discourse? Are there potential ethical conflicts? Are these conflicts being addressed? Surely, the ethics of those clinicians who watch surveillance video tapes of patients prior to providing "independent" assessment must be questioned. Ethical practice is suspect when physicians take an oath to "do no harm" yet send and read the opinions of others about an individual patient prior to administering a "second opinion." Is it not unethical for health care professionals to refrain from informing patients or clients that they are receiving monetary gain from providing information that can be used against the patient/client? These questions must become the focal point of contemporary medicine if the goals of medicine and the efficacy of the law are to be maintained.

Cultural Implications

The cultural implications concerning individual suffering in a modern, pluralistic, multicultural society are very important. How does legal discourse capture the rightness and/or wrongness of behaviour or the goodness or badness of human actions if the accepted standards of behaviour are not multiculturally based? Can these standards be multiculturally based and still fit the dialogue of the law and or medicine? What is the common understanding of the law and the process of medicine? In most North American societies, the law and medicine are held in considerable regard. Individuals from other countries may view the process of law and/or medicine very differently. Who explains the discourse, and how, to those who are vulnerable? Is it possible to have multicultural legal and medical discourse in a fast-changing postmodern world? Further, are the individual's spiritual traditions part of the dialogue, or are spiritual rights per se only considered? Do we simply respect diversity of beliefs but not incorporate them into the process of medical and legal dialogues? Would incorporation be prudent? These questions are challenges to be faced if optimal care for those who suffer is to be obtained. Medicine is attempting to address these questions through undergraduate education and through licensing requirements, but the assessment of effective transfer of knowledge into clinical practice is a challenge (14–17). In the legal system, while the process remains adversarial, there is now recognition that children and those who are mentally impaired require special consideration. This is considered to be a positive step in recognizing the importance of understanding the individual's felt experience.

All practitioners are challenged to consider the following question: If legal discourse serves the institution of the law, and medical discourse serves the institution of medicine, then who speaks to the patient's "felt" experience of suffering? In the past, the answer to the last question may have been the church. And to an extent, the answer remains true if suffering is defined within the constructs of religious teachings. In contemporary society, and especially in medicine, where suffering is not valued and is perceived to be a threat to an individual's idea of self and personhood, answers must be found within the dialogue and discourse of the professions of medicine and the law.

SUMMARY

The focus of this chapter was the importance of health care providers having a basic understanding of the history of the legal system under which their society operates. The British, American, and Canadian legal systems were used, in part, as examples to illustrate the need for understanding the impact of laws on human health. Legal and medical discourse were compared and contrasted to show how each impact on the power differential between individuals and professional helpers.

In this chapter, the processes of medical and legal discourse and their potential impact on suffering were discussed. Previous chapters have explored the importance of clearly defining suffering in medicine, outside the contexts of religion and spirituality. These discussions have been supported from evidence of scholarly theories and clinical practice. The following chapter provides research evidence that suffering is a measurable construct and illustrates key issues of concern in chronic illness.

CHAPTER 7 QUESTIONS

1 What are the basic historical precepts upon which the law is based?
2 What common misconceptions are held by patients and clinicians about the purpose of the law?
3 What was the purpose of the "Twelve Tables"?
4 Upon which code of law were the laws of Europe, the province of Quebec, and the state of Louisiana originally based?
5 What is the Napoleonic code?
6 Upon what legal tenets is the American Constitution based?
7 What is the purpose of common law?
8 What is the purpose of case law?
9 How do the principles of tort law affect health?
10 How does the "truth" in medicine differ from the "truth" in law?
11 How does medical and legal discourse impact on health?
12 What are the key ethical considerations relating to the health care professionals, the law, and the patient?

11 Identifying Those Who Suffer

NOW IS THE TIME TO KNOW

8 Power Differentials and Suffering

The need for personal autonomy and the impact that medical and legal discourse can have on personal power indicate that a complete assessment of individuals who suffer requires a comprehensive, objective measurement tool. The Measuring and Assessing Suffering Questionnaire (MASQ) is a clinical measurement tool to aid clinicians in determining those patients who are experiencing the process of suffering and to assist health care providers in planning effective, relevant, evidence-based treatment programs for those individuals who have a chronic illness. A more comprehensive treatment of suffering may have a positive effect on the management of pain and help prevent chronic disability.

This chapter presents: (a) the importance of obtaining informed consent from patients in both clinical and research environments, (b) the purpose of the MASQ and a review of key definitions to aid clinicians in data interpretation, (c) a description of the structural elements of the questionnaire, (d) a brief summary of validity and reliability values obtained from statistical analyses of the MASQ, and (e) collation of research findings. Examples of demographic data collection pertinent to the treatment of individuals with chronic illnesses such as arthritis, epilepsy, migraine headache, and spinal cord injuries are presented.

Informed Consent: Restoring Personal Power and Autonomy

Clinical Practice Requirements

Information Sheets · Patients with chronic illness who suffer often say that with the onset of illness or injury they find themselves in a foreign world, a social world that they no longer understand. When managing suffering in clinical practice, it is important that health care providers give patients the tools needed to help them understand their changed circumstances. Patients can be given information sheets that delineate the qualifications of the health care professional with whom the individuals will work as well as the philosophy of care and organizational policies of the health care facility. Information may be provided in written form, in concise, clear language that is free from professional jargon. These information sheets may be reviewed verbally with the patient prior to obtaining consent, and patients should be given time to consider the issues at hand. This type of information will show respect for the patient's autonomy because consent would be based on an ethical framework rather than on power. Patients are then more likely to form realistic expectations of their health care provider and the health care organization.

The goals of the relevant health care profession should be clearly described. In the example provided (see example 1), the profession of physiotherapy is briefly described. The types of specialized modalities are also described so that patients have a basic understanding of any procedures that may be used in their care. A brief outline of what is involved in the treatment plan is illustrated, and issues such as any clothing, hair products, creams, lotions, or other factors that may impact on the efficacy of the treatment or evaluation of the patient need to be described.

Patients are usually very concerned about whether they will experience pain, and if pain does occur, procedures that should be followed should be outlined. Estimates of rate of recovery and length of time for each treatment are also matters of concern to patients who are to start treatments. In private clinics or facilities where a fee for service may be immediate, fee structures should be made available to the patient prior to beginning treatments. Issues of how confidentiality will be maintained must be clearly stated. The patient is asked to sign the information sheet, indicating an understanding of the clinical process offered. Signatures are dated, witnessed by a third party, and countersigned by the attending clinician. A copy of the completed information sheet is given to the patient (see example 1).

After the patient has read the information sheet and has had the opportunity to discuss any issues of concern with the health care professional, the patient may take the information sheet home and discuss it with family members. If there are aspects of their care that patients believe will not be addressed in the proposed care plan, they can discuss their concerns with the clinician. If the issues presented are beyond the scope of practice of the clinician and the patient wants another health care professional's opinion, such referrals can be made free from prejudice. The process respects the personal power and autonomy of the patient, a factor critical to those who suffer. Often, the patient simply acknowledges his understanding of what will happen and is then asked for formal consent (example 2).

EXAMPLE 1 (CLINICAL EXAMPLE)

Brown Physiotherapy Practice Group

Mary Browne, R.P.T., M.C.P.A., C.A.F.C.I., B.A., Ph.D.

For Your Information*

Assessment of the Impact of the Illness/Disorder on the Patient

Introduction

Welcome to our clinic. *Mary Browne*, R.P.T., M.C.P.A., C.A.F.I., is a registered Physiotherapist with additional training in acupuncture. Our approach to rehabilitation encompasses a holistic (whole person) approach to health care delivery.

(If the health care professional has other credentials, they should be stated here.)

*This form is a guideline only.

Philosophy

A holistic approach involves considering the impact of illness and/or injury on the whole person rather than simply focusing on a body part. For example, if you were involved in a car accident and suffered many injuries, the treatment might involve not only exercises to improve muscle strength and range of movements but also might involve determining how the accident and the resulting injuries have impacted on your life (job, family relationships, school, etc). SUGGESTIONS (general advice) concerning the impact of your injuries on your coping mechanisms, diet, stress, and modifications to your home and/or work environments may be made. You might discuss these suggestions with your doctor, work place advisors, family, and any others you may choose to help you remain independent.

*What Exactly Is Involved in Physiotherapy?**

The practice of physiotherapy is the assessment of physical function and the treatment, rehabilitation and prevention of physical dysfunction, injury, or pain, to develop, maintain, rehabilitate or augment function or to relieve pain (the Physiotherapy Act).

You may be asked many questions about how your illness/injury affects you as a person, how it affects your work life and your family or leisure activities. Often these questions are presented in the format of written questionnaires to which there are not right or wrong answers. These assessment forms simply indicate areas for attention. Your physiotherapist will discuss the purpose and results of the questionnaires so that you will be fully involved in making decisions about your care.

What Is Acupuncture?

Acupuncture is a therapeutic treatment which consists of inserting fine needles into the body at specific points along energy pathways or meridians. The age-old practice, which is widely used to relieve the symptoms of some physical and psychological conditions, is often integrated by physiotherapists into the treatment of clients with pain or physical dysfunction (College of Physiotherapists of Ontario, Position Statement 1998).

(*If the clinician has expertise in other specialized modalities they should also be delineated*).

Treatment Plan

You may bring a friend/family member with you on any or all of your treatments.

What will my treatments consist of?

1 At each visit you will be assessed and treated. The initial visit may involve you answering questionnaires and being examined by the Physiotherapist. This may

*Physiotherapy is used simply to illustrate the need to inform patients of the professional scope of practice. The Physiotherapy Act 1991 cited is the Canadian Physiotherapy Act and is used for purposes of illustration only.

require the physiotherapist to observe your body while it is still and while it is moving. It will be necessary for the physiotherapist to touch your body and to move your body while assessing and treating your injuries and/or impairments.
2 Upon completion of your assessment, *Ms. Browne* will discuss the specific treatment plan recommended for you. Some of the following techniques and modalities may be used as part of the treatment plan: mobilization, massage, passive and active stretching, exercises, electrical muscle stimulation, transcutaneous electrical nerve stimulation (TENS), acupuncture, and acupressure. You are encouraged to ask questions at any time during the assessments and treatments. Any known complications, risks, benefits, and potential side effects will be discussed with you.
3 *Ms. Browne* will explain the general healing process of injury and illness. If the therapist considers the following to be appropriate for successful rehabilitation, suggestions may be made to help you cope with distress, diet, as well as home and workplace modifications. It is your responsibility to consider these suggestions and discuss them with your doctor and/or other appropriate health care professionals.

What Do I Wear?

1 If your injury is to your lower limbs only, shorts are required.
2 For upper limbs/shoulder area, female patients are required to wear a bathing suit/halter top constructed so that the injuries may be assessed.
3 For neck and/or low back injuries as well as hip injuries, a bathing suit or shorts for males and a bathing suit and/or shorts are required for females.

In some instances in which your illness or injury prevents you from managing activities of daily living (i.e., dressing, etc.), you are advised to wear clothing that permits the physiotherapist to assess your difficulties and help you learn ways to dress/undress. This may involve the physiotherapist watching you perform these activities. If at any time you feel uncomfortable, you must tell your physiotherapist. You may stop your treatments at any time.

Will I Have Pain? What Do I Do?

After the initial visit you may be sore because your joints and muscles are stretched. You must tell your physiotherapist if you have more pain or any other symptoms. If you are unable to reach your physiotherapist you must call your family doctor.

How Long Will It Take Me to Get Better?

Each person is different. Rate of recovery depends on many factors such as the nature of your illness, injury, age, general health, previous occurrences, motivation and opportunities for practicing exercises and treatment, medication, and pain tolerance. Your physiotherapist will give an approximate estimate of how many treatments you require before physiotherapy re-evaluation and/or possible referral to your doctor is required.

How Long Will Treatments Last?
Initial assessments may take from 1 to 2 hours depending on the nature and complexity of the illness/injury.

Treatment sessions initially may last from 30 minutes to 2 hours, depending on the severity of the illness/injury and the degree of education required so that you can perform the exercises safely on your own. Further treatments usually take 1 hour.

Discharge assessments usually take from 1 to 2 hours. If you have been referred by a doctor, a copy of the assessment will be sent to the doctor with your consent. If you have referred yourself, the discharge assessment is available upon request.

Fees

What Are the Fees?
Payment of fees is the responsibility of the patient.

Treatment costs are:
$XX for the initial assessment
$XX for each treatment session
$XX for the Discharge Assessment
Payments are to be made after each visit by cash or cheque.

What If I Cancel an Appointment?
A minimum of 24 hours notice to cancel an appointment is appreciated. Failure to attend 2 consecutive treatment sessions will constitute a discharge from treatment. Further treatment will involve a re-assessment fee of $XX.

Confidentiality

All medical/health records will be kept confidential and will not be released to anyone without your written consent except where required by law.

I have read and understood the above policies and agree to abide by these conditions.

____________________	____________	____________________
Patient Signature	(Date)	(Print signature)
____________________	____________	____________________
(Witness Signature)	(Date)	(Print signature)
____________________	____________	____________________
(Physiotherapist Signature)	(Date)	(Print signature)

❑ A copy of the information sheet was given to the client Date: ____________

EXAMPLE 2 (CLINICAL EXAMPLE)

Browne Physiotherapy Practice Group

Mary Browne, R.P.T, M.C.P.A., C.A.F.C.I., B.A., Ph.D.

Patient Consent*

I, ____________________, have had the philosophy, the treatment plan, fee structure, and confidentiality issues explained to me. I am aware that Mary Browne is a Registered Physiotherapist with additional training in Acupuncture. I understand that my treatments will involve a "holistic" approach to rehabilitation as outlined in the information sheet entitled "For Your Information" which I have received and read. I am free to withdraw from treatment without prejudicing future treatment. My medical records will be kept confidential as required by law.

Information pertaining to my health and/or rehabilitation may be obtained from or released to:

Family Doctor   My Lawyer   My Insurance Co.   Other

If other please indicate: ________________________________

I consent to the above and agree to participate.

Name:

________________________   ________________________

Print Name

Date: ____________

Witness:

________________________   ________________________

Print Name

Date: ____________

Physiotherapist:

________________________   ________________________

Print Name

Date: ____________

A copy of this consent form was given to the client ❑

Date: ____________

Consent Forms · Patient consent forms usually contain a brief paragraph stating that the patient acknowledges that the philosophy of care, the treatment plan, fee structure if applicable, and confidentiality issues have been explained. In addition, individuals also confirm that they understand the qualifications of the health care provider, the approach to care that will be offered, and the nature of the confidentiality requirements as determined by the law. Patients also acknowledge that

*This form is a guideline only.

they are free to withdraw from treatments without prejudicing future care. They also indicate who may receive information about their health. Signatures from the patient, witness, and health care professional are obtained and a copy of the consent form is given to the patient. Consent now becomes more than simply obtaining permissions. The process is a contractual agreement based on an ethical framework. For those who suffer, obtaining consent is another tool available to help patients understand the dynamics of the new world of illness or injury. When health care professionals conduct clinical trials, patients must be asked whether they would like to participate in this research. Additional information must then be provided and a research consent form is signed.

Clinical Research Requirements

Information Sheets · Clinical research requirements are determined by individual hospital and university research advisory committees. The information sheet given in example 3 is simply a guideline. If the research objectives are complex, more detailed information is provided to participants. The information sheet must state the purpose of the study, outline any potential benefits and risks to the participants, and assure people that their personal information will be kept confidential. Individuals must also know that any scientific publishing of results will not reveal their identity. People must know that they may withdraw from the study at any time without prejudice. This last point is essential, particularly if the clinical research is conducted with patients who might fear that if they do not agree to participate in the research, their future care will be compromised. Individuals must also know who they can call if they have further questions and who to contact in an emergency. A copy of the information sheet is given to the patient.

Consent Forms · The consent form, example 4, contains a brief paragraph that outlines the purpose of the study and confirms that the participant understands what is to occur. Issues of confidentiality and freedom to withdraw from the project are reiterated. The participant's signature is obtained and dated, as is that of the principal investigator and co-investigator if applicable. A copy of the consent form is also given to the individual.

Providing information sheets and consent forms does not totally nullify the fact that the health care provider must still ask for permission. Personal power and autonomy are partially restored because informed consent permits the patient to enter into a contractual agreement with the health care professional. As health care providers review the information provided, there is an opportunity for dialogue between the patient and health care provider which allows the patient to express his or her autonomy. The patient determines who may or may not receive information about them albeit within the confines of the law. Personal power is respected because the patient clearly understands the scope and limitations of his or her health clinician and the treatments proposed. Autonomy is improved because once the patient knows the purpose of the assessment from a whole-life perspective, discussions of any rehabilitation choices may be discussed with the clinician. For example, the patient may decide that it is more important to walk with braces and crutches than to ambulate using a wheelchair, even though the energy expenditure involved in walking is considerable, given the extent of the person's impairments. In such cases, while the therapist may know that the wheelchair will allow the patient more personal freedom, it is the therapist's role to advise the patient, but the patient is the one who makes the choice. The patient is the one with the power and the therapist is the one who strives to help achieve the patient's goals. This relationship is most common in rehabilitation facilities where patients have chronic illnesses or catastrophic injuries. Autonomy and personal power in outpatient clinics or acute care facilities may be compromised, particularly in fee-for-service facilities where volume of treatments becomes a priority. Health care professionals need to give priority to the patient's wishes but always within an ethical framework. To further address patient autonomy and personal power, the collection of demographic data may also provide an opportunity for clinicians to gather more information about the patient's idea of self and personhood.

EXAMPLE 3 (RESEARCH EXAMPLE)
INFORMATION SHEET: ASSESSMENT OF THE IMPACT OF THE ILLNESS/DISORDER ON THE PATIENT*

This study is designed to help us understand how you feel about having *Arthritis* and how your illness/disorder affects your life. Many researchers have discovered that if doctors, nurses, physiotherapists, and other persons who try to help people with chronic disorders are able to fully understand what impact the disorder has on the patient and his life, better more effective treatments can be used.

To find out how patients feel about their disorder, a questionnaire has been designed (MASQ) to try and find out which matters are of greatest concern to our patients. You will be asked a series of 30 questions which ask you to tell us how you feel *now*. There are no right or wrong answers. The questionnaire will be given to you before you begin your treatments in physiotherapy and just before you are discharged from your treatments. How you answer the questions will not affect your treatments now or in the future. You are free to withdraw from the study at any time. Your identity and how you respond to the questions will be confidential. Any information published from the study will not reveal your identity.

*This form is a guideline only and arthritis is used as an example. Clinicians are advised to contact the Research Advisory Committee of the hospital/university organization to which they are affiliated.

If you would like any further information at any time you may call (name) ______ at (phone number) ____, Monday–Friday, 9 a.m.–5 p.m. In case of emergency, please call your family physician for instructions.

A copy of the information sheet was given to the client ❑ Date: ____________

EXAMPLE 4 (RESEARCH EXAMPLE)
CONSENT*

I, ____________________, agree to participate in the "Assessment of the Impact of Illness/Disorder on the Patient" project. I have had the purpose of the study explained to me. I agree to fill in the MASQ questionnaire. I understand that all my answers will be kept confidential and that any public or scientific publications reporting the results of this project will not reveal my identity. My identity will be protected through an identity number.

I also understand that I am free to withdraw from the project at any time without prejudicing my care now or in the future.

I agree to participate in the study.

Name:

____________________________________ ________________________________
Print Name

Date: ______________

Witness:

____________________________________ ________________________________
Print Name

Date: ______________

Principal Investigator:

____________________________________ ________________________________
Print Name

Date: ______________

Co-Investigator:

____________________________________ ________________________________
Print Name

Date: ______________

A copy of this consent form was given to the client ❑ Date: ____________

The Value of Demographic Data and Patients Who Suffer

The purpose of collecting demographic data is to determine the nature of an individual's personhood. In example 5, we see that the MASQ collects information relating not only to epilepsy but also to the effects it has on patients. Questions

*This form is a guideline only. Clinicians are advised to contact the Research Advisory Committee of the hospital/university organization with which they are affiliated.

relating to factors that may contribute to an inability to work, ambulate, and/or live independently indicate factors that may impede the resolution of suffering. Patients are asked if they have experienced any additional losses in the past five years. This information helps clinicians determine whether grief and mourning due to death of a family member or friend are part of the patient's current distress. The experience of suffering due to chronic illness may be compounded by additional suffering related to the loss of loved ones. In the case of epilepsy, stigma is sometimes associated with a seizure disorder and is an important factor in patients who suffer.

In addition to the above questions relating to self and personhood, demographic data collection from patients with migraine headache also includes information on stress, both at home and in the workplace (example 6). In patients with spinal cord injuries and patients with arthritis, suffering has been found to be related to the inability to live and work independently (see examples 7 and 8). Issues relating to the family, interpersonal relationships, the ability to manage with poor support systems, feelings of isolation in the community and fears about the impact of ageing, disability pension regulations, and personal independence in the future are part of the qualitative data items described in the MASQ. All these factors need to be addressed by clinicians if comprehensive treatment and assessment of suffering in patients with chronic illness is to be achieved.

EXAMPLE 5

MASQ—EPILEPSY / SEIZURE DISORDERS

RELEVANT SURGICAL INTERVENTIONS

____

DO YOU HAVE ANY OTHER MEDICAL CONDITIONS WHICH WOULD PREVENT YOU FROM WORKING? ______________________________

____

LOSSES IN THE PAST 5 YEARS:

______________________________ DATE: ______________

____

HOW MUCH FORMAL EDUCATION DO YOU HAVE? ______________________________

____

AMBULATION: INDEPENDENT ____ INDEPENDENT WITH AID ____

SUPERVISION WITH AID ____ WHEELCHAIR ____ OTHER ____

DO YOU DRIVE? Yes ____ No ____

DO YOU TAKE PUBLIC TRANSPORTATION? BUS ____ TAXI ____ OTHER ____

DO YOU LIVE ALONE? Yes ____ No ____

DO YOU LIVE WITH SOMEONE BUT YOU ARE INDEPENDENT? Yes ____ No ____

DO YOU LIVE IN A GROUP HOME WITH PARTIAL SUPERVISION? Yes ____ No ____

DO YOU LIVE IN A LONG-TERM CARE FACILITY WITH SUPERVISION?

Yes ____ No ____

MEDICATIONS: 1. ____________ DOSAGE ____________

2. ____________ ____________

3. ____________ ____________

4. ____________ ____________

5. ____________ ____________

ARE YOU TAKING YOUR MEDICATION ON YOUR OWN? Yes ____ No ____

HOW OFTEN DO YOU MISS TAKING YOUR MEDICATION?

Sometimes ____ Never ____

____

HOW MANY SEIZURES DO YOU HAVE IN A DAY? ____ MONTH? ____________

WHEN DO THEY OCCUR?

____

____

SEVERITY ____________ TYPE ____________

____

WHEN WAS YOUR FIRST SEIZURE? DATE ____________ TIME ____________

WHEN WAS YOUR LAST SEIZURE? DATE ____________ TIME ____________

ARE YOUR SEIZURES CONTROLLED? YES ____ NO ____

Work History

1. DO YOU HAVE A PAID JOB NOW? Yes ____ No ____

IF YES, Full Time ____ Part Time ____

IF NO, Have you ever had a job in the past? Yes ____ No ____

IF YES, What was it? ____________

Why did you lose it? ____________

2. WHAT DO YOU DO IN YOUR JOB? ____________

____

____

3. HOW LONG HAVE YOU WORKED AT THE ABOVE JOB? ____ (months)

4. ARE YOU RECEIVING A DISABILITY PENSION? YES ____ NO ____

5. DO YOU HAVE AN UNPAID JOB OUTSIDE THE HOME? Yes ____ No ____

6. WHAT DO YOU DO IN THIS JOB? ____________

____

____

7. HOW LONG HAVE YOU HAD THE ABOVE JOB? ____ (months)

8. HAVE YOU EVER BEEN TRAINED TO DO A SPECIFIC JOB?

Yes ____ No ____

IF YES, WHAT WAS IT? ____________

9. DO YOU TELL PEOPLE AT WORK THAT YOU HAVE SEIZURES?

Yes _____ No _____

10. HAVE YOU TRIED TO FIND PAID WORK IN THE PAST 2 YEARS?

Yes _____ No _____

11. WHY WERE YOU NOT SUCCESSFUL? _______________

____

____

12. SUBJECT'S AFFECT: _______________

____

____

EXAMPLE 6

MASQ–MIGRAINE HEADACHES

OTHER MEDICAL CONDITIONS _______________

High B.P.? _______

SURGICAL INTERVENTIONS

____

DATE OF ONSET ___________

FAMILY HISTORY OF MIGRAINE Yes _____ No _____

DETAILS _______________

WHAT WAS THE CAUSE OF YOUR FIRST MIGRAINE

❑ INJURY ❑ FOOD ❑ STRESS ❑ LACK OF SLEEP ❑ ALCOHOL

❑ STREET DRUGS ❑ OTHER _______________

HOW OFTEN DO YOU HAVE A MIGRAINE? _______________

DATE OF LAST HEADACHE: ___________

Describe a Typical Headache

WHAT CAUSES YOU TO HAVE A HEADACHE?

____

____

____

HOW DO THEY START?

SHORTEST EPISODE ___________ LONGEST EPISODE ___________

____

____

____

LOCATION OF HEADACHE

____

____

____

AURA: Yes ____ No ____ DESCRIBE

____

____

____

SEVERITY: None (1) — A little (2) — Some (3) — A lot (4) — Sometimes unbearable (5)

DURATION ______________

WHEN DO THEY START? A.M. / P.M.

____

DO YOU HAVE MOST OF YOUR HEADACHES ON WEEKENDS?

Yes ____ No ____ Some ____

DO YOU HAVE HEADACHES ON VACATION? Yes ____ No ____ Some ____

How Do You Manage Your Headache

❑ MEDICATION ❑ ACUPUNCTURE ❑ MASSAGE ❑ HEAT/MASSAGE

❑ YOGA ❑ COUNSELLING ❑ STRESS MANAGEMENT ❑ REST ❑ OTHER:

____

MEDICATIONS

1. ______________ DOSAGE ______________ TIME ______________ EFFECT

2. ______________ ______________ ______________

3. ______________ ______________ ______________

OTHER EFFECTS

____

____

DO YOU HAVE ANY ALLERGIES?

____

ARE YOU BEING TREATED FOR YOUR ALLERGIES?

____

HOW MUCH DO YOU SMOKE? ______________________

HOW MUCH ALCOHOL DO YOU USE? ______________________

HOW MANY HOURS DO YOU SLEEP AT NIGHT? ______________________

HOW OFTEN DO YOU EXERCISE PER WEEK? ______________________

ACTIVITIES OF DAILY LIVING: ______________________

____

____

DO YOU LIVE ALONE? Yes ____ No ____

DO YOU LIVE WITH SOMEONE ELSE BUT ARE INDEPENDENT? ______________

DO YOU HAVE THE RESPONSIBILITY OF CHILDREN? ____ AGES? ________

DO YOU HAVE THE RESPONSIBILITY OF OTHER FAMILY MEMBERS?

____

DO YOU DRIVE? Yes ____ No ____

DO YOU TAKE PUBLIC TRANSPORTATION? BUS ____ TAXI ____ OTHER ____

Occupation

HOW WOULD YOU RATE THE DEGREE OF RESPONSIBILITY THAT YOU MUST ASSUME AT WORK:

None (1) —— A little (2) —— Some (3) —— A lot (4) —— A great deal (5)

EMPLOYMENT: FT ____ PT ____ OTHER ______________________________

HOW MUCH SICK-TIME HAVE YOU LOST BECAUSE OF YOUR HEADACHES?

____

HOW MUCH LEISURE TIME HAVE YOU LOST BECAUSE OF YOUR HEADACHES?

____

WHAT DO YOU DO IN YOUR JOB NOW? (tasks)

____

HAVE YOU RECEIVED SPECIAL TRAINING TO DO THIS JOB?

____

HOW LONG HAVE YOU BEEN DOING THIS JOB?

____

HAVE YOU EVER RECEIVED A DISABILITY PENSION BECAUSE OF HEADACHES? ______

DO YOU HAVE AN UNPAID JOB OUTSIDE THE HOME? (volunteer)

Yes ____ No ____

WHAT DO YOU DO IN THIS JOB?

____

____

HOW LONG HAVE YOU BEEN DOING THE ABOVE JOB? ______________________

DO YOU TELL PEOPLE AT WORK THAT YOU HAVE MIGRAINE HEADACHES?

____

WHAT ACTIVITIES DO YOU NOT DO BECAUSE OF YOUR HEADACHES?

____

____

SUBJECT'S AFFECT: ____

____

____

EXAMPLE 7

MASQ–SPINAL CORD INJURIES

DIAGNOSIS ____

____

DATE OF ONSET ________________________ CAUSE: ___________________

RELEVANT SURGICAL INTERVENTIONS

____

OTHER MEDICAL CONDITIONS _____________________________________

____

MEDICATIONS: 1. ____________ DOSAGE ____________

2. ____________ ____________

3. ____________ ____________

4. ____________ ____________

5. ____________ ____________

AMBULATION: INDEPENDENT WITH AID ____ SUPERVISION WITH AID ____

WHEELCHAIR ____ OTHER ____

DO YOU DRIVE? Yes ____ No ____

DO YOU TAKE PUBLIC TRANSPORTATION? BUS ____ TAXI ____ OTHER ____

DO YOU LIVE ALONE? Yes ____ No ____

DO YOU LIVE WITH SOMEONE BUT YOU ARE INDEPENDENT? Yes ____ No ____

DO YOU LIVE IN A GROUP HOME WITH PARTIAL SUPERVISION? Yes ____ No ____

DO YOU LIVE IN A LONG TERM CARE FACILITY WITH SUPERVISION? Yes ___ No ___

Work History

1. DO YOU HAVE A PAID JOB NOW? Yes ____ No ____

   IF YES, Full Time ____ Part Time ____

   IF NO, Have you ever had a job in the past? Yes ____ No ____

   IF YES, What was it? ____________

   ____

   Why did you lose it? ____________

   ____

2. WHAT DO YOU DO IN YOUR JOB? ____________

   ____

3. HOW LONG HAVE YOU WORKED AT THE ABOVE JOB? ____ (months)

4. ARE YOU RECEIVING A DISABILITY PENSION? YES ____ NO ____

5. DO YOU HAVE AN UNPAID JOB OUTSIDE THE HOME? Yes ____ No ____

6. WHAT DO YOU DO IN THIS JOB? ____________

   ____

   ____

7. HOW LONG HAVE YOU HAD THE ABOVE JOB? ____ (months)

8. HAVE YOU EVER BEEN TRAINED TO DO A SPECIFIC JOB?

   Yes ____ No ____

   IF YES, WHAT WAS IT? ____________

10. HAVE YOU TRIED TO FIND PAID WORK IN THE PAST 2 YEARS?

    Yes ____ No ____

11. WHY WERE YOU NOT SUCCESSFUL? ____________

    ____

    ____

    ____

12. ARE YOU INVOLVED IN A VOCATIONAL TRAINING PROGRAM? ____________

____

____

13. SUBJECT'S AFFECT: ____________________________

____

____

EXAMPLE 8

MASQ–ARTHRITIS

DIAGNOSIS: ____________________________

DATE OF ONSET: ____________

MEDICATIONS: 1. ____________ DOSAGE ____________

2. ____________ ____________

3. ____________ ____________

4. ____________ ____________

5. ____________ ____________

SURGICAL INTERVENTIONS: ____________________________

____

AMBULATION: INDEPENDENT ____ INDEPENDENT WITH AID ____

SUPERVISION WITH AID ____ WHEELCHAIR ____ OTHER ____________

ACTIVITIES OF DAILY LIVING:

____

____

LIVES INDEPENDENTLY: ______

LIVES WITH SOMEONE ELSE BUT IS INDEPENDENT: ______

LIVES IN A GROUP HOME WITH PARTIAL SUPERVISION: ______

LIVES IN A LONG-TERM CARE FACILITY WITH SUPERVISION: ______

DRIVES A CAR: ______

TAKES PUBLIC TRANSPORTATION: ____ BUS: ____ TAXI: ____ OTHER: ____

IS EMPLOYED: ____________________________

WORKS AT HOME: ____________________________

How to Use the MASQ

It is strongly recommended that students and novice clinicians read Section I of the text, entitled "Suffering: What Man Has Made of Man," to familiarize themselves with the concept of suffering as an entity separate from pain. The following presents for review a very brief synopsis of the concept of suffering. In addition, a quick reference summary of the results of validity and reliability testing of the questionnaire (MASQ) and the evidence obtained to support the hypothesis that suffering and pain are separate and only sometimes related phenomena in chronic illness are presented for review.

The MASQ

The MASQ is a self-administered, valid, and reliable tool to identify those who suffer. The MASQ identifies those who suffer and also highlights areas of most concern to individuals. The MASQ provides information that may facilitate the application of suffering-specific treatments to patients with chronic illnesses. It may also assist in the treatment of suffering of individuals who have chronic pain and enhance other treatment outcomes. Suggestions for the application of the MASQ in the patient setting are given based on findings obtained from our evaluations of over 300 patients with chronic illness.

The Value of Using the MASQ

The MASQ is an important clinical tool because it:

- Provides a quick method of quantifying patients' perceptions of threat to the self and personhood in chronic illness, a factor particularly found to be useful in the management of patients with chronic pain syndromes
- Provides quick "at a glance" quantified data analyses for treatment and discharge planning
- Is a useful clinical outcome measure
- Is a thorough and pertinent method for assessing the impact of illness and/or injury on self and personhood (suffering) and for making decisions about fiscal compensation in work place and/or motor vehicle insurance cases
- Assists in effective evidence-based decision making

Definitions

Suffering: A perception of threat to a person's idea of self and personhood.

Idea of Self: A person's internal beliefs about how he/she manages adversity and still maintains a sense of self.

Personhood: A person's perceptions about how he/she has dealt with adversity in the past, and how he/she will manage in the present and future. Perceptions are independent of external verification, and they focus on whether anticipated outcomes will be managed in a manner that is acceptable to the individual.

Pain: An unpleasant sensory and emotional experience associated with actual or potential tissue damage or described in terms of such damage.

Structure of the MASQ

The MASQ is a valid and reliable tool to objectively delineate the suffering component in chronic illness.

The MASQ is a fifty-three-item self-administered questionnaire. Each question is scored on a 5-point Likert-type scale with a rating of 5 indicating the most negative response. A response at level 1 has a numerical value of 1 point; a response at level 2 has a value of 2 points, etc. Time to complete the questionnaire is about ten to fifteen minutes. To minimize bias of response, individual subscales of the questionnaire are labeled alphabetically rather than indicating the content. Therefore, Section A refers to pain, Section B to suffering, Section C to work beliefs and Section D to self-efficacy. The pain scale (Part A) consists of five items, suffering (Part B) has nineteen items, work beliefs (Part C) has twenty items, and there are nine items in the self-efficacy scale (Part D). Subscale clusters are pain intensity and pain coping mechanisms for the pain scale. Relationships, idea of self, response to illness, and coping are suffering subscale clusters. Self and work, family influences, and coping beliefs are work beliefs subscales. Nine items related to physical ability (standing, walking, stair climbing, reaching, bending, kneeling, lifting, carrying 1 & 2) make up the self-efficacy subscale (20–23).

The suffering items in the questionnaire are based on many theoretical works such as those of Cassell (2004) and others (1–15). Work belief items are derived and modified from the Health Quality of Life Scales 9ESI-55 and SF-12 (16–18). The pain scale was derived from selected items in the McGill Pain Scale (18) and the self-efficacy items were chosen from the Functional Abilities Confidence Scale (19).

Summary of Validity and Reliability Analyses of the MASQ

Validity and reliability results were obtained from a sample of patients with arthritis as well as other patients with chronic illness to determine whether the relationship between suffering and pain was consistent across disease categories.

Validity · Scaling success was 97.3% as determined from a sample of 166 persons with arthritis tested on admission (T1) and on discharge (T2) and confirmed in samples of subjects with epilepsy $n = 113$, migraine headache $n = 79$, and spinal cord injuries $n = 23$. Floor and ceiling effects are minimal for all subscales (range of floor effects 0.0%–2.4% and ceiling effects 0.0%–6.6%). Subscales show no evidence of redundancy and are reproducible. The questionnaire was shown to be sensitive to change because the mean change over time is statistically significant. Even minor changes were detected as demonstrated by the narrow confidence intervals for each mean pair.

Reliability · Items are relevant to the hypothesized subscales with item reliability at $\alpha = 0.8637$, and item total correlations which are all greater than the acceptable criteria of 0.20. Scaling item reliability at T1 was $\alpha = 0.85$ and $\alpha = 0.90$ at T2 is excellent. There is no evidence of item redundancy. A Pearson Correlation Matrix showed that all item suffering pairs correlated weakly at $p < 0.6$.

The relationship between suffering and pain intensity: Correlation Coefficients provide evidence to support the hypothesis that *suffering and pain are separate and only sometimes related entities.*

Total suffering and pain intensity: Arthritic Sample, N = 166. Subjects were tested on two occasions, Time 1 (T1) on admission and Time 2 (T2) on discharge.

T1: $r = 0.343$, $p = 0.000$

T2: $r = 0.438$, $p = 0.0001$

This relationship is also confirmed in other studies of persons with epilepsy, migraine headache, and spinal cord injuries.

Total suffering and pain intensity in other studies in which testing was done on one occasion only:

Epileptic Sample, N = 100

$r = 0.500$

$p = 0.000$

Spinal Cord Sample, N = 23

$r = 0.576$

$p = 0.004$

Migraine Headache Sample, N = 77

$r = 0.210$

$p = 0.06$

SUMMARY

This chapter introduces the MASQ, designed to measure and assess suffering in a manual format. Justification for use of the manual is based on both research evidence and clinical experiences. Key definitions of suffering, idea of self, personhood, and pain are briefly reviewed and enhance the value of the MASQ as a clinical assessment tool. Research evidence is summarized in an "at a glance" style so that clinicians may quickly determine the validity and reliability of the MASQ. The questionnaire is presented in its entirety. Collation and scoring of both raw data and normative data are presented in the following chapters.

CHAPTER 8 QUESTIONS

1 What is the purpose of the MASQ?
2 Why is the MASQ an important clinical tool?
3 What is the theoretical basis of the MASQ?
4 How are items scored?
5 What is the scaling success of the MASQ?
6 What is the item reliability at T1 and T2?
7 What evidence is there that items in the MASQ are not redundant?
8 Is the MASQ a valid and reliable measurement tool?

9 How to Assess Suffering

Raw Data Collation and Interpretation of the MASQ

The aim of contemporary medicine is to provide optimal care to patients based on objective scientific evidence. Raw data, that is, the actual numerical value designated by the patient for a specific item or the mean of a group of subscores in a particular section of the MASQ, provides an opportunity to clearly identify those areas of greatest importance to patients.

The purpose of this chapter is to (a) illustrate the MASQ, (b) show how to calculate raw data scores, (c) explain criteria for use of either a "long" or a "short" form and, (d) show the usefulness of raw data scores in clinical practice.

Measuring and Assessing Suffering: The MASQ

The MASQ is a self-administered questionnaire designed to evaluate responses on a scale of 1 to 5. As discussed in chapter 5, a score of 5 on any item indicates the most negative response. The MASQ is designed to indicate distress in four domains: (1) Suffering, (2) Work Beliefs, (3) Self-Efficacy, and (4) Coping. Raw data results can be recorded using a comprehensive long format ("long form"), which indicates the responses for each item, or the short form, which presents a summary of the raw data for each of the domains. Further, if suffering per se is the only domain of interest/concern for the clinician, then a short form entitled "suffering summary" is available. In general, short forms are used when the prime clinical objective is diagnosis. When treatment planning is the goal, then the long form is most useful, for it clearly identifies not only the suffering component but also the impact of suffering on personhood issues such as work beliefs, self-efficacy, and coping beliefs. In some instances, a physician may wish to determine how a patient's scores relate to other persons with chronic illness. To do so, normative data scores must be calculated from a series of diverse patient samples. Clinicians can compare an individual patient's results to other comparable groups to best gauge the severity of response. Normative data scores are particularly important in those cases where it is evident that pain is not the prime concern. A description of how to score the results using a normative data analysis is provided in chapter 10.

Administering the MASQ

Patients are given an information sheet that describes the treatment plans to be administered and consent for treatment is given. If the information to be collected is to be used for research purposes, the purpose of the study and methods to be employed must be given to individuals both verbally and in written form. Patients are reassured that should they not wish to be part of the research, future care will not be compromised. Issues of confidentiality are clearly defined both in the clinical setting and research program. Consent forms designed specifically for treatment and others for research are signed and witnessed. Contact telephone numbers are provided in case of emergency or if patients have further questions. The instruction sheets are given to patients prior to the test day so that the patient may ask questions before agreeing to participate in the study. After these preliminary documents are explained and consent obtained, instructions for scoring the MASQ must be brief and concise. The following instructions to patients address this point.

Instructions to Patients

Patients are asked to circle the response to each question that best describes how they feel currently, to answer all the questions, and not to add up subscores. Clinicians are advised to not use the word "suffering" when introducing the questionnaire to patients because this terminology introduces the possibility of bias of response, as "suffering" per se has many doctrinal associations both religious and societal. The MASQ adopts a secular stance and as a result neither includes nor excludes past understandings of the concept of suffering. Scoring of the questionnaire usually takes between 10 and 15 minutes and provides the clinician with immediate results.

The Questionnaire

MASQ

I.D.# ______

NAME ____________________ DATE ____________

PHONE ____________ D.O.B. ____________ GENDER ______

ADDRESS ____________ CITY ____________ POSTAL CODE ______

DIAGNOSIS ______________________________

____

INSTRUCTIONS:

1. **Please answer all questions.**
2. **Only circle one response.**
3. **Circle the response that best describes how you feel now.**

Part A

Please select the response that most describes **how you feel now**. Circle the number on the scale for each question.

1) How **much pain** do you have?

none	a little	some	a lot	sometimes unbearable
(1)	(2)	(3)	(4)	(5)

2) Do you think you will have **more pain**?

no	not likely	maybe	probably	yes
(1)	(2)	(3)	(4)	(5)

3) If you had more pain, do you think you **could stand it**?

yes	probably	maybe	not likely	no
(1)	(2)	(3)	(4)	(5)

4) If you had **less pain** but it never went away, could you **manage satisfactorily**?

yes	probably	maybe	not likely	no
(1)	(2)	(3)	(4)	(5)

5) If you were to have **no pain**, do you think you would be the same person as you were before your **illness/injury**?

yes	probably	maybe	not likely	no
(1)	(2)	(3)	(4)	(5)

OFFICE USE ONLY

Total Subscore: sum of scores / # of Items = ____ / 5 = [ ]

Grand Total = [ ]

(same as total subscore)

Part B

Please select the response that most describes **how you feel now**. Circle the number on the scale for each question.

Section I

1) How much **worry/concern** do you feel that your illness will have a bad effect on your **personal life with children**?

none	a little	some	a lot	a great deal
(1)	(2)	(3)	(4)	(5)

2) How much **worry/concern** do you feel that your illness will have a bad effect on your **personal life with a partner**?

none	a little	some	a lot	a great deal
(1)	(2)	(3)	(4)	(5)

3) How much **worry/concern** do you feel that your illness will have a bad effect on your **personal life with friends**?

none —— a little —— some —— a lot —— a great deal
(1) (2) (3) (4) (5)

4) How much **worry/concern** do you feel that your illness will have a bad effect on your **personal life in the future**?

none —— a little —— some —— a lot —— a great deal
(1) (2) (3) (4) (5)

OFFICE USE ONLY

I. Total Subscore: ______ = ☐
# of Items **4**

Section II

1) How much **worry/concern** do you feel that your illness will have a bad effect on **you as you age**?

none —— a little —— some —— a lot —— a great deal
(1) (2) (3) (4) (5)

2) How much **worry/concern** do you feel about your **illness/injury**?

none —— a little —— some —— a lot —— a great deal
(1) (2) (3) (4) (5)

3) Do you think that your body works the same way as it did before your **illness/injury**?

The same	almost the same (¾ of what I was or what I think I should be)	half of what I was (½ of what I was or what I think I should be)	much less (¼ of what I was or what I think I should be)	not at all
(1)	(2)	(3)	(4)	(5)

4) Do you think that your emotional feelings are the same as they were before your **illness/injury**?

The same	almost the same (¾ of what I was or what I think I should be)	half of what I was (½ of what I was or what I think I should be)	much less (¼ of what I was or what I think I should be)	not at all
(1)	(2)	(3)	(4)	(5)

5) Do you think that you will ever be the **same person** that you were before your **illness/injury**?

yes —— probably —— maybe —— not sure —— no
(1) (2) (3) (4) (5)

OFFICE USE ONLY			
II. Total Subscore:	______	=	☐
# of Items	**5**		

Section III

1) Do you think that how you feel now is **"normal"** in spite of your **illness/injury**?

yes	probably	maybe	not sure	no
(1)	(2)	(3)	(4)	(5)

2) How much **anger** do you have because of your **illness/injury**?

none	a little	some	a lot	a great deal
(1)	(2)	(3)	(4)	(5)

3) How much **sadness** do you have because of your **illness/injury**?

none	a little	some	a lot	a great deal
(1)	(2)	(3)	(4)	(5)

4) What kind of **future hopes** do you have **for yourself**?

high	med. high	medium	low	very bad
(1)	(2)	(3)	(4)	(5)

5) How concerned are **other people** about the fact that you have your illness/injury?

A great deal	a lot	some	a little	not at all
(1)	(2)	(3)	(4)	(5)

OFFICE USE ONLY			
III. Total Subscore:	______	=	☐
# of Items	**5**		

Section IV

1) How much **worry/concern** do you feel that your illness will have a bad effect on your **job**?

none	a little	some	a lot	a great deal
(1)	(2)	(3)	(4)	(5)

2) If the problems with your life that you have now never got better, could you **manage satisfactorily**?

yes	probably	maybe	not likely	no
(1)	(2)	(3)	(4)	(5)

The next question is about support systems. A support system is those people (family, friends, neighbours, co-workers, and/or other people) whom you can talk to about your private feelings.

3) What **kind** of **support system** do you have?

good ——— average ——— fair ——— poor ——— very bad
(1) (2) (3) (4) (5)

4) Do you feel that you are **managing** your illness/injury **alone**?

not alone ——— sometimes alone ——— almost alone ——— nearly alone ——— always alone
(1) (2) (3) (4) (5)

5) How much are you able to be **part** of your **community**?

A great deal ——— a lot ——— some ——— a little ——— not at all
(1) (2) (3) (4) (5)

OFFICE USE ONLY

IV. Total Subscore: ________ / **# of Items** = ______ / **5** = ☐

Grand Total = (sum of all subscores) / **4** = ☐

Part C

PLEASE TELL US WHAT YOU BELIEVE ABOUT YOUR ABILITY TO WORK

Please circle the answer that most describes **how you feel now**. Circle only one answer.

Section I

1. Do you think that you have **enough education** to get a job?

yes ——— probably ——— maybe ——— not sure ——— no
(1) (2) (3) (4) (5)

2. Do you think that you **have to** have a **job** in order to be just like everyone else?

yes ——— probably ——— maybe ——— not sure ——— no
(1) (2) (3) (4) (5)

3. Do you believe that people who work are **more respected** than people who do not work?

yes ——— probably ——— maybe ——— not sure ——— no
(1) (2) (3) (4) (5)

4. Do you believe that the **only thing** that stops you from living on your own is the fact that you do not have a job?

N/A ——— yes ——— probably ——— maybe ——— not sure ——— no
(0) (1) (2) (3) (4) (5)

5. How much do you like being around people that you do **not** know well?

a lot — a little — some — not much — not at all
(1) (2) (3) (4) (5)

6. How much **worry/concern** do you have that **other people** will be **afraid** when they **see you** having an illness/injury?

a lot — a little — some — not much — none
(1) (2) (3) (4) (5)

OFFICE USE ONLY

I. Total Subscore: ______ = ☐
# of Items 6

Section II

1. How many **chores** do you do in your home?

a lot — a little — some — not many — none
(1) (2) (3) (4) (5)

2. How many **close** friends do you have **outside** your family?

very many (10–20) — many (5–10) — some (3–4) — not many (1–2) — none (0)
(1) (2) (3) (4) (5)

3. How **happy** are you **helping** your family at home?

N/A — very happy — a lot — moderately — a little — not at all
(0) (1) (2) (3) (4) (5)

4. Do you think that **your family** would be **afraid** that you would get **hurt** if you had a **job**?

No Family Contact — no — not sure — maybe — probably — yes
(0) (1) (2) (3) (4) (5)

5. Do you think that **your family** would rather **you did not work** outside the home?

No Family Contact — no — not sure — maybe — probably — yes
(0) (1) (2) (3) (4) (5)

6. If you **lost** your **pension benefits**, could you **manage** satisfactorily?

Not on Pension — yes — probably — maybe — not sure — no
(0) (1) (2) (3) (4) (5)

OFFICE USE ONLY

II. Total Subscore: ______ = ☐
# of Items 6

Section III

1. If you had a job, would **you** be **afraid** you might get **hurt**?

no	not sure	maybe	probably	yes
(1)	(2)	(3)	(4)	(5)

2. Do you think that you might **hurt others** because of your illness/injury **while working**?

no	not sure	maybe	probably	yes
(1)	(2)	(3)	(4)	(5)

3. Can you get to work **on time** every day?

yes	probably	maybe	not sure	no
(1)	(2)	(3)	(4)	(5)

4. Do you think that you can get **transportation** to work **every day**?

yes	probably	maybe	not sure	no
(1)	(2)	(3)	(4)	(5)

5. Do you think that if you had a job, you would be able to **get home** every day **by yourself**?

yes	probably	maybe	not sure	no
(1)	(2)	(3)	(4)	(5)

6. Do you think that you would be able to take your medication **on time** at work?

yes	probably	maybe	not sure	no
(1)	(2)	(3)	(4)	(5)

7. Do you **worry** that your **illness/injury** would **affect** how you did **your job**?

no	not sure	maybe	probably	yes
(1)	(2)	(3)	(4)	(5)

8. Do you **worry** that you might **lose** some of your **pension benefits** because of **working**?

Not on Pension	yes	probably	maybe	not sure	no
(0)	(1)	(2)	(3)	(4)	(5)

OFFICE USE ONLY

III. Total Subscore: ________ / **# of Items** = ______ / **8** = ☐

Grand Total = (sum of all subscores) / **3** = ☐

Part D

We would like to know **how confident you are that you can do things**. Circle the number on the scale that best describes your level of confidence that you could perform the activity **today**. If you do not do an activity, please rate how confident you would be if you had to do these things.

1. How much **confidence** do you have that you can **stand** for as long as you want or need to?

   a great deal ——— a lot ——— some ——— very little ——— none
   (1) (2) (3) (4) (5)

2. How much **confidence** do you have that you can **walk** as long as you need to?

   a great deal ——— a lot ——— some ——— very little ——— none
   (1) (2) (3) (4) (5)

3. How much **confidence** do you have that you can **climb up and down stairs** safely?

   a great deal ——— a lot ——— some ——— very little ——— none
   (1) (2) (3) (4) (5)

4. How much **confidence** do you have that you can **reach above your head** without losing your balance?

   a great deal ——— a lot ——— some ——— very little ——— none
   (1) (2) (3) (4) (5)

5. How much **confidence** do you have that you can **bend down** and return to a standing position without falling?

   a great deal ——— a lot ——— some ——— very little ——— none
   (1) (2) (3) (4) (5)

6. How much **confidence** do you have that you can **kneel down** and return to a standing position?

   a great deal ——— a lot ——— some ——— very little ——— none
   (1) (2) (3) (4) (5)

7. How much **confidence** do you have that you can **carry a small box**?

   a great deal ——— a lot ——— some ——— very little ——— none
   (1) (2) (3) (4) (5)

8. How much **confidence** do you have that you can **carry a large box**?

   a great deal ——— a lot ——— some ——— very little ——— none
   (1) (2) (3) (4) (5)

9. How much **confidence** do you have that you can **lift a box from the floor** without losing your balance?

   a great deal ——— a lot ——— some ——— very little ——— none
   (1) (2) (3) (4) (5)

OFFICE USE ONLY

Total Subscore:	______ =	☐
# of Items	9	
Grand Total	=	☐

(same as total subscore)

Thank you for answering these questions.

Scoring the Questionnaire

Step 1: The maximum score per question is 5 points.

Example: If the patient scores the following two questions as indicated below:
Question 1: How much worry . . .

(1)	(2)	(3)	(4)	(5)
none	a little	some	a lot	a great deal

Question 2: How much worry . . .

(1)	(2)	(3)	(4)	(5)
none	a little	some	**a lot**	a great deal

Then, question 1 = 1 point and question 2 = 4 points.

Step 2: Please add up the value for each question and divide by the number of questions in each section. Therefore, the subscore for the above example would be:

Subscore = $\frac{\text{sum of the values for each question } (1 + 4) = 5}{\text{divided by the number of items } (2)} = 2.5$

Step 3: At the end of each major subsection entitled Part A, B, C, or D please enter the sum of all subscores obtained for each major subsection divided by the number of sections. To achieve the Grand Total Score:

Grand Total Score = $\frac{\text{sum of all sub-scores}}{\text{number of sections}}$

Data Collation

All professional jurisprudence regulations require health care personnel to keep accurate records of client assessments, treatment regimens, and outcomes. Further, multidisciplinary health care delivery programs depend on accurate, concise communication methods between health care professionals. Comprehensive record keeping is critical not only to monitor patient progress but also to the development of more efficacious interventions.

Data from the questionnaire may be collated in two ways. Raw data (grand totals and/or subscores) may be recorded as described in the following section of this chapter or the raw data may be converted to normative scores and plotted as described in the section "Normative Data Collation" in chapter 10.

Raw Data Collation

Long-Form Instructions

On page 1 of the long-form record (figures 9.1–9.4), the grand total scores obtained from the questionnaire for pain (Part A of the questionnaire), suffering (Part B), work beliefs (Part C), and self-efficacy (Part D) are outlined. Record the date of testing at the bottom of each section. Under the comments section, write a brief interpretation of the results.

On the second, third, and fourth pages of the long form, record the subset results for each section. Part A (pain) has subscores for pain intensity and pain coping. Part B (suffering) has four sections. Record the subscores for relationships, idea of self, and response to illness and coping. Under the comments section, key points for special attention are noted. Part C (work beliefs), has three sections. Section I refers to "self," section II, "family," and section III "coping." Part D (self-efficacy) reports the subscores for confidence in standing, walking, stair climbing, reaching, bending, kneeling, carrying small box (carry 1) and large box (carry 2), lifting. Examples of how data may be interpreted clinically are also presented in figures 9.1–9.4.

Long-Form Scoring and Collation

Step 1: Plot the grand total scores on page 1 of the data summary chart for long form (see figure 9.1).

Step 2: Plot subset scores on pages 2, 3, and 4 of the data summary chart for long form (see figures 9.2–9.4).

Review of page 1 of the data summary sheet clearly indicates potential areas of concern. Pages 2 and 3 of the data summary sheet indicate, more specifically, areas of distress determined in each part of the assessment.

Application of Long-Form Data: Integration of Suffering in Clinical Practice

The development of patient information documents is an important component of successful integration of the construct of suffering into the treatment planning of those who suffer. Figure 9.1 is an example of a summary of the raw data scores obtained from a patient assessed using the MASQ. This form can be placed at the front of the patient's chart to alert other clinicians to the patient's difficulties. In the summary (see figure 9.1) a mean score of 4 indicates that the patient is very concerned about the issues assessed. In this example, the patient's degree of concern relating to pain and pain management would be described as "moderate." The patient is not impaired because of adverse work beliefs and describes a great deal of confidence in physical abilities with mean scores of 2. From this summary sheet all health care professionals would be aware that suffering is a main problem that should be addressed by all health professionals.

Figures 9.2, 9.3, and 9.4 are the detailed scores for each of the domains. In figure 9.2, Part A, pain intensity is moderate and the patient expressed a moderate concern about his/her ability to cope with pain (scores of 3).

The main issues of concern in figure 9.2, Part B, are related to idea of self and ability to cope (scores of 4 and 5 respectively). With scores at level 5 indicating severe distress, clinicians know that these issues are of prime concern to the patient and require immediate investigation.

Figure 9.3, Part C, deals with work beliefs and raw data scores are in the low end of the scale indicating a lesser degree of worry. Attention would be paid to issues relating to family, as it is the area in which the patient is most concerned (scores of 3). In Part D, confidence is lacking in ability to climb stairs and in reaching for objects above the patient's head (scores of 4). In figure 9.4 there is also a moderate degree of concern that the patient believes he/she will have difficulty carrying objects of various sizes and weights (score of 3).

Raw data collation as depicted above is particularly useful for all health care professionals. For example, nurses are aware that patients may need additional care and support after family visits. Physiotherapists have a clear idea of how to design treatment interventions that will improve not only physical performance but also foster integration into the family and community at large. Occupational therapists, psychologists, social workers, and chaplains will all have a clear indication of where to begin to dialogue about the concerns of the patient and have insight about the impact of chronic illness on ideas of self and personhood. In our studies, the importance of raw data collation was found to be clinically relevant when a large number of patients, after taking the test, approached our researchers to inquire about how and where they could get help.

Short-Form Instructions

There are two short-form formats available (figs. 9.5 and 9.6). One, format "short form" (complete) provides summary information about pain, suffering, work beliefs, and self-efficacy. The second format entitled "short form" (suffering component only) is useful when only information about the suffering component

EXAMPLE

LONG FORM

DATA SUMMARY (RAW SCORES)

MEASURING AND ASSESSING SUFFERING QUESTIONNAIRE

NAME: ____________________ DATE: __________

ASSESSOR: ____________________

Likert-Type Scale: (1 - 5) 5 = Worst Response.

I. GRAND TOTAL SCORES

	PART A PAIN		**PART B** SUFFERING		**PART C** WORK BELIEFS		**PART D** SELF-EFFICACY
Max. Pain (5)		Max. Distress (5)	X	Negative Beliefs (5)		No Confidence (5)	
(4)		(4)		(4)		(4)	
(3)	X	(3)		(3)		(3)	
(2)		(2)		(2)	X	(2)	X
No Pain (1)		(1)		Positive Beliefs (1)		Total Confidence (1)	
	Patient's score:		Patient's score:		Patient's score:		Patient's score:
	Date:		Date:		Date:		Date:

COMMENTS:

1) Suffering is the most significant issue (a lot of distress).
2) Pain is moderate.
3) Work beliefs are very good.
4) Self-efficacy is very good.

Therefore, suffering may be a factor which will negatively impact on treatment outcomes.

Figure 9.1

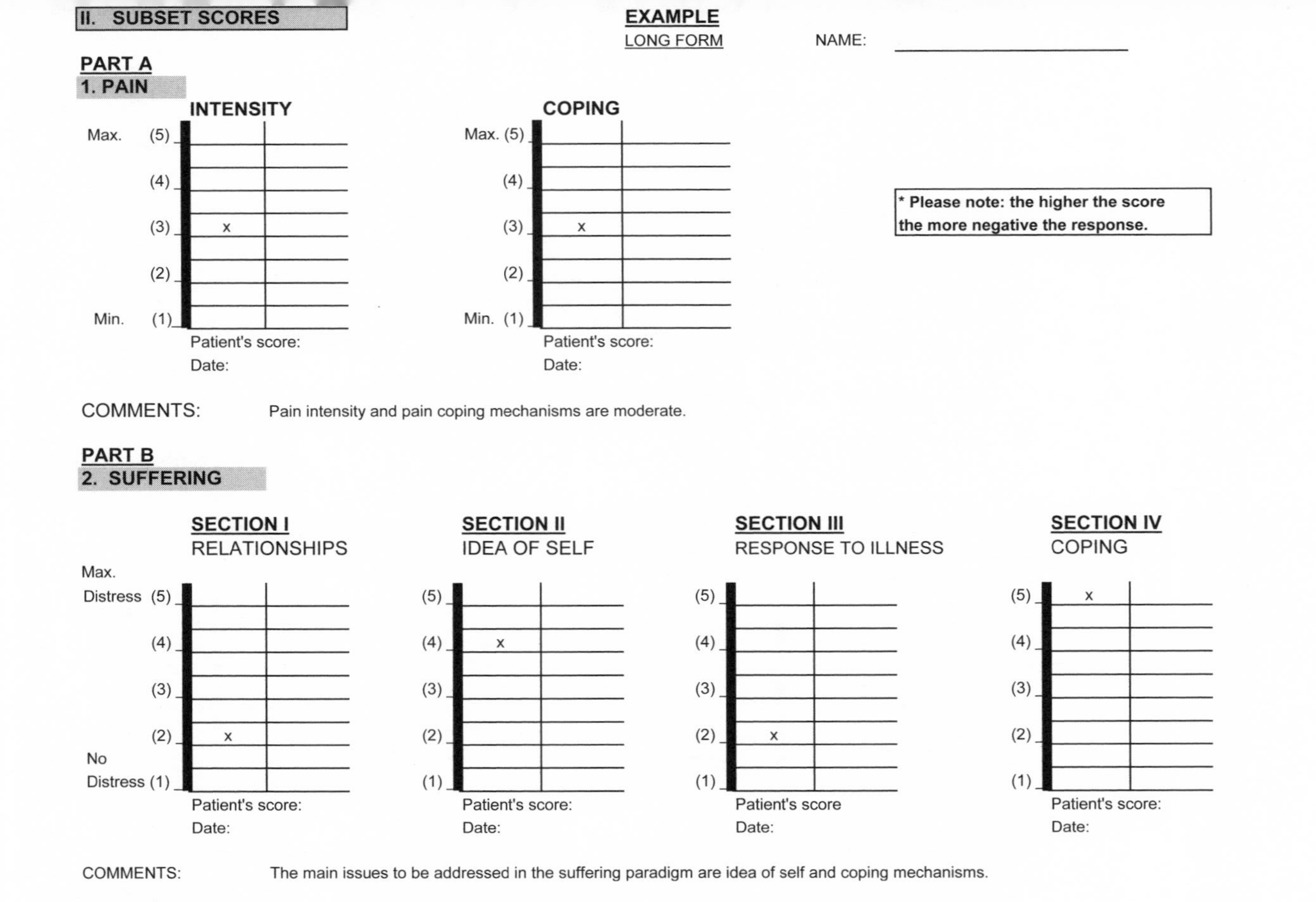

II. SUBSET SCORES

EXAMPLE
LONG FORM

NAME: ____________________

PART A
1. PAIN

INTENSITY

Max. (5)
(4)
(3) x
(2)
Min. (1)

Patient's score:
Date:

COPING

Max. (5)
(4)
(3) x
(2)
Min. (1)

Patient's score:
Date:

*** Please note: the higher the score the more negative the response.**

COMMENTS: Pain intensity and pain coping mechanisms are moderate.

PART B
2. SUFFERING

SECTION I
RELATIONSHIPS

Max. Distress (5)
(4)
(3)
(2) x
No Distress (1)

Patient's score:
Date:

SECTION II
IDEA OF SELF

(5)
(4) x
(3)
(2)
(1)

Patient's score:
Date:

SECTION III
RESPONSE TO ILLNESS

(5)
(4)
(3)
(2) x
(1)

Patient's score
Date:

SECTION IV
COPING

(5) x
(4)
(3)
(2)
(1)

Patient's score:
Date:

COMMENTS: The main issues to be addressed in the suffering paradigm are idea of self and coping mechanisms.

Figure 9.2

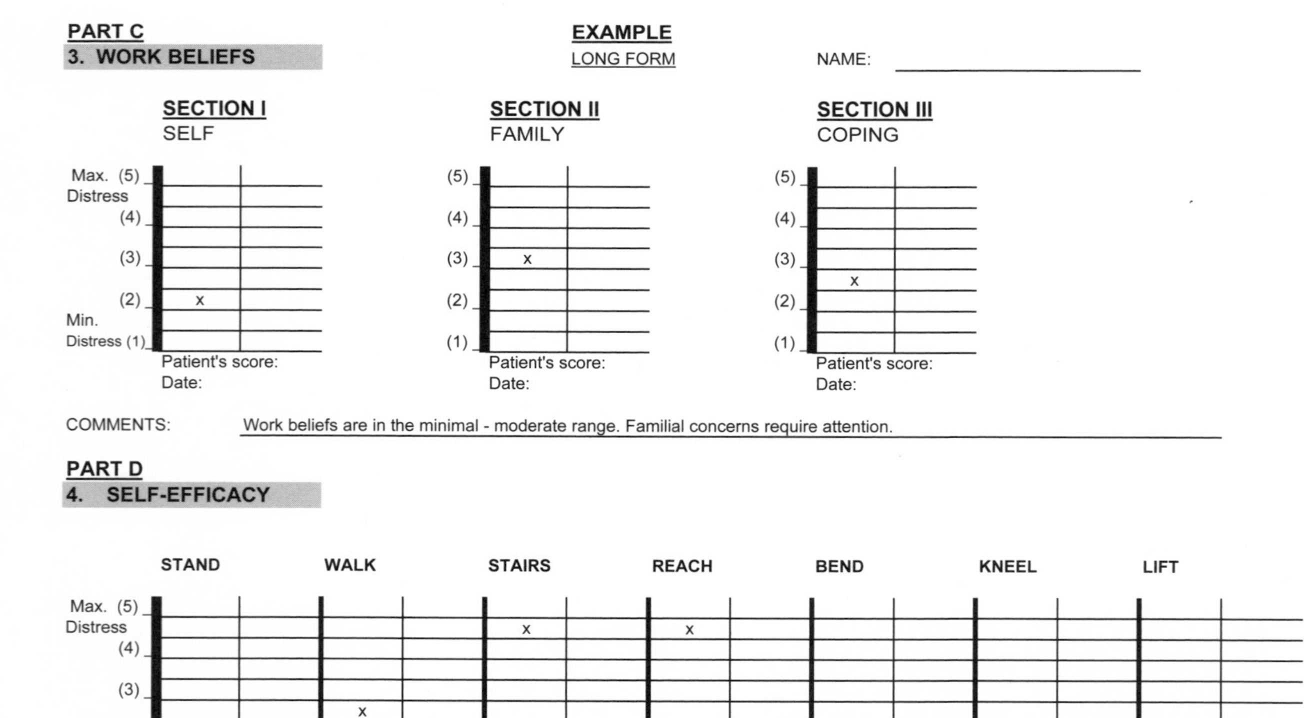
PART C
3. WORK BELIEFS
EXAMPLE
LONG FORM
NAME:
SECTION I
SELF
SECTION II
FAMILY
SECTION III
COPING
Max. (5)
Distress
(4)
(3)
(2)
Min.
Distress (1)
Patient's score:
Date:
COMMENTS:
Work beliefs are in the minimal - moderate range. Familial concerns require attention.
PART D
4. SELF-EFFICACY
STAND
WALK
STAIRS
REACH
BEND
KNEEL
LIFT
Score:
Date:
COMMENTS:
Confidence is lacking in ability to climb stairs and in reaching for objects above head.
Balance may be an issue. There is some concern regarding carrying objects. (see next page)

Figure 9.3

EXAMPLE

LONG FORM

NAME: ______________________

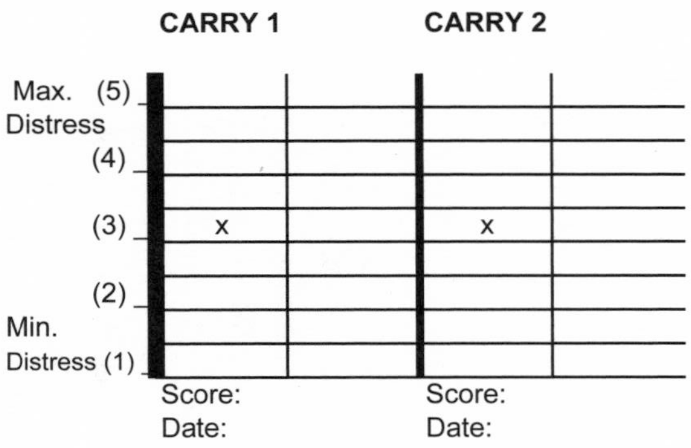

	CARRY 1	CARRY 2
Max. Distress (5)		
(4)		
(3)	x	x
(2)		
Min. Distress (1)		
	Score:	Score:
	Date:	Date:

COMMENTS: The key factors that may negatively influence performance and work re-entry are related to suffering (the perception of threat to a person's idea of self and personhood) and self-efficacy and physical performance (climbing stairs, reaching above head, carrying objects).

Assessor Signature: ______________________

Date: ______________________

Figure 9.4

of the MASQ is required. In this form, the grand total score for suffering is recorded as well as the subset score for Section I (relationships), Section II (idea of self), Section III (response to illness), and Section IV (coping). There is space for the assessor's comments and signature at the bottom of the form. This format provides a quick "at a glance" method of indicating areas of concern and is particularly helpful in confirming diagnosis and referrals for treatment, as well as when summary data information is required from auxiliary agencies (insurance companies, workplace evaluations). Examples of scoring and clinical interpretation of data are also given in figures 9.5 and 9.6.

Short-Form Scoring and Collation · In certain circumstances, a quick "at-a-glance" summary of patient responses is required. The complete short form is most useful when a summary of responses is required and placed in the patient's medical record to alert physicians and others of the patient's difficulties. In this situation, the person who administered the MASQ would be available for clarification and further elaboration of findings.

Short Form (Complete)

Step 1: Plot the grand total scores for pain, suffering, work beliefs, and self-efficacy (see figure 9.5).

Step 2: Record clinical interpretation of the data results in the space provided at the bottom of the form.

If the information about suffering only is of prime concern, the short-form (suffering only) data summary sheet is used.

Short Form (Suffering Only)

Step 1: Plot the grand total score for pain (see figure 9.6).

Step 2: Plot the subset scores for section I (relationships), section II (idea of self), section III (response to illness), and section IV (coping).

Step 3: Record clinical interpretations of data results in the space provided for comments.

Application of Short-Form Raw Data: Integration of Suffering in Clinical Practice

The use of short-form raw data analysis is particularly useful to insurance adjusters and in cases involving workplace analyses. In such instances, summary data may be all that is required initially. From this summary, insurance adjusters can quickly ascertain the area of major concern and lawyers are quickly alerted to the fact that in this case there is no evidence of malingering, as the patient has shown that he/she possesses good work beliefs and self-confidence in physical abilities (score of 2). These data indicate that factors relating to suffering that involve ideas of self and personhood are of considerable concern to the patient

EXAMPLE
SHORT FORM (COMPLETE)

DATA SUMMARY (RAW SCORES)

MEASURING AND ASSESSING SUFFERING QUESTIONNAIRE

NAME: ____________________ DATE: __________

ASSESSOR: ____________________

Likert-Type Scale: (1 - 5) 5 = Worst Response.

I. GRAND TOTAL SCORES

PART A PAIN		PART B SUFFERING		PART C WORK BELIEFS		PART D SELF-EFFICACY	
Max. Pain (5)		Max. Distress (5)		Negative Beliefs (5)		No Confidence (5)	
(4)		(4)	X	(4)		(4)	
(3)	X	(3)		(3)		(3)	
(2)		(2)		(2)	X	(2)	X
(1)		(1)		Positive Beliefs (1)		Total Confidence (1)	
	Patient's score: Date:		Patient's score: Date:		Patient's score: Date:		Patient's score: Date:

COMMENTS: 1) suffering is the most significant issue (a lot of distress). 2) pain is moderate. 3) Work beliefs are very good.
4) Self-Efficacy is very good. Therefore, suffering may be a factor which will negatively impact on treament outcomes.

ASSESSOR SIGNATURE: ____________________

Figure 9.5

EXAMPLE

SHORT FORM

*(SUFFERING COMPONENT ONLY)

DATA SUMMARY (RAW SCORES)

MEASURING AND ASSESSING SUFFERING QUESTIONNAIRE

NAME: ______________________ DATE: ______________

ASSESSOR: ______________________

Likert-Type Scale: (1 - 5) 5 = Worst Response.

I. GRAND TOTAL SCORE

II. SUBSET SCORES

	PART B SUFFERING	SECTION I RELATIONSHIPS	SECTION II IDEA OF SELF	SECTION III RESPONSE TO ILLNESS	SECTION IV COPING
Max. Distress (5)	•		•	•	
(4)					
(3)		•			•
(2)					
No Distress (1)					
	Patient's score:	Patient's score:	Patient's score:	Patient's score:	Patient's score:
	Date:	Date:	Date:	Date:	Date:

COMMENTS: This patient has a high total suffering score. Problem areas focus on perceptions of threat to "ideas of self" due to the illness and/or injury. The patient's response to the illness (anger, sadness, concerns about managing alone, never showing desired improvement, etc.) is very high (negative). However, the patient's coping skills only are moderately impaired. Referral for counselling and/or incorporation of strategies to address the above into nursing care, physiotherapy and family therapy are appropriate depending on the nature of the illness/injury.

ASSESSOR SIGNATURE: ______________________

Figure 9.6

(scores of 4 and 5). In the example cited above, the personnel involved would then be able to explore with the patient factors that may cause the suffering.

In figure 9.6, the summary of raw data scores refers only to the items on the MASQ that relate to suffering. Figure 9.6 shows that the key issues of concern are associated with ideas of self, response to illness, and ability to cope (scores of 4 and 5). Using the example cited, insurance adjusters are able to clearly see the effects of the illness and/or injury on the whole person and determine the degree of compensation available, thus avoiding causing further harm to the patient that may occur due to current adversarial investigative methods.

SUMMARY

This chapter has illustrated the usefulness of collating raw data and the importance of providing patients with clinical and/or research information prior to beginning treatments or enrollment in research trials. Examples of information packages and consent forms are provided to aid the clinician in the development of appropriate materials for their own specific areas of practice. Criteria for long-form as opposed to short-form raw data collation formats are given.

Examples of clinical interpretation of data results are also given. Raw data scores are useful for long-term treatment planning because details of specific areas of distress are identified. Sometimes, clinicians require information about where the patient's responses fall in comparison with other persons with chronic illness. In such cases, normative data results are essential. An example of when this type of information is useful may be in circumstances where monetary compensation is required. Chapter 10 provides instructions for converting raw data into normative scores.

CHAPTER 9 QUESTIONS

1 In figure 9.2, the main issues to be addressed are "idea of self" and "coping mechanisms." How would you begin to address these issues with a patient?
2 How might the degree of concern expressed in figure 9.2, Part B, interact with results reported in Part D (self-efficacy) in figure 9.3?
3 How might raw data scores depicted in figure 9.5 be useful in assessing a patient's ability to return to work?
4 How would the data presented in figure 9.6 aid in medical legal evaluations of a patient's ability to return to work?
5 What is the value of patient information documents?
6 Are consent forms necessary to quality of care? Explain.
7 How may objective and subjective data contribute to patient-centered, cost-effective care?

Normative data are obtained from tests and scales and are used for comparison of results from one group or individual to the means and standard deviations of another group or to individual sets of measures. They delineate that which usually occurs in a specific population at a specific point in time and are an important treatment guide, particularly when specific treatment interventions such as drug therapy are being considered. Normative data are important in developing standards of care. The ability to "place" patients along a continuum of response or clinical outcome, for example, is useful when clinicians must make determinations of when to refer patients to other health care professionals or to track significance of specific interventions. Normative data information about suffering is essential after patients are involved in accidents or when it is important to determine the significance of chronicity, in situations involving litigation or disability compensation, or when crisis intervention is required (1–9).

The purpose of this chapter is to: (a) demonstrate the need for comparative data, (b) report the normative data results of suffering and pain scores obtained from a sample of 166 persons with arthritis and 100 individuals with epilepsy, (c) provide instructions about how to calculate normative scores from raw data, and (d) present examples of clinical interpretation of normative data.

How Does the Patient Compare with Persons Who Have Similar Disorders?

Normative data scoring methods are used when a clinician wishes to compare an individual patient's scores with those of a larger sample or a similar comparison group. To date, only complete data sets for the construct of suffering for persons with epilepsy and those with arthritis are available (10). These illnesses are representative of the extremes of the suffering and pain experiences (epilepsy—less suffering, and arthritis—severe suffering): therefore, it is possible to "place" other persons along this continuum. Normative data scoring is important because its interpretation is thought to be more useful clinically than raw data scores, and allows health care professionals to better ascertain the dimensions of an individual's clinical complaints. To date, there is no gold standard for suffering per se, but preliminary descriptive inferential statistics (mean, standard deviation, and resultant Z scores) have been derived from the 166 patients with arthritis and 100 persons with epilepsy introduced earlier. Z scores are useful because they indicate how many standard deviations an element is from the mean. If a patient's score is below the mean of that of the reference sample, i.e., a negative Z score, the results are rated as favourable (little or no distress). A Z score of zero indicates moderate distress and a Z score above the mean, a positive Z score, indicates that the patient is in severe distress and requires immediate attention.

How Is the Z Score Calculated?

The Z score is simply computed as follows:

$\mathbf{Z} = (x - \bar{x}) / SD$

Where:

x = the individual patient's suffering score from one of the MASQ subscales

x̄ = the mean suffering subscale score based on an established sample

SD = the standard deviation based on an established sample

The following values, obtained from two sample groups that are representative of the problems of suffering and pain can be used for comparison purposes. The arthritis sample represents comparative values for individuals with chronic illness who usually experience considerable suffering. The epilepsy sample is representative of persons who have chronic illness but usually experience little suffering. The information below is needed to convert raw data results into normative scores.

Reference Scores

TABLE 10.1 · Arthritic Sample Results

Arthritis (N = 166)	Mean/x̄ ± SD
Total suffering score	3.27 ± 0.655
Total pain score	2.89 ± 0.597
Total work beliefs score	N/A
Total self-efficacy score	N/A

Note: N = total number of individuals in the sample.

TABLE 10.2 · Arthritis (N = 166) Suffering Subscale Scores

Suffering subscale	Mean / x̄ ± SD
Idea of self	4.01 ± 0.742
Relationships	3.29 ± 0.952
Response to illness	3.01 ± 0.808
Coping with life	2.78 ± 0.724

TABLE 10.3 · Epilepsy Sample Results

Epilepsy (N = 100)	Mean/x̄ ± SD
Total suffering score	2.31 ± 0.837
Total pain score	3.51 ± 0.631
Total work beliefs score	4.02 ± 1.01
Total self-efficacy score	2.40 ± 0.451

TABLE 10.4 · Epilepsy (N = 100) Suffering Subscale Scores

Suffering Scores	Mean / x̄ ± SD
Idea of self	2.56 ± 1.15
Relationships	2.25± 1.19
Response to illness	2.39 ± 0.82
Coping with life	2.04 ± 0.74

Instructions for Converting Raw Results into Normative Data Scores

There are six basic steps to follow to determine how patients compare with similar groups:

Step 1: Administer the nineteen-item suffering component of the MASQ. Each item is scored on a scale of 1 to 5, where a low score is best.

Step 2: Compute a mean score for the pain items and each of the four suffering subscales as indicated on the questionnaire to obtain a **Total Subscore** for each section.

Step 3: Calculate the **Grand Total Scores** as indicated on the questionnaire. When scores have been previously collated on the raw data forms, the values may be simply transposed into the following transformation formula as indicated in figure 10.1.

Step 4: The last step is to compute a Z (standard) score that will put the patient's suffering state into a clinical context based on a referent sample of patients with the same or similar disorder. If the clinician is uncertain as to which group the patient is most similar, then two Z scores are calculated, one from the most severely involved group and one from the least involved group.

Step 5: Plot the new values on either the long or short forms (normative data). You will notice that the scales of these forms are different from those of the raw data sheets in that the Y-axis depicts the **Z score values** rather than the mean values obtained from the 5-point Likert-type scales. Please see examples 1–3 (figures 10.3 to 10.5).

Step 6: Record the clinical interpretation of the Z score results in the space provided.

How To Obtain **Total Subscore** & The **Grand Total** For **Each** Part of The MASQ

PartB
Section IV

1) How much **worry/concern** do you feel that your illness will have a bad effect on your **job**?

none ----------- a little ---------- some ---------- ***a lot*** ---------- a great deal
(1) (2) (3) ***(4)*** (5)

2) If the problems with your life that you have now never got better, could you **manage satisfactorily?**

yes ---------- probably ---------- maybe ---------- ***not likely*** ---------- no
(1) (2) (3) ***(4)*** (5)

The next question is about support systems. A support system are those people (family, friends, neighbours, co-workers, and/or other people) who you can talk to about your private feelings.

3) What **kind** of **support system** do you have?

good ---------- ***average*** --------- fair ---------- poor ---------- very bad
(1) ***(2)*** (3) (4) (5)

4) Do you feel that you are **managing** your illness/injury **alone**?

not alone ----- ***sometimes alone*** ----- almost alone ----- nearly alone ------ always alone
(1) ***(2)*** (3) (4) (5)

5) How much are you able to be **part** of your **community**?

A great deal ---------- a lot ---------- some ---------- a little ---------- ***not at all***
(1) (2) (3) (4) ***(5)***

$$\textbf{Total Subscore: } \frac{17}{\textbf{\# of items } 5} = 3.4$$

$$\textbf{Grand Total: } \frac{4.25 + 4.6 + 2 + 3.4}{4} = 3.56\ ^*$$

*These values are obtained from Part B Sections I, II, III, IV

Figure 10.1

How to Obtain Z Score Values for One Component of the MASQ

For Comparison with a Severely Involved Patient Group (Arthritis)

For example, if a patient scores the MASQ, Part B, Subsection II, which related to "idea of self," as shown in figure 10.2, first calculate the Total Subscores and for "idea of self." Then, calculate the Z score for the suffering subscale idea of self. In this case the value is

$x = 4.6$ (see figure 10.2).

Therefore, comparison of the patient's score with those obtained from research studies would be

$x = 4.6$ (mean of the patient's raw data scores [see figure 10.2])

$\bar{x} = 4.01$ (mean from the arthritic sample "idea of self" subscale [see Reference Scores section at the beginning of this chapter]).

$SD = 0.742$ (standard deviation from the arthritic sample "idea of self" subscale [see Reference Scores section at the beginning of this chapter]).

Z (for idea of self) $= (4.6 - 4.01) / 0.742 = 0.795$ (score to be used by comparison).

Interpretation of Findings · Transformation of the raw data to normative scores indicates that this patient has a Z score 0.79 standard deviation units above the mean, relative to the arthritis sample. This information tells the clinician that the patient in question is experiencing slightly more distress than a comparable group of patients with arthritis.

For Comparison with a Less Involved Patient Group (Epilepsy)

Calculate the Z score for the suffering subscale idea of self. In this case the values are as follows:

$x = 4.6$ (mean of the patient's raw data scores [see figure 10.2])

$\bar{x} = 2.56$ (mean from the epilepsy sample [see Reference Score section at the beginning of this chapter]).

$SD = 1.15$ (standard deviation of the epilepsy sample [see Reference Scores section at the beginning of this chapter]).

Z (for idea of self) $= (4.6 - 2.56) / 1.15 = 1.77$ (score to be used for comparison).

Interpretation of Findings · Transformation of the raw data score shows a patient score that is 1.77 deviations above the mean relative to the epilepsy sample.

How to obtain the **Z-Score** values for **one** component of the MASQ

PartB
Section II

1) How much **worry/concern** do you feel that your illness will have a bad effect on **you as you age**?

none ----------- a little ---------- some ---------- a lot ---------- ***a great deal***
(1) (2) (3) (4) ***(5)***

2) How much **worry/concern** do you feel about your **illness/injury**?

none ----------- a little ---------- **some** ---------- *a lot* ---------- a great deal
(1) (2) **(3)** *(4)* (5)

3) Do you think that your body works the same way as it did before your **illness/injury**?

The same------almost the same ------- *half of what I was* -------- much less ---------**not at all**
(3/4 of what I was or what I think I should be) *(1/2 of what I was or what I think I should be)* (1/4 of what I was or what I think I should be)
(1) (2) *(3)* (4) **(5)**

4) Do you think that your emotional feelings are the same as they were before your **illness/injury**?

The same------- almost the same ------- *half of what I was* ------- much less ------- **not at all**
(3/4 of what I was or what I think I should be) *(1/2 of what I was or what I think I should be)* (1/4 of what I was or what I think I should be)
(1) (2) *(3)* (4) **(5)**

5) Do you think that you will ever be the **same person** that you were before your **illness/injury**?

yes ---------- probably ---------- *maybe* ---------- not sure ---------- **no**
(1) (2) *(3)* (4) **(5)**

Total Subscore: 23 = 4.6
# of items 5

Figure 10.2

The clinical interpretation of these normative data is that the patient is experiencing more suffering than the patients who are expected to have considerable suffering (arthritis patients) as well as those who are expected to have less suffering (epilepsy patients). In this way the patient being evaluated is "placed" and determinations of whether referrals to a specialist in psychological care as well as application of suffering-specific strategies by all team members will result in optimal treatment outcomes or whether basic team approaches are sufficient. Normative data results do not provide all the answers needed to resolve an individual's problems but when considering the relationship between suffering and pain, they are useful indicators of the dimensions of distress. The last step is to plot the values obtained.

Clinical Application of Normative Data

To date, unlike pain, there are no substantive theories that delineate suffering. Consequently, the MASQ has been designed to objectively identify the perception of suffering in patients. In addition to determining the degree of worry or concern individuals have that their illness/injury will have a negative effect on ideas of self and personhood, health care professionals must have an indication of the significance of these perceptions to an individual's health.

The mean values for the arthritic and epilepsy study groups are listed at the bottom of each section for clinical comparisons.

Example 1 (see figure 10.3) is a summary of the normative data obtained from each of the subsections (pain, suffering, work beliefs, and self-efficacy) of the MASQ for patient X. In this example, one can quickly determine the areas of greatest distress.

The Z scores of the patient are calculated for each main category using the data from the Grand Total Scores (see figure 10.1) and compared with results from data of the referent groups, epilepsy and arthritis. On the graph * indicates Z scores based on the arthritis referent sample and • indicates scores based on the epilepsy referent sample. This format does not delineate the key item issues of concern but rather indicates the general areas requiring attention. Comparative data for the factors, work beliefs, and self-efficacy are only available for the epilepsy group. More research is needed to determine the impact of suffering on these components of personhood.

In this example, when the patient is compared with the arthritis referent sample, the patient is experiencing more pain and suffering than the arthritis group. When the patient is compared with the epilepsy referent group, suffering issues still predominate. The patient's pain, work beliefs, and self-efficacy concerns showed less distress than the referent epilepsy group.

Normative data analyses provide the guide. Our research studies have shown that data from arthritis patients are a valid indicator of severity response and data from epilepsy patients indicate less concern.

Example 2 (see figure 10.4) shows how the normative data scores may be collated if only the suffering component is required. In this short form, the Z scores were tabulated for the factors "total suffering," relationships, idea of self, response to

SHORT FORM (COMPLETE)

NORMATIVE DATA SUMMARY (Z SCORES)

MEASURING AND ASSESSING SUFFERING QUESTIONNAIRE

NAME: ____________ DATE: ____________

ASSESSOR: ____________

- Z SCORE:	LESS DISTRESS.
0 Z SCORE:	DISTRESS LEVEL COMPARABLE TO MEAN OF ESTABLISHED GROUP.
+ Z SCORE:	MORE DISTRESS.

CALCULATIONS: $Z = \frac{(\bar{x} - X)}{S.D.}$

NOTE:
$\bar{x}$ = patients' mean score
X = mean of sample subscore
SD = standard deviation of sample

Likert-Type Scale: (1 - 5). 5 = Worst Response.

I. GRAND TOTAL SCORES Z-score: The number of Standard Deviation Units above or below the mean.

Z-score

COMPARISON GROUPS:

	PAIN	SUFFERING	WORK BELIEFS	SELF-EFFICACY
Arthritis:	$\bar{x}$ = 2.89 ± 0.597 SD	$\bar{x}$ = 3.27 ± 0.655 SD	N/A	N/A
Epilepsy:	$\bar{x}$ = 3.51 ± 0.631 SD	$\bar{x}$ = 2.31 ± 0.837 SD	$\bar{x}$ = 4.02 ± 1.01 SD	$\bar{x}$ = 2.40 ± 0.451 SD

COMMENTS: * if comparing person to the arthritic sample both pain and suffering show that patient is experiencing more pain and suffering compared with the mean of the arthritic group. ● If comparing person to the epilepsy sample, the suffering issues predominate, pain score indicates little distress, work beliefs and self-efficacy results show less distress than the group to which the patient is being compared.

ASSESSOR SIGNATURE: ____________

Figure 10.3

EXAMPLE 2
SHORT FORM
* (SUFFERING COMPONENT ONLY)
NORMATIVE DATA SUMMARY (Z SCORES)
MEASURING AND ASSESSING SUFFERING QUESTIONNAIRE

NAME: ______________________ DATE: ____________

ASSESSOR: ______________________

- Z SCORE:	LESS DISTRESS.
0 Z SCORE:	DISTRESS LEVEL COMPARABLE TO MEAN OF ESTABLISHED GROUP.
+ Z SCORE:	MORE DISTRESS.

CALCULATIONS: $Z = \frac{(\bar{x} - X)}{SD}$

NOTE:
$\bar{x}$ = patients' mean score
X = mean of sample subscore
SD = standard deviation of sample

Likert-Type Scale: (1 - 5). 5 = Worst Response.

I. GRAND TOTAL SCORES

Z-score: The number of Standard Deviation Units above or below the mean.

PART B (total subscale scores)
SUFFERING

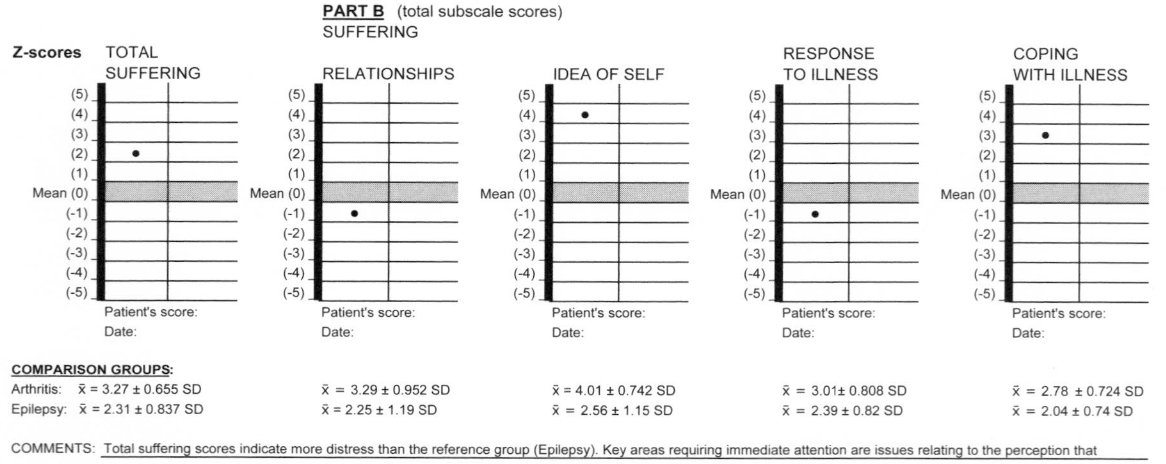

COMPARISON GROUPS:

	TOTAL SUFFERING	RELATIONSHIPS	IDEA OF SELF	RESPONSE TO ILLNESS	COPING WITH ILLNESS
Arthritis:	$\bar{x}$ = 3.27 ± 0.655 SD	$\bar{x}$ = 3.29 ± 0.952 SD	$\bar{x}$ = 4.01 ± 0.742 SD	$\bar{x}$ = 3.01± 0.808 SD	$\bar{x}$ = 2.78 ± 0.724 SD
Epilepsy:	$\bar{x}$ = 2.31 ± 0.837 SD	$\bar{x}$ = 2.25 ± 1.19 SD	$\bar{x}$ = 2.56 ± 1.15 SD	$\bar{x}$ = 2.39 ± 0.82 SD	$\bar{x}$ = 2.04 ± 0.74 SD

COMMENTS: Total suffering scores indicate more distress than the reference group (Epilepsy). Key areas requiring immediate attention are issues relating to the perception that the person's illness/injury is having a negative impact on issues relating to idea of self and coping strategies.

Figure 10.4

illness, and coping with illness. This short form provides more detailed information about the key factors contributing to the patient's suffering. In this example, the clinician can quickly compare the patient's scores with the reference groups (epilepsy and arthritis). While the total suffering of the patient is considerably more than the referent groups (2 standard deviations from the mean), the key issues of concern to the patient are "idea of self" (4 standard deviations from the mean) and "coping with illness" factors (3 standard deviations from the mean).

Referent means are 2.31 ± 0.837 SD (epilepsy) and 3.27 ± 0.655 SD (arthritis).

Example 3 (See figure 10.5) illustrates the usefulness of determining normative data when assessing patients and developing treatment plans. Example 3 is the summary sheet of the Z scores calculated for all four domains (pain, suffering, work beliefs, and self-efficacy) of the MASQ. Z scores are compared with least-suffering patients (epilepsy) and most-suffering patients (arthritis).

In example 3, if the patient is compared with the arthritis sample, the patient's score indicates more severe pain and suffering than the referent group. When compared with the epilepsy sample, suffering issues still predominate. Referent scales for work beliefs and self-efficacy still need to be developed for the arthritis group. Results indicate that concerns expressed by the patient over work issues and self-efficacy are less than the epilepsy referent group.

The following examples, 4 (figure 10.6), 5 (figure 10.7), 6 (figure 10.8), and 7 (figure 10.9), outline the degree of pain, suffering, work beliefs, and self-efficacy. The long form is very useful when applied at initial assessment. The clinician can then determine key areas that may have considerable significance in determining the outcome of treatments. Reassessing the patients at discharge and determining normative scores at that time will objectively indicate the effectiveness of treatments, a factor of considerable importance in cases involving compensation and/or litigation.

Record Keeping

Once again there is the option to report normative data using either a short or long format. The criteria for selecting one method over the other are the same as that explained in the previous chapter. The Y-axis of the graphs indicates the Z score values so that the distance of the patient's score from the mean of the comparison group is clearly delineated. The equation used to calculate the Z score appears at the top centre of the page, with the codes for the calculations needed placed to the right-hand side of the formula. Guidelines for interpretation of the Z score results are shown in the box to the left of the equation. Comparison-group means are found beneath the graphs. There is space for comments and the assessor's signature.

The design of the long form parallels the raw data format, but the information required to calculate the normative data is also provided. Criteria for when

EXAMPLE 3

LONG FORM

NORMATIVE DATA SUMMARY (Z SCORES)

MEASURING AND ASSESSING SUFFERING QUESTIONNAIRE

NAME: ______________________ DATE: __________

ASSESSOR: ______________________

- Z SCORE:	LESS DISTRESS.
0 Z SCORE:	DISTRESS LEVEL COMPARABLE TO MEAN OF ESTABLISHED GROUP.
+ Z SCORE:	MORE DISTRESS.

CALCULATION: $Z = \frac{(\bar{x} - X)}{SD}$

NOTE:
$\bar{x}$ = patients' mean score
X = mean of sample subscore
SD = standard deviation of sample

Likert-Type Scale: (1 - 5). 5 = Worst Response.

I. GRAND TOTAL SCORES

Z-score: The number of Standard Deviation Units above or below the mean.

Z-score

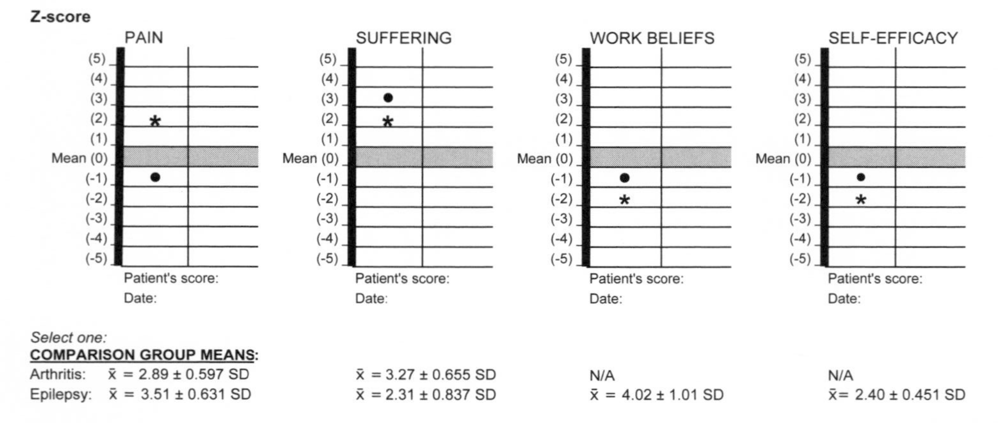

Select one:

COMPARISON GROUP MEANS:

	Pain	Suffering	Work Beliefs	Self-Efficacy
Arthritis:	$\bar{x}$ = 2.89 ± 0.597 SD	$\bar{x}$ = 3.27 ± 0.655 SD	N/A	N/A
Epilepsy:	$\bar{x}$ = 3.51 ± 0.631 SD	$\bar{x}$ = 2.31 ± 0.837 SD	$\bar{x}$ = 4.02 ± 1.01 SD	$\bar{x}$ = 2.40 ± 0.451 SD

INTERPRETATION: * If comparing person to the arthritic sample both pain and suffering show that the patient is experiencing more pain and suffering compared with the mean of the arthritic group.

• If comparing person to the epilepsy sample, the suffering issues predominate, pain score indicates llittle distress, work beliefs and self-efficacy results show less distress than the group to which the patient is being compared.

Figure 10.5

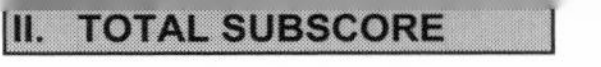

EXAMPLE 4
LONG FORM

PART A
1. PAIN

NAME: ____________________

INTENSITY | **COPING**

Z-score

Z-score	Intensity	Coping
(5)		
(4)		
(3)		
(2)	*	
(1)	●	●
Mean (0)		
(-1)		
(-2)		*
(-3)		
(-4)		
(-5)		

Patient's score:
Date:

Patient's score:
Date:

* Please note: the higher the score the more negative the response.

COMPARISON GROUPS:

	Intensity	Coping
Arthritis:	x̄= 2.99 ± 0.83 SD	x̄= 4.50 ± 0.708 SD
Epilepsy:	x̄= 3.55 ± 0.92 SD	x̄= 3.50 ± 0.829 SD

COMMENTS

* If comparing the patient to the arthritic sample, the person experiences greater pain intensity than the reference group but coping mechanisms are better.
• If comparing the patient to the epileptic sample, the person experiences greater pain and suffering than the reference group because the Z-scores are calculatedfrom the mean and standard deviation of the comparison group.

Figure 10.6

PART B

2. SUFFERING

EXAMPLE 5

LONG FORM

NAME: ____________________

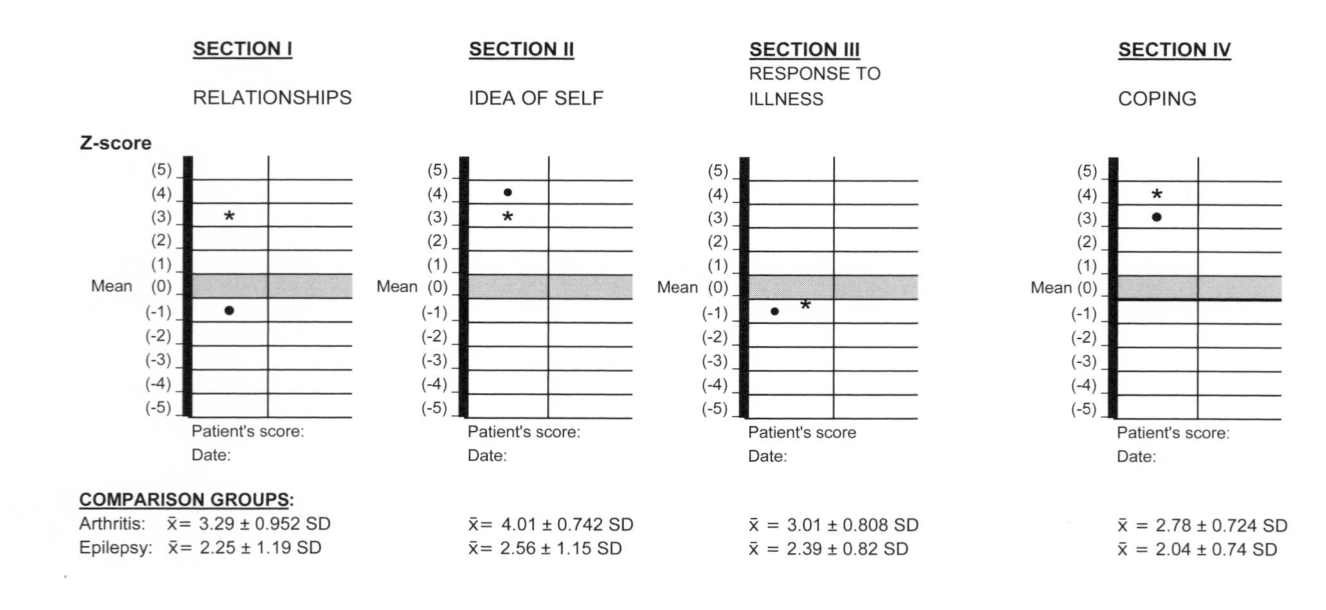

COMPARISON GROUPS:

	Section I	Section II	Section III	Section IV
Arthritis:	$\bar{x}$ = 3.29 ± 0.952 SD	$\bar{x}$ = 4.01 ± 0.742 SD	$\bar{x}$ = 3.01 ± 0.808 SD	$\bar{x}$ = 2.78 ± 0.724 SD
Epilepsy:	$\bar{x}$ = 2.25 ± 1.19 SD	$\bar{x}$ = 2.56 ± 1.15 SD	$\bar{x}$ = 2.39 ± 0.82 SD	$\bar{x}$ = 2.04 ± 0.74 SD

COMMENTS * If comparing person to the arthritic group, the patient has considerably more distress when dealing with relationships and with "Idea of Self" and coping mechanisms. Response to illness results show less distress than the compared group.

• If comparing person to the epileptic group, results indicate less distress in areas of relationships and response to illness bu more distress (than the referent epilepsy group) for idea of self and coping strategies.

Figure 10.7

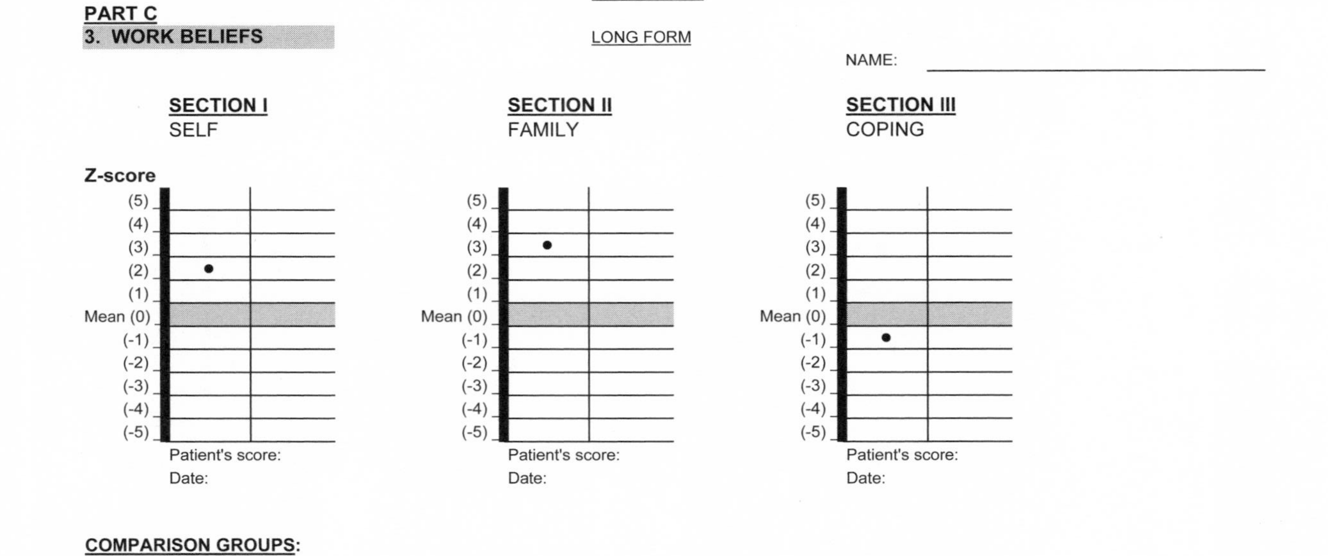

EXAMPLE 6

PART C
3. WORK BELIEFS

LONG FORM

NAME: ______________________

	SECTION I SELF	**SECTION II** FAMILY	**SECTION III** COPING
Z-score			
(5)			
(4)			
(3)		●	
(2)	●		
(1)			
Mean (0)			
(-1)			●
(-2)			
(-3)			
(-4)			
(-5)			
	Patient's score:	Patient's score:	Patient's score:
	Date:	Date:	Date:

COMPARISON GROUPS:

	SELF	FAMILY	COPING
Arthritis:	N/A	N/A	N/A
Epilepsy:	x̄= 2.55 ± 0.789 SD	x̄= 2.44 ± 0.633 SD	x̄= 2.25 ± 0.583 SD

COMMENTS:

- When comparing the individual to persons with epilepsy, results indicate that the person experiences more distress in work beliefs relating to the self and family but is still able to cope with less distress than the referent group.

Figure 10.8

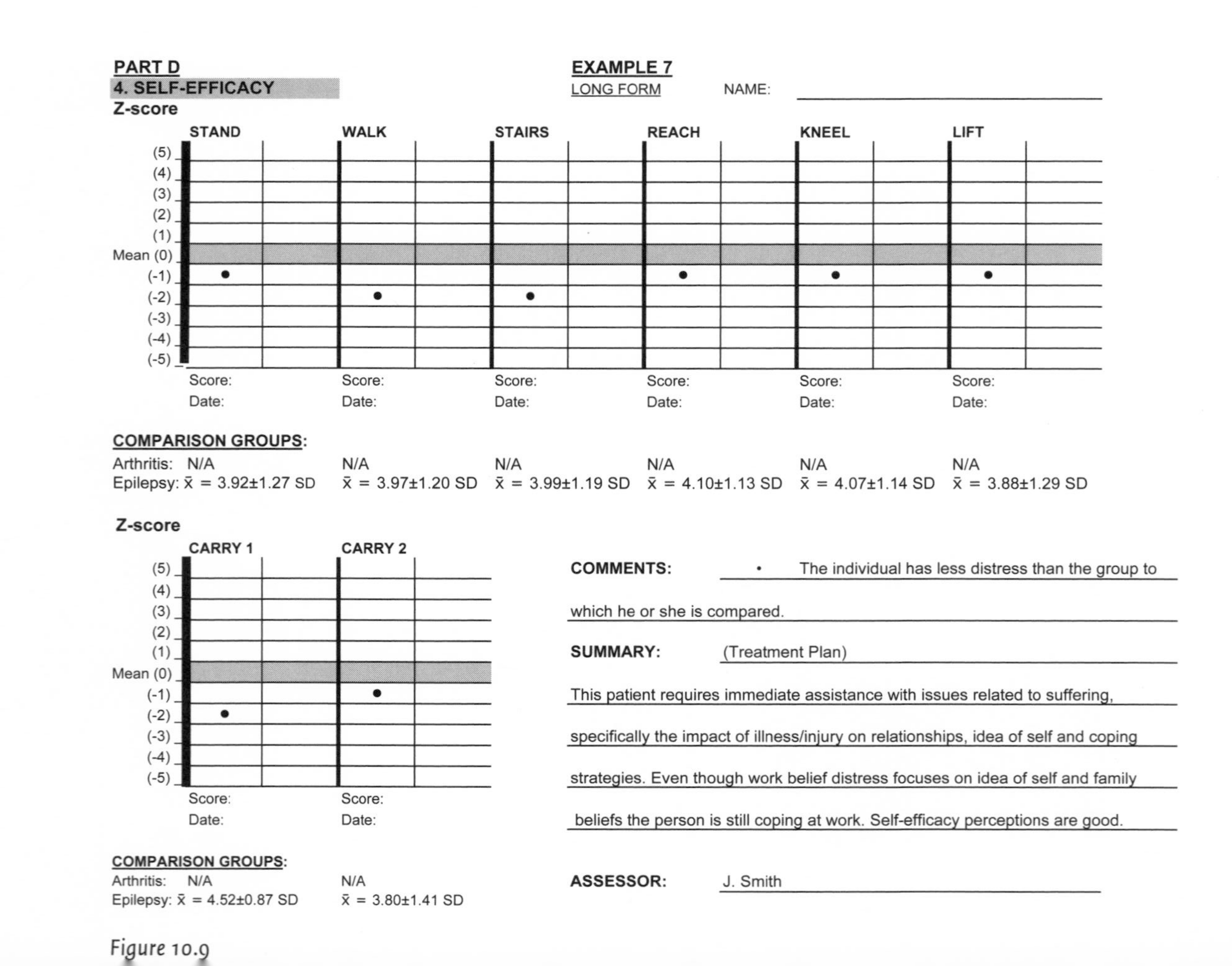

PART D
4. SELF-EFFICACY

EXAMPLE 7
LONG FORM — NAME: ______

Z-score

Z-score	STAND	WALK	STAIRS	REACH	KNEEL	LIFT
(5)						
(4)						
(3)						
(2)						
(1)						
Mean (0)						
(-1)	●			●	●	●
(-2)		●	●			
(-3)						
(-4)						
(-5)						
	Score: Date:	Score: Date:	Score: Date:	Score: Date:	Score: Date:	Score: Date:

COMPARISON GROUPS:

	STAND	WALK	STAIRS	REACH	KNEEL	LIFT
Arthritis:	N/A	N/A	N/A	N/A	N/A	N/A
Epilepsy:	$\bar{x}$ = 3.92±1.27 SD	$\bar{x}$ = 3.97±1.20 SD	$\bar{x}$ = 3.99±1.19 SD	$\bar{x}$ = 4.10±1.13 SD	$\bar{x}$ = 4.07±1.14 SD	$\bar{x}$ = 3.88±1.29 SD

Z-score

Z-score	CARRY 1	CARRY 2
(5)		
(4)		
(3)		
(2)		
(1)		
Mean (0)		
(-1)		●
(-2)	●	
(-3)		
(-4)		
(-5)		
	Score: Date:	Score: Date:

COMPARISON GROUPS:

	CARRY 1	CARRY 2
Arthritis:	N/A	N/A
Epilepsy:	$\bar{x}$ = 4.52±0.87 SD	$\bar{x}$ = 3.80±1.41 SD

COMMENTS: • The individual has less distress than the group to which he or she is compared.

SUMMARY: (Treatment Plan)

This patient requires immediate assistance with issues related to suffering, specifically the impact of illness/injury on relationships, idea of self and coping strategies. Even though work belief distress focuses on idea of self and family beliefs the person is still coping at work. Self-efficacy perceptions are good.

ASSESSOR: J. Smith

Figure 10.9

to use the long form is the same as the raw data collation. The advantage of the normative data format is that it "places" the patient in comparison with others with chronic illness and consequently provides the opportunity to quickly develop more comprehensive treatment plans.

SUMMARY

The need for normative data and methods used to convert raw data scores into normative data was illustrated. Methods of transcribing raw data into a normative data format were given with examples of how to do the required calculations. Normative data can be displayed using either a long or short format. The main difference between plotting the raw data scores and the normative data is that raw data scores are the mean values for each section displayed on a graph and the normative data represents the Z score values. A Z score indicates how far an individual's score is from the mean value obtained from a much larger sample. The research data presented for comparison are from two divergent groups. The first group is persons with epilepsy and is depicted as the "least impaired" end of the spectrum, while the arthritis patients, who are most impaired from the perspectives of pain and suffering, are at the other end of the spectrum. Clearly, more research is needed to more accurately "fix" patients along the continuum, but the comparative data represent results from over 300 patients with chronic illness.

Examples of the clinical interpretation of the Z scores are provided to demonstrate how the normative data may be used in clinical decision making. Use of the MASQ aids in the attainment of a more comprehensive assessment of the individual's health problems in comparison with others who have chronic illnesses. The next step would be to develop suffering-specific treatment strategies. The following chapters report the key components of suffering as determined from a group of over 300 individuals with chronic illnesses.

CHAPTER 10 QUESTIONS

1. Of what value to clinicians are normative scoring methods?
2. Why was data obtained from arthritis patients as a referent sample?
3. What is the purpose of a Z score?
4. How are raw data scores converted to normative data?
5. How are Z scores calculated?
6. How are Z scores interpreted clinically?
7. How could the normative data illustrated in examples 1 (figure 10.3) and 2 (figure 10.4) in this chapter affect your care plan for the patient?
8. Based on example 3 (figure 10.5), the long form, how and when would you use this form to enhance care? Consider issues of idea of self and personhood.

11 Key Components of Suffering in Chronic Illness

The universal characteristics of suffering are a loss of central purpose, unresolved self-conflict, and impaired interpersonal relationships. The differentiation of suffering from pain responses is challenging because patients often talk about pain intensity and suffering at the same time. Research results as discussed in chapter 2 show clearly that suffering and pain are separate entities. Further, many expressions of suffering such as anger, crying, and sadness are common to those who are in pain and those who also suffer. While the process of suffering has universal characteristics, it is the expression of suffering not the process per se that is idiosyncratic and influenced by pre-morbid factors such as personality, anxiety, depression, and environment. It is therefore critical that clinicians are aware of common issues of most concern to those who suffer. The Measuring and Assessing Suffering Questionnaire (MASQ) not only identifies those individuals who suffer but also reveals which issues are of greatest concern to patients. Our results of studies of patients with chronic illnesses such as epilepsy, arthritis, spinal cord injuries, and migraine headache provide insights into key issues that are held in common by most patients with chronic illnesses. Results show that suffering is not disease specific. The ability to identify key factors of concern in suffering will assist all clinicians.

The purpose of this chapter is to: (a) briefly describe the characteristics of four major chronic illnesses—arthritis, epilepsy, migraine headaches, and spinal cord injuries; (b) present a brief description of results obtained from a research study that used the MASQ to assess suffering; (c) compare research results across disease categories that show that key factors of suffering are not disease specific; and (d) review principles of professional communication competencies needed to achieve a comprehensive assessment of suffering. The focus of the discussion is to identify key suffering issues.

Suffering in Patients with Arthritis

Arthritis is a condition in which there is an inflammation of the joints. The joints of persons who have arthritis may be painful, hot, red, and swollen due to inflammation, infection, and/or trauma. There are many classifications of arthritis. Osteoarthritis and inflammatory arthritis (rheumatoid) are the most common. The management of patients with arthritis is complex, involving anti-inflammatory drug polytherapy, surgery, physiotherapy, occupational therapy, psychology, voca-

TABLE 11.1 · Arthritis Subjects by Age and Diagnostic Category

Disease category	N	Mean ± SD
OA	80	62.74 ± 13.13
RA	63	60.75 ± 13.77
Other	23	49.30 ± 19.30
Total	166	60.31 ± 14.23

Note: OA = Osteoarthritis; RA = Rheumatoid arthritis.

tional counselors, and chaplaincy services. In the midst of numerous assessments and interventions, the issue of suffering as an entity separate from pain may be overlooked.

The results from a study of 166 patients with arthritis have been reported elsewhere in considerable detail (1, 2). The beliefs of patients in this study are presented to show the relevance to treatment planning.

The MASQ was given to a group of 166 persons who had arthritis and were attending a hospital-based outpatient clinic. Individuals were tested on admission and just prior to discharge. The total time frame selected was three weeks because it was thought to be an appropriate interval required to meet the criteria for test-retest reliability (3) and because a great change in suffering scores over such a short time frame is not expected. This was not a randomized control study with interventions and control groups. Simply, every patient who attended the clinic was asked to participate. Thirteen people who were initially tested later withdrew from the project. Patients received physiotherapy, occupational therapy, educational information, social work, and psychological counseling as determined by the health care team. The mean age was 60.31 ± 14.23 SD years. There were 127 females in the study. Duration of illness was 10.83 ± 11.16 SD years. There were 80/166 people with osteoarthritis and 18/80 were males. Sixty-three (63/166) people had inflammatory arthritis and 16/63 were males. Twenty-three (23/166) individuals were categorized as "other," 5 of whom were males. There were no statistically significant differences between the age of those with osteoarthritis and those with inflammatory arthritis. Subjects in the "other" category were younger than those patients in the previous categories (see table 11.1).

Other disorders include mechanical low back pain, myofascial pain, avascular necrosis, pseudo gout, and chronic soft tissue pain. No specific interventions to address suffering were applied. Because these patients were involved with the initial development and testing of the MASQ, there were no specific work belief questions asked. The work beliefs section was added after the initial validity and reliability testing of the MASQ was performed. Patients with arthritis were only asked to report the degree of worry or concern they had that their illness would negatively impact on work. Only those persons with epilepsy, migraine headache, and spinal cord injuries were also assessed for specific work belief items.

As has been previously stated in chapter 2, the relationship between suffering and pain is not strong and provides evidence that suffering and pain are only sometimes related entities. Significant ($p = 0.000$) key issues of concern for persons with arthritis tend to focus on the amount of worry or concern individuals have that their illness will damage their relationships with their children, partner, and friends. The desire for a personal life is perceived as being threatened. Practical concerns about having a job and work performance were important concerns for 52% of the patients interviewed on admission. The impact of illness with ageing, feelings of sadness, anger, and beliefs that pain would return were all key issues. Twenty percent (20%) of the patients believed that they would never be the person they once were and 56% stated that they were not able to participate in their communities.

It is important for clinicians to be aware that measures of suffering differ from quality-of-life issues and that different treatment interventions are needed to resolve the respective problems. Quality-of-life scales measure abilities and opportunities, while measures of suffering address perceptions of threat to self and personhood. Suffering is a measure of an individual's beliefs about how the self should behave in times of adversity.

Clearly, addressing suffering issues is a critical component of the effective management of patients who have arthritis. During the course of obtaining this data, patients asked the researchers where they could get help with their concerns. Patients stated that the issues raised in the questionnaire were ones that were causing considerable difficulty but those matters were not being addressed by the patient's current health care providers. Patients reported a reluctance to raise suffering concerns with clinicians for fear of being thought "weak" or socially impotent. More resources are needed to help patients with matters relating to suffering. It was most encouraging to note that while suffering per se was not addressed in the treatment plans, on discharge, fewer people expressed as much distress over the above issue as they did on admission (see table 11.2). However, items relating to perceptions of self were still seen as a major concern for many people. It is also interesting to note that perceptions of pain severity decreased prior to discharge (see table 11.3). Many factors may influence perceptions of improvement, especially the fact that patients were in a safe environment where they believed that they would receive help. While clinical practice results support the need to address suffering as separate from pain, future studies are needed to determine whether treating suffering per se results in even greater improvements in chronic pain.

TABLE 11.2 · Areas of Concern in Patients with Arthritis (%)*

Item	T1**	T2***
Job	52.7	33.8
Children	43.7	26.5
Partner	43.1	25.2
Friends	44.3	21.9
Personal life	79.0	48.9
Ageing	81.4	60.9
Degree of worry	70.7	45.0
Body mechanics	74.9	63.3
Emotional stability	59.9	45.0
Restoration of self	71.3	66.2
Feel normal	64.1	48.3
Anger	34.7	32.5
Sadness	47.3	30.5
No community involvement	56.9	38.4

*Responses reported indicate areas of most concern. **T1 = admission. ***T2 = discharge.

TABLE 11.3 · Individuals with Arthritis Who Rated Pain at the Most Severe Levels

Item	T1* (%)	T2** (%)
Pain intensity	77.7	37.7
Recurrence	50.3	43.7
Endurance	31.7	24.5
Less but persistent	21.6	23.2

*T1 = admission. **T2 = discharge.

Suffering in Patients with Epilepsy

Epilepsy is a term used to describe a seizure disorder (4–7). "Primary seizures" are also known as idiopathic, essential, or cryptogenic seizures and have no known cause. Some people inherit a tendency for primary seizures. In these cases, the first seizure occurrence is usually before twenty years of age. Primary seizures may occur after this age, but they are usually due to causes such as stroke, tumors, or trauma.

"Secondary seizures" are also termed "organic" or "symptomatic" and have a defined etiology. Some possible causes are head injuries, alcohol abuse, tumors, cerebral vascular disease, or congenital abnormalities of the brain. Seizure activity may be focal or generalized involving the sensory-motor system. Seizure activity is unpredictable, but there are often pre-seizure warning signs that patients may experience prior to seizure onset.

Management of seizures may involve anticonvulsant polytherapy medications, neurostimulation (pacemakers), and surgical removal of parts of the brain in which seizures begin. Many people with epilepsy are well controlled with these interventions, but may experience considerable impairment due to medication side effects. Some common side effects are tremor of the limbs, slow motor reaction times, and poor balance and coordination. Other individuals may have intractable seizures, which result in chronic disability. The issue of the amelioration of suffering in epilepsy is of considerable concern.

One hundred thirteen (113) individuals with epilepsy were assessed. There were 58 females. The mean age of the sample was 41.56 ± 11.42 SD years. Illness duration was 22.8 ± 12.96 SD years. Mean seizure frequency was 8.38 ± 30.06 SD seizures/month. Sixty percent (60%) of the patients assessed were seizure free. Forty-nine percent (49%) had complex partial seizures, 46% were classified as tonic-clonic, and 5% were unclassified. Thirty-seven percent (37%) of the subjects had more than 1 seizure per month and 63% had less than one seizure per month. Less than 1% of the patients assessed were uncertain about the number of seizures experienced. One-third of those persons sampled reported pain, rating it as severe (levels 4 and 5). Pain was not related to seizures per se but rather to a variety of accompanying complaints such as arthritis, trauma, and previous surgical procedures.

Of the 56 people who worked, 12 had one or more seizures per month and 43/56 who worked were seizure free. Fifty-seven (57/113) people did not work. Of those individuals, 29/57 had more than one seizure per month. All patients were on anticonvulsant drug polytherapy.

Issues of prime concern to people with epilepsy focus on concern that epilepsy will have a negative impact on job performance, relationships with children, aging, idea of self, being perceived as "normal," and being able to participate in their community (see table 11.4). Other issues of concern focused on pain severity, work beliefs, and self-efficacy (see tables 11.5–11.7).

Both the patients with epilepsy and those with arthritis have many suffering items in common even though the patients with arthritis were older, with most patients acquiring the disease in midlife as opposed to persons with epilepsy, who often have had epilepsy since childhood.

Assessing Suffering in Patients with Migraine Headaches

Migraine headache is thought to occur when a traveling wave of hyperexcitable nerve cells passes across the brain, leaving in its path a trail of hypoactivity. The

TABLE 11.4 · Areas of Concern in Patients with Epilepsy

Item	Response (%)*
Job	31.8
Children	24.3
Partner	18.7
Friends	15.9
Personal life	26.2
Ageing	28.0
Degree of worry	29.9
Body image	21.5
Emotional stability	22.4
Restoration of self	48.6
Don't feel "normal"	34.6
Anger	20.6
Sadness	19.6
Not part of community	25.2
Others not concerned	29.9

*Responses reported indicate greatest concern.

TABLE 11.5 · Individuals with Epilepsy Who Rate Pain at the Most Severe Levels

Item	Response (%)
Pain intensity	26.3
Recurrence	32.5
Endurance	28.8
Less but persistent	30.0

hyperactive cells are thought to act on nerves and blood vessels in both the autonomic nervous system and the central nervous system, producing severe pain often experienced on one side of the head.

There are many classifications of migraine headache, such as those determined by the International Headache Society classification system, which aid physicians in treatment planning. Management of migraine headache ranges from medications to control pain, to transcranial magnetic stimulation of the brain. Because the process of headache development is complex, many motor and sensory signs (double vision, hemi-paresis, etc.) may be experienced by patients. Further, the frequency and intensity of headache may impact on an individual to such an extent that disability is incurred (8–10).

Suffering in migraine is usually thought to be the secondary component of pain

TABLE 11.6 · Key Issues Relating to Work: Epilepsy

Item	Response (%)*
Importance of work	58.3
Enough education	23.3
Work equals respect	27.5
Work does not equal independence	40.8
Family fears work injuries	52.5
Patient fears work injuries	63.3
Patient fears others will be hurt	56.7
Family doesn't favor work	70.0
Poor work performance	44.2
Poor social confidence	26.7
Fear stigma	32.5

*Responses reported indicate greatest concern.

TABLE 11.7 · Confidence in Physical Abilities: Epilepsy

Item	Response (%)*
Prolonged standing	66.7
Walking	67.5
Stair climbing	70.8
Reaching above head	75.0
Bending	71.7
Kneeling	66.7
Carrying a small box	88.3
Carrying a large box	67.5
Lifting box from floor	66.7

*Responses reported are the most positive.

and that if pain is eliminated, suffering stops, but many of our patients state that they can endure pain but the suffering that is experienced because of the impact of migraine on self is the greater problem.

Seventy-nine (79) individuals were assessed. Two people did not meet the inclusion criteria. The mean age of those assessed was 42.77 years ± 12.22 SD. There were 66/77 females. The mean duration of headaches was 20.51 ± 11.98 SD hours. All subjects were employed outside the home. Only 6.3% of the people assessed complained of headache at the time of testing. Seventy-two percent (72%) of the patients had full time employment, 16% part-time. Fifty-nine percent (59%) were trained on the job, and 76% reported that they had a great deal of responsibility at

TABLE 11.8 · Key Suffering Items in Patients with Migraine

Item	Response (%)*
Job	49.9
Children	36.7
Partner	44.3
Friends	27.8
Personal life	51.9
Ageing	51.9
Degree of worry	53.2
Restoration of self	31.6
Sadness	25.3
Managing alone	29.0
No community involvement	21.5
Concern of others	31.6

*Responses reported indicate greatest concern.

TABLE 11.9 · Key Issues Relating to Work: Migraine

Item	Response (%)*
Job performance	54.4
Physical work increases pain	26.6
Poor emotional workplace	26.6
Work equals respect	50.6
Fear of job loss	15.2
Loss of promotion	12.7
Job selection	17.7
Medications	27.8
Believe job is in jeopardy	13.9

*Responses reported indicate greatest concern.

work. Only 1% of persons interviewed received a pension. Individuals reported a mean of 9.52 ± 18.66 days/year of sick time and a mean of 32.2 ± 44.8 days/year in lost leisure time.

Key issues of concern to individuals with migraine headaches focused on the fear that migraine would negatively affect job performance; relationships with children, partners, and friends; personal life; and aging (see tables 11.8–11.10). These patients had high levels of worry, and many felt they would never be the people they once were. The potential negative impact of headache on job performance was of considerable concern. Persons with migraine believe that people who work

TABLE 11.10 · Pain Status and Beliefs: Migraine Patients

Item	Response (%)*
Pain intensity	6.3
Pain recurrence	20.3
Endurance	29.0
Less pain but persistent	24.0

*Responses indicate greatest concern.

are more respected than those who do not. Over 25% of those assessed stated that their physical work and emotional work environment tended to increase headache frequency. Many people felt that they were managing alone, others did not care about them, and how they felt at the time was not normal. Twenty-nine percent (29%) said they could endure more pain, and 24% believed that if their current experience of pain never changed, they would manage satisfactorily. Only 6% of patients rated pain at the highest level of discomfort.

Assessing Suffering in Patients with Spinal Cord Injuries

Spinal cord injuries may be due to trauma, infection, congenital defects, or inflammation. The end result may be partial or complete paralysis of muscle and denervation. Considerable impairments occur, and patients are often totally disabled or severely impaired. Surgical interventions, medications, and rehabilitation treatments are the interventions of choice. Successful rehabilitation outcomes require months and sometimes years before they are considered optimal. The restoration of the self (suffering) is long and complex with varying concerns throughout the rehabilitation process (11).

We report key issues obtained from a group of 23 people who have been labeled as having reached their maximum physical potential. Diagnoses include paraplegia, quadriplegia due to transections of the cord, herniated discs, cervical stenosis, spina bifida, and Brown-Sequard Syndrome. Injuries were sustained due to falling and to motor vehicle, diving, hockey, stabbing, and gunshot accidents. The mean age of people assessed was 46.21 ± 8.54 SD years. There were 16 males and 7 females. Of the total sample, 18 individuals complained of pain at the time of testing. Mean illness duration was 10.95 ± 11.91 SD years. Nine (9) of the patients lived alone, 14 did not. Of those living alone only 4 of the 9 considered themselves to be living independently. None of the individuals tested lived in a group home or a long-term facility. Eight of the patients (8/23) worked full time.

The relationship between total suffering scores and total pain scores was a sig-

TABLE 11.11 · Key Suffering Items in Patients with Spinal Cord Injuries

Item	Response (%)*
Job performance	30.4
Relationship with children	21.7
Relationship with partner	26.1
Relationship with friends	21.7
Personal life	30.4
Ageing	43.5
General worry	34.8
Body mechanics	69.6
Emotional stability	30.4
Restoration of self	60.9
Don't feel normal	21.7
Low participation in community	34.8
Concern of others	30.4

*Responses reported indicate greatest concern.

nificant but weak inverse relationship ($r = -0.219$, $p = 0.02$) Correlation analyses of the total sample was $r = 0.320$, $p = 0.320$. Again values indicate a weak relationship between total suffering and total pain scores in which one could account only for 9% of the variance. Pearson correlation coefficient results between pain intensity and total suffering for the whole sample was $r = 0.575$, $p = 0.004$ which, while stronger, still only accounted for 25% of the variance.

Key suffering issues as well as aspects of pain in spinal cord–injured patients were similar to those in persons with other chronic illnesses. Major differences focused on work beliefs that related to the mechanisms of work such as transportation, and punctuality. Issues relating to ideas of self and personhood were the same as those for individuals who had arthritis, migraine headache, and epilepsy (see tables 11.11–11.13).

Comparison of Experimental Results

Comparison of key suffering items remains consistent across illness categories. The values reported are the number of individuals expressed as a percentage of all respondents who expressed the most worry or concern about the various issues. These individuals scored items at level 4 or 5 (most negative) on the MASQ scale. The patients with arthritis expressed the most overall concern. These findings may be due to the fact that these people were older and had been living with chronic illness for a long time. The belief that the individual would never be the same person

TABLE 11.12 · Key Work Beliefs in Patients with Spinal Cord Injuries

Item	Response (%)*
Enough education	17.4
Work equals acceptance	73.9
Work equals respect	34.8
Number of close friends	26.1
Work equals independence	21.7
Work at home	26.1
Family fears work injuries	73.9
Patient fears injuries	91.3
Fear others will be hurt	91.3
Family doesn't favor work	69.6
Punctuality	30.4
Job performance	39.1
Loss of benefits	30.4
Depends on pension	47.8
Stigma	60.9

*Responses indicate greatest concern.

TABLE 11.13 · Key Pain Items and Beliefs in Patients with Spinal Cord Injuries

Items	Responses (%)*
Pain intensity	39.1
Pain recurrence	26.1
Cope with more pain	52.2
Less pain but persistent	60.9
No pain equals same person	30.4

*Responses indicate greatest concern.

or the person they wished to be was consistent across categories. This item is one of the critical tenets of suffering as a perception of threat to ideas of self. It is also interesting to note that despite repeated interactions with medical personnel, patients repeatedly reported the belief that they were managing alone and that no one cared about them. It is also important to note that a large percentage of people expressed a great deal of sadness rather than anger about their illness (table 11.14).

There are many items of common concern in patients tested for work beliefs. Patients with epilepsy, who often have seizures from early childhood and who are dependent on family for care, and spinal cord–injured people, many of whom

TABLE 11.14 · Comparisons of Areas of Concern across Illness Categories

Item	Responses (%) (scored at level 5, the most negative)			
	Arthritis	Epilepsy	Migraine	Spinal cord
Job performance	52.7	31.8	49.9	30.4
Relationship with children	43.7	24.3	36.7	21.7
Relationship with partner	43.1	18.7	44.3	26.1
Relationship with friends	44.3	15.9	27.8	21.7
Personal life	79.0	26.2	51.9	30.4
Ageing	81.4	28.0	51.9	43.5
Degree of worry	70.7	29.9	53.2	34.8
Body mechanics	74.9	21.5	31.6	69.6
Emotional stability	59.9	22.4	19.0	30.4
Restoration of self	71.3	48.6	31.6	60.9
Don't feel normal	64.1	34.6	29.1	21.7
Anger	34.7	20.6	16.5	4.3
Sadness	47.3	19.6	25.3	13.0
Lack of community involvement	56.9	25.5	21.5	34.8
Others not concerned	22.2	29.9	31.6	30.4
Managing alone	28.1	15.0	29.0	17.4

experienced significant trauma resulting in disability, have work beliefs clearly related to limitations imposed by the pathophysiology of their respective diseases/disorders. Patients who had migraine headache were usually more concerned with job performance and termination issues and factors contributing to stigma in the workplace. Patients tested strongly believed in the value of work and believed that people who worked were more respected than those who did not (table 11.15).

Comparisons of pain levels were consistent across illness categories (see figure 11.1). More research is needed because sample sizes were variable across categories. Clinically, attending physicians were surprised to find that persons with epilepsy reported such high levels of pain and that this pain was not reported to clinicians on clinic visits. Subsequent follow-up interviews with patients in our research study revealed that patients did not speak about their pain because they said that the purpose of the clinic visit was to talk about their seizures. The relationship between pain intensity and pain occurrence in epilepsy is unknown. These interviews add support to the theory that patients know what language health care providers understand and to the hypothesis that many people talk about pain when they really are describing suffering.

TABLE 11.15 · Comparisons of Work Beliefs in Chronic Illness

	Responses (%)*	
Item	Epilepsy	Spinal Cord Injuries
Importance of work	58.3	73.9
Not enough education	23.3	17.4
Work equals respect	24.5	34.8
Work does not equal independence	40.8	21.7
Family fears work injury	52.5	73.9
Patient fears work injury	63.3	91.3
Fear others will be hurt	56.7	91.3
Family doesn't favor work	70.0	69.6
Poor work performance	44.2	39.1
Poor social confidence	26.7	13.0
Stigma	32.5	60.9

*Responses indicate greatest concern.

The MASQ was found to be a useful tool to identify those patients who suffer and to delineate key issues that contribute to an individual's experience of suffering. The challenges of managing suffering in clinical practice involve not only understanding the language of suffering and its relationship to patient autonomy and personal power, but also an awareness of issues of prime importance to patients. While the MASQ provides information to foster dialogue between clinicians and patients, there are many factors that may impinge on effective communication.

Communication and Suffering

The Role of Language

Effective health care delivery depends a great deal on the communication skills of both the patient and the clinician. Language is used to express ideas, feelings, and emotions and is a method in which information is exchanged between professionals, patients, and families. Language is also a way of conveying responses to given information and for providing directions to manage health care problems. Language is a very powerful negotiating tool between individuals. In addition to the spoken word, body language—that is, body and facial postures—may reflect one's reactions to situations and others' words. Body language may vary from culture to culture (11, 12).

The ability to understand another depends on one's ability to recognize that there are many barriers to communication based on different language struc-

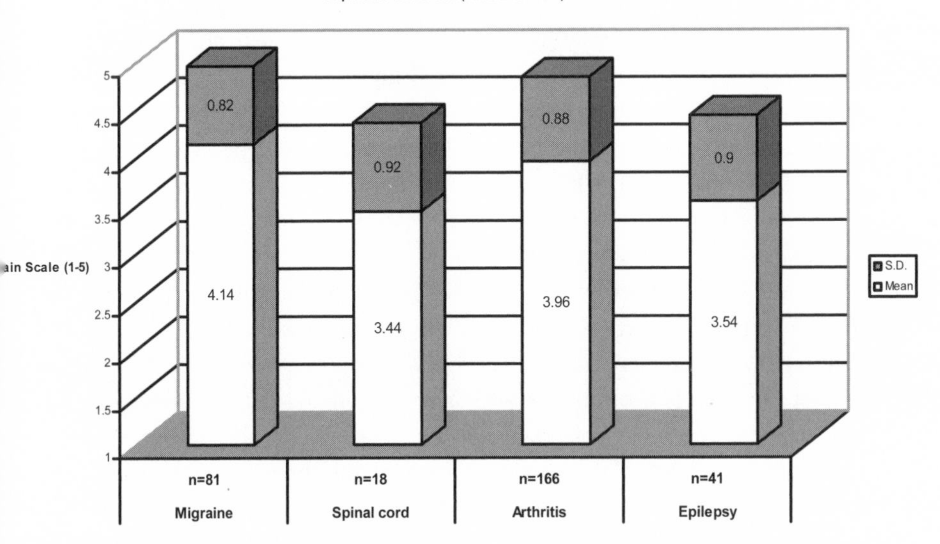

Figure 11.1

tures. What is being said may be misunderstood if the speaker's and listener's everyday language structures differ. For example, if the therapist is of Japanese cultural background, formality of language and communication styles may be very important, while North American methods are less formal, both in words used and style of speech. Cultural attitudes relating to age and gender often influence communication between individuals. Older people may prefer to be addressed by their surname, while the first name may be the choice of younger individuals. The challenge to health care practitioners is to be aware of cultural, age, or gender preferences and to realize that in contemporary society, individuals may incorporate both old-world and contemporary beliefs. The clinician needs to be able to communicate with sensitivity while avoiding stereotyping.

Expressiveness

Emotional expressiveness, volume of voice, tone, and pitch may mean different things, depending not only on personality or pathology but also on cultural habits. Some individuals are naturally more expressive in the manner of delivery of language. For example, North Americans of African or Southeast Asian descent may normally speak louder and more quickly than North American aboriginal peoples, and immigrant individuals new to a country may speak very softly and with hesitation. Interpretations by health care providers of an individual's intellectual abilities or compliance with instructions must be understood within the context of illness concerns, personality, and cultural differences.

Some cultures value expressions of politeness more than others. If patients are perceived as "not getting to the point quickly enough," when describing their health problems, the listener must understand that, in some cases, such hesitant approaches are culturally based. The use of silence may also be a communication barrier if misunderstood. Silence may be interpreted as an indication of hostility or noncompliance, but silence may also indicate a need for personal privacy or in some instances a sign of agreement.

Gestures and facial expressions also convey important information. Expressions of surprise, anger, or displeasure may be expressed through the eyes and mouth. However, some Asian cultures do not look favourably on persons making direct eye contact. The meaning of what is being said must be interpreted not only through the words expressed but also by the body language that accompanies the language. Knowledge of this duality is particularly important when discussing suffering with patients.

Competencies

Effective communications depend on one's abilities to know when to start a conversation. As we saw with the patient Laura, in chapter 6, whose family died in a car crash, many medical staff did not know how to start the conversation with her about possible suffering. Some of us were uncomfortable talking about suffering outside the context of pathology. Perhaps this occurred because we were psychologically wounded by events in our own lives and were afraid to venture into the discomfort of suffering with our patient. It is easier to be the authority figure who analyzes and prescribes than to engage in the process of another person's suffering. This approach is not useful when addressing suffering.

Because suffering is not always understood outside the perspective of pathology, health professionals may fail to acknowledge and respond to patients' gestures and questions. While many of us were aware that Laura was probably suffering, we simply ignored the issue and told ourselves that suffering was outside the scope of our respective clinical practice. Effective communication depends not only on how empathetically clinicians listen to individuals' concerns but also how clearly they understand the power of patients' belief systems on these concerns.

Much has been written about the various cultural and religious beliefs individuals hold about death and dying, and medicine has been able to incorporate a variety of treatment interventions into the prevailing medical models of care. Suffering, on the other hand, is still often thought of as the secondary component of pain in medicine. In contemporary society, any hardship may be labeled as suffering.

These past attitudes are not useful in contemporary medicine. New approaches to care need to be developed.

SUMMARY

This chapter has illustrated the results of applying the MASQ to identify those who suffer in groups of people with a variety of chronic illnesses. Patient responses to questionnaire items clearly showed perceptions of threat to ideas of self and personhood to be of great concern to all individuals.

All groups scored high on items relating to concern that their illness would have a negative effect on restoration of the self; relationships with family and friends; job and community performance; and personal life. The belief that they were managing alone and that others were not concerned were also key factors. These findings provide evidence to support the arguments that suffering involves perceptions of threat to self and personhood.

The need for effective communication and the potential impact of culture on understanding patient stories was also reviewed. Much more work is needed before suffering can be optimally managed in clinical practice. Some basic strategies to assist those who suffer are offered in the following chapter.

CHAPTER 11 QUESTIONS

1. What is the MASQ?
2. What are the key components of suffering in patients with arthritis?
3. What factors are of concern relating to work in patients with epilepsy?
4. What are the current theories about the pathology/physiology of causation of migraine headache?
5. What are the key issues relating to work in patients who have migraine headache?
6. What are the key personhood concerns of patients who have sustained a spinal cord injury?
7. What constitutes expressiveness in patient/clinician communications?
8. What are the key concepts relating to professional communication competencies needed to address suffering in clinical practice?

III Caring for Those Who Suffer

WHEN THE WORLD IS TOO MUCH WITH US

Me, myself and you
I see you, love you, and hate you, like you
Care, cheer, fear for you.
But I don't know you
Know you, know you
Little soul of me.

Fragrant flower, hiding, hiding
Lone, lonely shadows
Dancing, dance, dancing.
Scarlet flashes on barren plains
Salty teardrops
Dripping.

Little spirit
Brave and true?
Crushed beneath some careless heel.
Whispers, whispers,
Sacred shadow swinging wildly
Silver silence haunts the night.

Earthly footsteps
Creeping, closer
Night thieves stealing.
Lost forever!
Calling, calling.

Softly, softly, never fear.
Secret whispers
Play, play, playing
Screeching, raging, ripping, roaring
Swirling mists and numbing fog.
Calling, calling, calling.

Squinting darkness, you, small self
Fumbling, stumbling, heart to heart.
Drumming, strumming
Strains of music
Faintly,
Humming.

Monstrous mania writhes in horror.
Flings my being,
Crushing, smashing.
Searing, screaming
A thousand stars to smear the sky
Blinking.

Confused and helpless
Comes the dawn.
I remember.
I remember you.
You
Brave little soul.

Laughing, fighting, loving
I remember you
Dancing, swirling, lightly glancing
I remember you
Remember you
May I?

Some may interpret the above expressions of suffering using the semantics of psychic or psychological pain. But the poem is perhaps better interpreted as expressing the characteristics of suffering in which there is a perception of threat to the individual's idea of self, a loss of central purpose expressed by the unanswered "calling, calling," and finally the individual's remembering the old self and the invitation to healing, as expressed by the words "may I?" Exploration of suffering, defined as the potential impact of perceptions of threat to an individual's idea of self and personhood, has revealed that suffering and pain are separate constructs that are only sometimes directly related. Religious, spiritual, and cultural traditions influence suffering across the life span as does the effect of legal and medical discourse. These factors have the potential to either negatively or positively affect individuals' sense of personal power and autonomy. Effective clinicians who hear and understand the language of suffering need to have high communication skills and a basic understanding of the factors that may impact on individuals who suffer. Research evidence shows that it is possible to identify those individuals who experience suffering as well as key factors common to all patients with chronic illnesses (1–6). Interviews with patients reveal that patients often speak of suffering using the language of pain because they are aware that health care practitioners may be unfamiliar with the language of suffering (4, 5).

In medical practice, comprehensive problem identification involves analyses of patient stories about their illness and/or injury. For this task more extensive methods of problem identification are required than the usual empirical style in which the clinician listens for specific signs indicative of disease. While the thrust of this text is to advocate for the implementation of suffering-specific awareness and interventions across all health care practice dimensions, specific psychological interventions, in cases of unresolved suffering, are the province of mental health care providers and are beyond the scope of this book.

The purpose of this chapter is to: (a) explore a variety of methods to identify the nature of suffering through analyses of common types of stories patients tell that indicate suffering, (b) to explore the dynamic of storytelling and its relationship to self, and (c) to provide some guidelines to assist clinicians in managing the issues of suffering as it relates to restoration of self and personhood in everyday clinical practice.

Detecting Suffering, Separate from Pain: Hearing the Story

A key theme in the language of suffering is the expression of a lost self. Patients may describe themselves as being lost in a world in which they no longer believe they have a place or in which they are unable to create a world that is acceptable to them. They may perceive themselves as being irrevocably changed and "invisible" in the world they once knew. They may express a loss of innocence and the need to hide away from the world. One patient spoke of feelings of shame and guilt; "If only I had paid more attention, then this terrible event wouldn't have happened to me." He also expressed feelings of isolation and anger; "People come to me and tell me their horror stories; don't they realize that I can't help them, that I don't have the energy to help them? I can't help them, I need help." Another young man spoke of being trapped in a sorrow so profound that he believed that there was no way of recovering. Sometimes people who suffer speak of the feeling that they are not understood. Clinicians who understand will not try to convince the patient to the contrary, but will simply affirm the belief. It is possible to know about someone's experience, but it is not possible to know another's felt experience.

Individuals may express feelings of not belonging anywhere, of searching for a place of comfort or safety. They may also express feelings of victimization and an overwhelming fear that there is more adversity in the future. The language of suffering also involves individuals asking "why" they were selected for such trauma. This question is often rhetorical and not an indication that there is a lack of understanding of current events. Often there is a strong need to keep telling the story of catastrophe, illness, or injury over and over again.

In situations in which the threat is less powerful, patients may only refer to these themes in an oblique way. It is important for clinicians to recognize that storytelling from which a diagnosis is obtained is different from the storytelling that describes the depth of an individual's suffering (7–13).

The Dynamics of Storytelling

Storytelling is a way an individual can navigate through life (7). With serious illness, there is a loss of old stories and the ways people formerly managed their lives. Patients are forced to tell a new story, that is, develop a new map about how they can live life. These stories are not simply about the sick body but rather about the impact the sick body has on the person's idea of self and personhood. People constantly tell stories about themselves to others as well as to themselves. Stories help repair the damage an illness or event has done to people's idea of self and to their perception of where they are placed in life and where they feel they may be going. Stories reveal patients' general disposition, as well as the things they value and perhaps hold sacred, how they view life and the place of humankind in the cosmos. Does the patient believe that there is a special place for him/her in the universe? Can a new place be imagined now that health and lifestyle are changed? What is the individual's worldview? Clinicians may also obtain important clues about patients' self-identity, idea of self, and beliefs about the role of adversity in human experience from their stories. As with the other types of stories being told, the health clinician's role is to hear what patients want and to help them achieve those goals. Health care providers need to be aware of the types of stories that are told and to affirm patients' interpretations of their accounts. Common story genres include restitution, chaos, and quest stories.

Restitution Stories

In restitution stories, things get better. There are expressions of the belief that there will be a happy ending because the illness or event is transitory. These stories are usually about the triumph of medicine and are not really about the triumph of the self over adversity. Restoration stories are a way of convincing the self that all is not lost. Clinicians usually like to hear restitution stories because they confirm professional beliefs. Patients try to oblige the health care provider by telling stories that indicate that they are following the "rules." Such patients are often compliant and undemanding of health care resources. Consequently, personal and potentially painful introspection on the part of the clinician about the effects of illness, injury, or death is avoided. Both patients and health care providers tell restitution stories. Clinicians may tell restitution stories when they want to motivate patients.

Chaos Stories

In contrast to restitution stories, chaos stories are about situations that never get better. These stories are told as the experiences occur, and they are usually told without any expression of causality or any sequencing of the narrative events. These stories produce considerable anxiety because they express the patient's vulnerability, futility, and impotence. Chaos stories are about being trapped by the disasters occurring in the person's life. While these stories are acutely about the self, the self is not heard by others. Such stories are often very difficult for health care professionals to hear because they may feel a need to solve the problem rather than simply listen to what the patient is saying. They may have the need to tell the patient how to objectively solve the problem and avoid ever becoming personally engaged in the story. Without personal engagement in the individual's story, the solutions provided by caregivers will be ineffective. Chaos stories are told because the patient is trying to find the power of the self by repeating the story in the hope that a new resolution to the problem will somehow be revealed.

Health professionals may inadvertently contribute to the chaos story when they bombard patients with "facts" relating to the probability of restoration and/or adverse treatment side effects. Chaos stories told by clinicians have the potential to do considerable harm, as patients put their trust in professional abilities. It is a challenge to present a realistic picture of health problems without destroying hope.

Quest Stories

Patients who tell quest stories use the narrative in an attempt to manage the chaos in their lives created by illness or traumatic events. The patient has a voice and tells the story from a personal perspective. In such situations the illness/injury is embraced and used to develop a new life map of survival. Quest stories help the patient manage fears of being powerless and not having any personal autonomy. These stories allow the patient to move forward through feelings of living in a lost life to being alive in the present. Quest stories are sometimes thwarted by health care providers who insist the patient "accept" the illness and/or disability and then proceed with social customs such as making wills, and preparing for future catastrophes based on health care provider opinion. The major problem with this approach is that "acceptance" implies that the person had a choice of whether to be ill/disabled or not. Nonacceptance implies that they have made the wrong choice. Insistence on acceptance thwarts the quest for a future, even if that future is possible only for a few hours. Sometimes, all people want is to have someone confirm their reality and offer comfort and understanding.

Hearing Stories in Clinical Settings

Individuals tell stories for two main reasons. The first is simple survival and the second is to be a witness to that which is generally unrecognized. In the first instance, where survival is the goal, there are no moral responsibilities other than survival. In the second situation people who tell stories of illness or injuries become witnesses who turn those events into a moral responsibility. The telling of any story forces the listener into an obligation to hear the essence of the message.

The challenge for health care providers is to listen and hear the thrust of a patient's story without passing judgment (14). This requirement is often difficult for those health care providers who have been trained to listen for specific information that fits into a preset dialogue that reveals clues necessary for the formulation of a differential diagnosis. Much has been written documenting that often clinicians do not listen to the whole story being told because they are only listening for specific signs that reveal illness characteristics. It is only when such clues are heard that the clinician asks patients specific questions. When considering the phenomenon of suffering all health care professionals must be aware of the specific "clues" available from the main story types, as these stories are indicators of the status of the patient's inner world. By carefully listening to the stories of those who suffer, the clinician can determine if the main concerns are about a loss of central purpose, impaired relationships, and self-conflict.

The restoration narrative reveals the patient's will to live, to cure and to be cured. Chaos stories are presented as a testimony that is only true at the moment the story is being told. Quest stories search either for ways of being well or of other ways of being ill. What relationship the events in the story have to each other may provide very important information to clinicians, information that can be used to help the patient.

Stories are coloured by the individual's culture, religious/spiritual beliefs, and the society in which the person lives. Expressions of suffering vary and are related, in part, to an individual's personality. The challenge of health care clinicians is to hear the stories with both empathy and intelligence and to assist with the individual's restoration and/or maintenance of the self as determined by the patient. Clinicians need to understand the difference between empathy and sympathy. Sympathy is having feelings of pity and sorrow for someone else's misfortune. Empathy is the ability to understand and share the feelings of others.

Empathetic listening also involves the ability to recognize that it is the patient's story and that the central theme of the story reveals the patient's perception of threat to idea of self and personhood. This approach is in stark contrast to the current empirical method in which the patient's story is heard within the context of obtaining the scientific evidence for cause and effect of disease/injury (15). Empathy requires that the listener be able to share, on a human level, their own stories which may confirm or reflect an intuitive awareness and experience of thoughts and feelings that are the same or similar to those expressed by the patient. Empathetic listening helps patients feel less isolated, allows the testing of ideas and strategies, and provides much needed comfort to those managing traumatic life events. Empathetic listening respects the nature of the story and validates the person's idea of self. Sympathy, on the other hand, may be perceived by the patient as pity. Pity may diminish the individual's sense of self and may make the patient feel isolated from his/her community. It may, at times, be a difficult task for clinicians who are strongly rooted in evidence-based practice, or those who are very rigid about the rightness and wrongness of how life should be lived, to introduce an element of ceremony into their practice. Yet cost-effective, ethical care requires such an approach.

Patients and health care professionals form relationships based on knowledge and experience. While the clinician uses clinical skills and personal experience to aid those who suffer, patients also strive to preserve and restore the self. The dynamic of self preservation is often not taught in the medical education of health care professionals (16, 17).

Self Preservation

All individuals have a sense of separateness from others (16). That is, we each have a sense of a unique self. People believe the integrity of their own experiences and have a sense of a private world. We each are able to determine which events in life concern us and which do not. Having a perception of personal continuity over time, we are the same person now that we were one hour ago. While circumstances change, we do not. How individuals perceive their personal history is central to personal ideas of self.

While people usually are not a victim of their life history, they may become a victim of their life events, depending on how they interpret their stories. Usually, individuals believe they have choices and a purpose in life and that they are responsible for their actions. Consequently, people believe they are identified by their choices. They see themselves in relation to others, believe the experience of others is comparable to their own, and assume that others have a sense of personal self. People become aware of themselves through reflection on experiences. In most situations, they know what has happened to them, what they have to deal with as a result of these events, and how their thoughts and feelings are likely to impact on future events. Sometimes they need help in achieving goals that they have defined for their life.

Strategies to Preserve the Idea of Self

People have a view of human nature from which they are able to explain themselves and their behaviour. They judge themselves in relation to others, and they react to people in a way that is congruent with their view of them. An individual has many social roles and consequently many "selves." However, central to this variety of roles, are behaviours that are perceived as acceptable to the individual.

For example, a man may believe that he must keep his feelings to himself when in distress and as a reward for this behaviour considers himself to be a good, courageous individual, regardless of the cost in terms of poor health or economic status. If this belief system fails, the individual may find himself in crisis.

While our early family experiences teach us how to negotiate with others, we may realize that there may also be times when these early teachings are not useful. It is important to be able to set aside these early views so that new ways of functioning can be developed. For example, it is important also to recognize that our understanding of our past is actually based on an erratic memory of past events, and it is often possible to "rewrite" or "see" our history from another perspective, which then may make it more compatible with our present circumstances.

Strategies to preserve the idea of self also require support from our external world. Patients who suffer often find that while they have many people who care about them and are willing to help, few, if any, know what to do. The impersonal/personal relationship of the health professional provides an opportunity for fears and feelings to be validated without the patient having to be concerned that his/her story has made listeners feel bad. Comfort, reassurance, and empathic listening to stories of grief, loss, anger, and rage without judgment may be useful.

Sometimes help is needed to preserve or restore idea of self. While individuals have a tremendous human capacity for creativity, which can be used to restore the idea of self, there are many obstacles to self-knowledge.

Obstacles to Self-Knowledge

Perceptions of Individuals

Self-knowledge is a necessity of life and in order to plan their lives and make choices, people have to be able to anticipate their behaviour in the future. People like to know what to expect in changed circumstances. When individuals become aware of the dangers of change, they may take refuge in rigid and inflexible notions of themselves as persons. Sometimes, a belief cannot be abandoned because the belief is central to the way individuals view themselves and others. One cannot abandon a belief if one sees no alternatives. Health care providers can help patients with alternative ways of interpreting beliefs of self.

Attitudes in Medicine

There is a prevailing attitude among some health care providers that is sometimes shared by postmodern society at large that science answers all of mankind's problems. Consequently, if there is no scientific evidence for a phenomenon, then it must not exist. Medical practice often adopts the stance that it is the responsibility of medicine to control and validate the patient's felt experience.

Third-party interpreters of the patient's stories such as nurses, medical residents, social workers, and therapists, without confirmation from the patient, determine relevance of events and intensity of experience. The patient's felt experience may be dismissed as "catastrophizing," and patients are advised to "reframe" their experience, often to suit prescribed medical criteria. In other instances, issues such as suffering are disregarded because they don't fit with the health care professional's model of practice. Because suffering is often seen as the secondary component of pain, questionnaires may be erroneously deemed to be measures of anxiety or depression or considered replicas of existing anxiety and depression scales. Suffering then becomes anxiety and/or depression, symptoms to be remediated with pharmacological agents. Suffering may not be considered to be a normal life experience, but rather, simply a pain behaviour. The impact of such attitudes is that patients with unresolved suffering may be advised to "smarten up," or "get on with it," or be told "you can't cry over spilt milk, so forget it and move on." While such messages may be delivered more subtly than this, the message to patients is that they must either follow such advice or keep quiet. The end result is an escalation of suffering. Often, such behaviours on the part of health care providers stem from unresolved personal issues of suffering, death, and bereavement in the clinician's life.

Another prevailing attitude is to tell patients that their efforts to cope with their illness are "heroic." The label suggests superhuman courage and strength. Such a label, when applied to an individual with a devastating physical and/or mental disability, offers no comfort, especially if the heroic act involves tasks that the nondisabled perform with ease. This approach escalates the suffering of patients because it isolates the person from the society to which he once belonged. The patient now becomes part of a group regarded by the greater community as damaged or unfortunate and whose very existence depends on being heroic. This approach distances the clinician from the patient and places the patient in a subordinate role. Such management methods of patients who suffer calls into question the ethic of medicine that purports to do no harm.

While health professionals have varying degrees of expertise in human behaviour, the methods presented above, while not useful, are not based on malicious intent but rather on a desire to be kind and compassionate. Knowledge of the patient as a unique individual coupled with an understanding of the process of suffering will more effectively enhance clinical care of sufferers.

Specialized skills may be required when stories reveal deep-seated emotional disturbances. In such cases, a team approach where mental health care providers lead the team is critical. Suffering per se must be addressed by all persons caring for the patient, within the limitations of professional expertise. To be helpful to sufferers, it is important to have at least a basic understanding of the process of restructuring the self (10).

Steps to Restructuring the Self

Step 1: To change the self, individuals must first of all have some understanding of who they perceive themselves to be. When faced with adversity, illness, or injury, patients are encouraged to think about meditating on "self." What am I like? How do others see me? What is my history? Do I believe what I have been taught about myself from early childhood experiences? What roles do I play? Do these roles conflict with my natural inclinations? What conflicts in these beliefs do I encounter? What changes need to occur? Are my evaluations of my present situation accurate? Probable? Health care professionals can help patients find answers to these questions.

Step 2: To change past beliefs, an individual must have a goal. It is helpful for the person to be able to imagine what he/she will be like after going through a change. It is useful to try to act the role of this new self even though, initially, the individual really does not believe he/she is that person. Eventually, however, the patient can become the new person. To effectively rebuild the self, one belief at a time is removed and then quickly replace with another belief. Clinicians may find that patients report feelings of guilt when they begin to experience the dislodgement of the self from an old belief set. These feelings of guilt usually arise from feelings of violating the old pictures of self rather than a violation of the patient's moral or social code.

Step 3: Often patients experience obstacles to this change of self that must be overcome. Other people may have an idea of us that they do not want to see changed. To change ourselves may be a very threatening experience because we may, in fact, become something unpredictable to ourselves. It is helpful to remind patients that we are all involved in a life process where facets of ourselves are revealed to us. We often reinterpret the meaning of our life in a way that reveals our long-standing but hidden dimensions.

Step 4: Once issues of self are addressed, this new self must be able to visualize itself in its current situation. How will individuals manage the world of work, of personal relationships, now and in the future? Clinicians must be able to listen to patients' stories as they evolve from perhaps tales of restitution, to chaos, to quest, or from quest to chaos. Assistance may be needed in the development of new stories of personhood that help the patient achieve his/her new life goals. The journey through change is determined by the patient and not the clinician. If the journey becomes impossible, an "I told you so" attitude is not useful or warranted. No one knows what is possible for someone else. Health care professionals only know the probability of a set of events occurring. It is not necessary to repeatedly inundate the patient with this type of information unless specifically requested to do so. This task is particularly difficult for health care providers who have been trained to be paternalistic and authoritative in their approach to patient care.

Step 5: Clinical reports from patients on the resolution of suffering indicate that patients are successful if they believe they have a good support system, are autonomous in decision making, and are able to be creative in determining their new world (8, 9). Creativity, in the sense of its relationship to suffering may occur when patients discover a special way of being independent, of caring for family in spite of limitations due to disability, or by aiding heath care practitioners in ways of workplace and home modifications. There are several studies that report the benefits of patients' expressions of loss and grief in which keeping a journal and/or other artistic endeavors are helpful (10–12). Health care practitioners need to encourage and assist patients in determining and expressing their human creativity. Multidisciplinary teams in medicine may provide the consistency of support that is required as well as act as an educational resource for the family and community at large.

The range of expressions of suffering is vast and highly idiosyncratic. The characteristics of suffering that involve a loss of central purpose, impaired interpersonal relationships, and self-conflict are constant. The list of questions, outlined below, may be posed to patients to give clinicians a quick indication of which patients might benefit from answering the MASQ test, and to identify those who need immediate mental health care interventions. The questions listed below are offered as starting points for dialogue between patients and health professionals. The characteristics of suffering appear in parentheses.

Quick Clinical Checklist

1. What does this illness and/or injury mean to the patient? Sometimes back pain is simply back pain. At other times, for example, it may mean that a father cannot be the parent he believes he should be, and consequently, the person is in a great deal of distress (loss of central purpose).

2. What does this injury mean to the patient's family, employer, and friends? The patient's family may be concerned about potential financial loss, and the patient's employers are concerned about the impact on profit margins due to the absence of a key employee who may end up requiring a long-term disability pension (impaired interpersonal relationships).

3. What are the patient's expectations of recovery? The patient may believe that full recovery is not possible at the time, while the therapist believes that with

special modifications of home, car, or the workplace, the patient may continue with life events that are currently enjoyed (self-conflict).

4. What does the patient think is probable? On the other hand, the clinician may know that the likelihood of full recovery from an accident or illness is not likely. However, medical practice is filled with many unexpected results, and while a reasoned response to patient's inquiries must be fulfilled, it is not necessary to advocate the abandonment of hope (self-conflict).

5. Is patient autonomy maintained? A practice in many rehabilitation clinics is the development of contracts where the patient and clinician determine priority of goals and how outcomes of success will be determined. For example, is it reasonable and satisfactory to the patient if he/she is able to walk within the home but use a wheel chair outside? Telling people that they have accepted their situation only serves to demean the patient and enforce the power of the clinician (impaired interpersonal relationships).

6. Are patients receiving comfort within the boundaries of ethical practice? Due to the prevalence of litigation and the potential for accusations of abuse, health care providers are extremely cautious about offering any behaviours (physical or emotional) that may be misconstrued. However, simple behaviours such as remembering the names of the patient's family or remembering a patient's vocational interest are simple ways of helping people feel they are still part of a world of which they may feel they are no longer a member. Further, one of the most powerful methods of offering patients comfort is to reassure them that you will work with them until their goals are achieved and that you will not give up on them even if the journey is very rough. The only factor that will deter you is if their goals conflict with your professional code of ethics (loss of central purpose).

7. Is the patient receiving the assistance required to make necessary changes to ideas of self and personhood? What are the barriers to change? Are they primarily internal, or due to external forces and events? What is the patient's disposition? How is life viewed? Is life a place of adversity and hardship that must be overcome or worked through? Does the patient believe that every person is unique and has a value? Does the patient think that he/she will be able to manage now that physical and/or emotional impairments may have altered the person he/she once was? How are these views perceived to be threatened? (loss of central purpose).

8. Are there clear indicators to determine when to refer to another health care professional? Health care providers must be very clear about the skills and competencies they possess and those they do not. The excuse of not enough time to care for the patient or "it's not my job" are unacceptable because suffering must be addressed to varying degrees by all health care providers who are involved in the care of the patient (impaired interpersonal relationships, self-conflict).

9. How will I avoid feelings of abandonment in my patients if I refer them to

others for psychological help? Often patients are comfortable with a referral to another colleague within a discipline or externally if they are assured that their current health care provider will be available for advice. An approach where clinician and patient "learn together" from a referral source may be very successful (loss of central purpose).

While the above questions quickly alert health care providers to suffering, they do not identify the precise areas of concern. Application of the MASQ will not only help patients identify key areas of concern but will also help health care professionals determine the scope and intensity of patient concerns. Patients and clinicians may then be better able to work together, prioritize the issues, and try to resolve suffering.

SUMMARY

This chapter has briefly outlined challenges involved when incorporating suffering as an entity separate from pain into clinical practice. The significance of storytelling and the clinical information revealed from restitution, chaos, and quest narratives were reviewed. Self-preservation techniques and effective strategies to maintain ideas of self were outlined as were common obstacles to self-knowledge. Clinical guidelines indicate the steps that clinicians may follow to help those who suffer restructure the self.

There are many psychological schools of thought concerning the dynamics of self. For example, personal construct theories, trait theory, and stimulus-response theories are approaches with which some clinicians may wish to become familiar to improve their existing skill set. Elements of these theories have been mentioned in the previous sections. It is not an expectation that every health care clinician will be able to manage all the complexities of suffering that people may experience throughout the lifespan, but all clinicians have the responsibility to identify those who suffer when assessing patients referred for care and to provide appropriate interventions. Incorporation of suffering into clinical practice has the potential to: (a) affect the impact of the illness/injury on the individual's idea of self, (b) time limit the experience of suffering, (c) contain the problems presented, (d) result in more efficacious treatments, and (e) decrease fiscal expenditures and enhance human potential. While all clinicians have the obligation to hear and assist in the resolution of the stories of suffering, not all clinicians have the same skill set. The following chapters will discuss expectations of specific health professionals by both patients and health care organizations, and will very briefly describe the specific roles of each profession with regard to suffering. The expectations of patients, health professionals, and health care organizations need to be in concert if individuals who suffer and have chronic illness are to be helped.

CHAPTER 12 QUESTIONS

1. What are some common themes that emerge when stories of suffering are told?
2. What are the three major types of stories told by those who experience suffering?
3. What is the difference between sympathy and empathy?
4. What is the therapeutic value to those who suffer of empathetic listening by health care providers?
5. What constitutes the concept of self-preservation?
6. How may those who suffer survive emotionally?
7. What obstacles prevent those who suffer from attaining self-knowledge?
8. How may current attitudes in medicine hinder a patient's ability to maintain or restore "idea of self"?
9. What are the steps an individual can take to restore his/her idea of self?
10. What are the key questions a health care provider must ask patients prior to a full assessment of the individual's experience of suffering?

13 The Roles of Health Care Professionals

The challenges of managing the experience of suffering in modern medicine occur throughout treatment from the acute stage of illness or injury to either complete restoration of health or, in some cases, permanent chronic disability. Initially, the doctor is the first health care professional to encounter the suffering of the patient. Issues of concern that focus on the impact of the disorder on the person's physical body soon expand to include fears of a threat to the individual's idea of self.

Patients look to health care providers to help them survive the trauma of these events. If patients understand the role and scope of practice of their professional caregivers, treatment expectations are realistic and efficacious. More importantly, individuals have a greater sense of control when they know who in the health care system may have the expertise to address specific problems.

The purpose of this chapter is (a) to illustrate the nature and challenges of modern health care environments on health care professionals and the impact of these factors on suffering from the perspectives of professional responsibility and autonomy and (b) to examine the specific roles and potential suffering-specific treatment strategies of physicians, nurses, and chaplains. The profession-specific challenges and the barriers to effective care are the focus of this chapter.

Most people believe they know the role of the doctor, but few are aware of the environmental constraints under which doctors practice. Adequate understanding of the relationships between personal responsibility, autonomy, and accountability in the delivery of care is a critical factor in the management of suffering. The role of the physician in the management of the experience of suffering as an entity separate and only sometimes related to pain is complex and sometimes quite limited.

The Physician

Professional Responsibility and Autonomy

In contemporary practice, doctors have the ultimate moral, ethical, and often legal responsibility for the patient. Consequently, professional autonomy is of paramount significance to all physicians in a society where policy objectives to contain health care delivery costs may conflict with the ethics of providing adequate health care to patients (1). Other health care providers work in concert with physicians and are also bound by legislative rules and regulations as well as professional standards of autonomy and accountability.

Professional autonomy is the foundation of accountability because accountability demands the ability to understand and evaluate what is at stake when choices are made and the effect such choices may have on the society at large (2). Professional autonomy, on the part of doctors, demands that doctors protect patients from the power of the technological imperative and shield them against third-party pressures to not only provide less than optimal care but actually undertreat. The mandate of all health care professional organizations protects the public from malpractice. Past struggles to avoid losing the balance between the art and science of medicine are, for the most part, lost, and many contemporary clinicians are enmeshed in the dichotomy between technology and materialism. It is against this background that doctors must work to help those who suffer, for whom they still have the ultimate legal authority and responsibility.

Ethical Considerations

The objective of postmodern medical bioethics is based on a desire to rescue human values from the throes of technology in a society in which there is no longer an overriding moral imperative but rather a prevailing materialism. As a result, science and statistics may be seen as the adversary of compassionate care. In science, the body is an object of study and use. Daily news reports are filled with details of medical studies that involve, for example, organ transplants and in vitro fertilization. These procedures are not without risk, and when not successful, the state assumes fiscal responsibility. Autonomy in medicine has become a politic of free choice without a real moral imperative. Personhood of individuals, as discussed in chapter 7, is often disregarded and instead is defined by clinicians as moral competence and autonomy. Personhood becomes the province of the law and is really a form of "contractualism" (3). Patients either agree to health care contracts such as those concerning consent to care, specific treatment interventions, and end-of-life codes or they do not. In these latter cases patients must either seek help elsewhere or turn to the courts for legal determinations of ethical responsibility. Issues of patient competency are determined by third-party evaluations often based on cultural and religious views not held by the involved individual.

Traditionally, beneficence—that is, doing good—and professional autonomy, two fundamental tenets of medical practice, resulted in modes of treatment that are paternalistic in nature (4). The self of individuals was not considered to be autonomous, and patients relied on clinicians to "do no harm." In contemporary medicine, bioethics is now driven by the law, materialism, and consumerism. Patients have "rights" and "entitlements," and malpractice suits flourish. In some arenas, patients are even referred to as clients, customers, consumers, and service users. Personhood is often redefined as a determinant of social "normality," entitlement, and financial restitution rather than being based on individuals' integrity and personal ethics. Clinicians who adhere to the principles of beneficence and fiduciary responsibility may find themselves in a constant state of conflict as they try to balance the goals of providing evidenced-based cost-effective scientific interventions with compassionate care. Clearly, the environment of contemporary health care delivery is complex and ever changing. In countries where health care is sustained by public tax dollars, the system is often more highly regulated in terms of personal autonomy and accountability than in those systems based on fee-for-service. In both instances, the real danger is that decision making is based primarily on fiscal considerations rather than on medical ethics and scientific evidence. Because of these social changes, professional accountability is a pressing social need in modern life.

This environment is one in which all health care providers must not only diagnose, prognosticate, and intervene, but, in the area of human suffering, must develop a morality based on the force of their own personal will, beliefs about liberty and freedom, and notions about human good. Many changes in clinician-patient relationships have evolved from the paternalistic methods of the past that were based on the ethics of beneficence and fiduciary responsibility. Considerable confusion persists about the ethics of modern-day health care practice.

Physician-Patient Relationship: Challenges

Contemporary patient-doctor relationships are also very complex. There is often a dichotomy between doctors' perceptions of their scope of practice and that of their patients and colleagues. Patients rarely understand the environmental expectations placed on physicians, and patients' own cultural or even generational expectations of health clinicians are extensive and variable. In general, issues of rights and freedoms are not well understood and articulated in contemporary society (5). Not everyone in a multicultural society has the same cultural rights. Differences are based on whether individuals are born in the country in which they live or whether they are new immigrants. Rights are usually formulated on the beliefs of a nation's founding culture. Usually, all individuals have the same rights under the law, as well as the right to fight for individual beliefs and practices, but the implementation of practices that are not held by the mainstream society is not an entrenched right. Sometimes complex communication problems arise because issues of rights, responsibilities, and freedoms are not well understood in medicine. The fiduciary relationship between doctors and patients can be lost not only because of environmental constraints but also because of patients' and doctors' ignorance of each others' cultural expectations. Further, physicians may not do what is in the optimal interests of patients simply because of time and fiscal constraints. Consequently, patient-doctor relationships may become more adversarial than complimentary. In addition to differing cultural expectations, technological advances may, unfortunately, impact negatively on doctor-patient relationships (6–8).

In this technological age, patients sometimes think that the Internet is a source of knowledge when in fact it is merely a source of information. Consequently, patients may demand treatments, medications or tests that they have heard about on the Internet or a newscast. When advised against such actions by doctors, individuals may feel they are being discriminated against or that their "rights" have been denied. Further, health care providers may, in the spirit of adhering to personal rights to self-determination, expect patients to make medical and ethical decisions based on knowledge they do not possess. Patients usually do not have degrees in medicine, nursing, or philosophy. Currently, the role of physicians is to determine the nature of the illness, confirm the differential diagnosis with appropriate tests, determine the best interventions, explain findings to the patient, and institute care. The responsibility of patients is to concisely tell their doctors the story of their complaints, be sure they understand the doctor's advice, recognize that their doctor's responsibility to them is based on legal and ethical regulations, appoint the doctor to act on their behalf, and then follow the doctor's instructions. Postmodern medicine demands a new relationship of beneficence, fiduciary responsibility, and trust between physicians and patients based on respect for individual and cultural differences. Because past methods combined with recent technological advances have enhanced care, there has been an escalation of health care costs. It becomes clear that one solution to the maintenance of care while controlling health care delivery costs is to address suffering as an entity separate and only sometimes related to pain, because both entities contribute to the development of chronic disability. The medical and social costs of disability are great both in economic and human terms. Those who suffer expect that the physician will enter into the relationship of suffering. We have also seen from the research evidence presented in chapter 2 that it is likely that pain outcomes will improve if suffering is addressed.

The expectations and restrictions on doctors to still practice both the art and science of medicine are great, and some clinicians control time constraints by resorting to methods in which the objective is only to improve technological findings. For example, if there is evidence on a magnetic resonance imaging machine (MRI) that there has been a positive change, the patient is considered to be cured and is discharged from care, even though the individual is not able to resume a reasonable life.

It is beyond the scope of this text to suggest resolutions to all these social difficulties. The main objective of the discussion is to argue that in spite of the environmental, professional, and ethical pressures on the modern day physician, most doctors are committed to preserving and restoring both the health and the human dignity of those seeking medical attention. It is imperative that suffering is clearly defined as a perception of threat to idea of self and personhood so that appropriate suffering-specific interventions may be developed based on the technical and clinical skills of specific health care providers.

The Role of the Physician and Suffering

Some authors argue for the need to enhance physicians' skills of empathetic listening (9), but medical school admissions criteria do not necessarily screen for applicants who have these skills. Those who suffer expect the doctor not only to be empathetic but also to provide hope for the best physical outcome and to assist individuals in the achievement of their optimal emotional restoration (10). This expectation has been explored in terminal illness but not for those who suffer from chronic illness or injury (11). Patients want doctors to be aware that during suffering, the central purpose of the patient's life may be lost or at best changed. The role of the doctor is to validate the patient's concerns, hear and share their stories, and advise patients as they would their own family. Patients need to know that their doctor will support and assist them in attainment of their goals, even if the route they have chosen is not one that the doctor would choose for himself/herself under the same circumstances. Patients depend on their doctor to help them get the best scientific medical care, to advocate for them when necessary, to help successfully navigate the medical system, and to protect them from external sources such as insurance and legal hindrances. The challenge for some physicians is to achieve these goals in the face of social and environmental limitations (12, 13). Fear of litigation can result in physician behaviours that can destroy all hope for the patient and family in an attempt to be sure that statistical risks are delineated. Failure to explain to the patient what these numbers mean in relationship to everyday living escalates the perception of threat to self and personhood. Some physicians may believe that the patient is not thinking "right" and it is their duty to correct the patient. This approach, without a full exploration of the patient's understanding of the nature of the illness and natural history of the illness or disorder, may lead to a loss of patient autonomy and personal power. In medicine, it is expected that the doctor will maintain the patient's sense of autonomy. This is particularly true in North American society, where autonomy is seen as an end product of civil rights. Respect for the individual is the dominant factor in North American democracy and is a key factor in all judicial and legal precepts. When patients suffer, they depend on doctors to help them make decisions under the rules of beneficence. Doctors who help those who suffer must also be concerned with justice and malfeasance, because patient autonomy may now become a matter of patient competency.

Effective problem identification includes measures of suffering and an exploration of the nature of the patient's perceptions of threat to self and personhood.

Successful outcomes are based on patient determinations of restoration of their lives as well as the management of physical and/or emotional illness.

Suffering is a complex construct, often fraught with religious, spiritual, and cultural overtones. If doctors are to advocate for patients who suffer, they must address issues of loss of self, loss of an individual's central purpose in life, and the impact of existential loneliness on health. Doctors who are not emotionally able to explore and examine these issues in their own life may prematurely label patient behaviour as being pathological. When pragmatic perspectives on the part of the doctor overrule human compassion and empathy, suffering of patients and their families is increased.

To the patient, the doctor is the ultimate authority and recipient of their trust. Because courses in cultural practices and philosophy are often not part of routine medical education, the busy doctor is further challenged to engage in continuous postgraduate education in these areas or be able to relinquish some of the professional prestige involved with being the ultimate authority or power figure and admit to not knowing. The patient and doctor can then form a mutually interactive relationship in which each learns from and trusts the other. This approach to the management of health requires an ability and willingness to enter into the patient's experience of suffering. Many doctors practice successfully in this way and patients do not feel abandoned or victimized. Hope, trust, and mutual respect are maintained. Allied health care practitioners such as nurses, chaplains, therapists, social workers, and psychologists can assist physicians in their treatment of patients who suffer. Unfortunately, their additional expertise is often unavailable in this age of diminishing health care fiscal resources.

The Nurse

Professional Responsibility and Autonomy

While physicians may have the ultimate legal responsibility for the patient, nurses also are legally responsible for their actions and behaviours. Scope of practice and professional standards established by colleges of nursing govern nursing practice. Nurses are responsible not only for maintaining and upgrading their professional nursing skills and techniques, but also for the health of individuals under their care. Superimposed on these responsibilities are the administrative obligations of health care organizations for whom the nurse works.

The challenge between best practice and cost containment is enormous. Further, cost containment has resulted in the use of less comprehensively trained nurses, who are paid considerably less money than registered university-trained nurses, to care for patients in hospital wards and hospital clinics. Often clinics are now managed by administrators who are skilled in business administration but not in the care of the sick. In the community, unskilled personnel are used to perform nursing care duties in the home that do not involve the use of drugs. Further, nurse practitioners are being trained to assume duties that were previously performed by physicians. The role of the nurse as healer, patient advocate, and protector of the patient is being undermined by systematic changes that favour a materialistic, impersonal approach to health care delivery. The modern nurse must struggle with the challenges of upholding the responsibilities of the nursing profession and its culture of holistic care in an environment of business-driven objectives of health care organizations and political mandates.

In terms of personal autonomy, the nurse's job is often the most complex of all the health care professionals. The nurse has absolute autonomy in the administration of specialized nursing skills and techniques, but in most instances must still follow and enforce the instructions of the doctor and other health care providers. Further, nurses must also foster the empowerment and autonomy of patients (15). Autonomy and accountability in nursing are closely intertwined. Nurses are accountable to doctors, administrators, patients, and their families, as well as to the nursing profession per se. To effectively meet all these challenges, nurses must be well educated not only in nursing but also in the fields of administration, bioethics, and sociology. The advent of nurse specialists who also act as resources to frontline nurses addresses these concerns. Unfortunately, economic constraints often eliminate these specialists from the health care team in favour of less costly personnel with less training. As a result, continuity of care from hospital to home to clinic and eventually to the workplace is lost, as is the evolution of care from acute stages of illness to chronic care. The ethical challenges to nurses are significant in such environments.

While the nursing profession has been proactive in responding to technological advances and the resulting escalation in health care costs, on decision-making boards, nurses often find they are the lone voices advocating for the autonomy of nurses and patients, and for the administration of ethical care.

Ethical Considerations in Nursing

Nurses are confronted with many conflicts in the delivery of ethical care. They must be able to determine and differentiate between everyday problems and ethical dilemmas (16). In contemporary society, where there is no longer a unifying moral imperative, determination of what is or is not an ethical dilemma, a situation in which there is a conflict between moral imperatives, is based on individual moral principles. Nurses face many challenges in this regard. For example, if a clinical measure is deemed to be morally right but the outcome of such action is likely to have a bad effect, then a dilemma exists. A nurse is often faced with conflicting moral imperatives established by institutions, the society at large, patients' individual cultural and religious beliefs, and the nurse's own personal principles. The nurse not only must be able to personally navigate these sometimes conflicting views but must also help patients make the best ethical decisions about their health. Further, unlike members of hospital bioethics committees, whose role is to advise and provide guidelines, nurses are accountable for their influence on patient decision making. Rarely does the process of ethical decision making result in easy answers (17).

Because of the nature of personal autonomy in nursing, the nurse may be faced with administrative decisions that are in conflict with nursing codes of practice. For example, premature discharge of a patient, without full determination of community resources available to aid the patient, has the potential to result in further impairments, disability, and even death. It is the nurse who must argue on behalf of the patient against administrators and sometimes even doctors who want early discharge of patients in order to free up beds in hospital settings without regard for the impact on the patient (18).

The nurse is also the gatekeeper of quality care (19–23). Nurses are the health care professionals who must monitor the quality of care administered by other nurses, nursing assistants, doctors, students, and other health care professionals. It is the nurse who most often must report inappropriate care practices to nursing and/or administrative supervisors. The onus of such ethical responsibility usually falls to nurses because they have the most contact with patients and those who interact with them. Frontline nurses are the managers of the health care system per se. Consequently, ethical nursing care demands highly trained professionals.

Further, nurses play a critical role in infection control and the prevention of the spread of disease, not only within the hospital but also the community at large. This responsibility includes the care and management of the physical hospital buildings. Unfortunately, contemporary society has significantly decreased its concern for hospital and home caregivers' hygiene. Hospital personnel no longer change their clothing, wash their hands, or practice sterile technique to the extent that was once common. Hospital staff are often seen in restaurants and university buildings wearing hospital surgical garments as they "slip out for a coffee." Also, hospital buildings are often very unclean, and the general public receives little education about the possibility or probability of contracting diseases when visiting hospitals. Young infants are placed on the floor to have diapers changed, and others are left to play unrestricted in hospital corridors. The relaxation of basic principles of hospital hygiene presents a further challenge to nurses. Their valuable time is taken away from immediate care by such issues, and they must struggle with what modern society considers the rights of individuals over the rights of those who are ill. Clearly, nursing leadership is paramount to optimal health care delivery.

In managed-care situations, there is an even greater challenge to the nurse who must advocate for ethical care to patients in the face of strict insurance company restrictions. To be effective, nurses must establish relationships that will meet not only the expectations of patients but also that of the health care system in general. The nurse's prime commitment is to the patient.

The Nurse-Patient Relationship: Challenges

For patients, it is a given that the nurse is technologically proficient. Individuals expect nurses to care about them personally, to advocate on their behalf, and to treat them with the dignity and respect they would give to their own loved ones. The nurse is the person patients trust with their secret fears and vulnerabilities. Patients turn to nurses for their skill, compassion, and understanding. They trust nurses to safeguard not only their health but also their human dignity. Nurses are the people who are most skilled in transcultural care. Patients know that nurses will try to accommodate differences in cultural practices should they arise between individuals and the health care organizations. Patients can assist nurses by being informed about the nature and limitations imposed on and by health care organizations and by having realistic expectations of the power of the nurse.

When patients realize that cultural misunderstandings are simply misunderstandings and not an infringement of personal rights or entitlements, then health care delivery improves. Mutual respect is critical to the nurse-patient relationship. Patients must also recognize that nurses are highly skilled professional health care practitioners whose prime objective is to heal and facilitate healing of the whole person (23–26). They are not hospitality workers.

The Role of the Nurse in Suffering

Nurses are usually the first health care professionals to assess the patient. Initially, the nurse obtains information about the nature of the illness or injury to determine the severity of the complaints and whether immediate treatment is needed. If the situation does not require emergency care, the nurse continues to obtain information about the whole person. When addressing suffering, the nurse explores the impact of the illness or injury on the patient's idea of self and personhood. Enquiries are made about how the patient's cultural, religious, and spiritual beliefs impact on his/her perception of threat to self and personhood. The nurse is often the first and sometimes the only person who hears the complete story of the patient's illness/injury and its significance to the patient and the patient's family. As we have discussed in the chapter on storytelling, the nurse is the first health care professional who will hear the story in its unedited form. As patients encounter other clinicians, their stories often become modified to meet their perceptions of health care providers' needs. Listening to and interpreting the stories demands considerable skill and knowledge about the nature of suffering. Care must be taken when recording patient responses to avoid misinterpreting suffering as mental illness. Suffering is a life experience that may affect health. It is not a disease.

In the process of caregiving, the nurse can assist the patient through the experience of suffering. The nurse may be the only person the patient feels able to repeatedly tell the story of suffering to until there is no longer a need for further narrative. The nurse is the health care provider who is able to help the patient heal the self even though the illness may remain. Nurses know that thoughts have a great influence on the body and that the body stores emotions. Many nursing care techniques such as massage, Rolfing, and reflexology address these difficulties. Nurses are aware also of the relationship between the human mind, body, and spirit. It is often the nurse who alerts the physician to the possibility that the patient might benefit from more advanced spiritual or psychological care than the nurse is trained to provide.

When addressing suffering, nurses can support patients' need for care beyond organizational care plans and often are the first to help patients recognize that a new central purpose for their life is possible. Through the nurse's validation of the patient's story, the patient may start to resolve issues of self-conflict. Clearly, the nurse is critical to identifying those who suffer, validating their stories of suffering and providing empathy and compassion as they try to cope with perceptions of threat to ideas of self and personhood.

The nurse is also the health care team member who can facilitate and enhance clinical education to other health care providers about the nature of suffering and treatments that are likely to facilitate restoration of self and personhood in those who are chronically ill. The management of suffering in clinical practice always involves close collaboration between health care professionals, and this is especially so between the professions of nursing and chaplaincy.

The Chaplain

Professional Responsibility and Autonomy

Often there is confusion about the professionalism of chaplaincy in contemporary medicine. Professionalism usually relates to membership in a group based on educational standards, self-governance, and legislative regulations. To date, there is considerable diversity in the educational requirements and certification programs of chaplains. This situation is not unique to chaplaincy, for there are other accepted and well-integrated health care professionals in hospital organizations who do not have legislative standing. In North America, chaplains usually have postsecondary education in religious studies or the humanities and receive extensive training in pastoral counseling, crisis intervention, and family and marital therapy. Chaplains are certified in Canada by the Canadian Association for Pastoral Care and in the United States by the Association of Professional Chaplains. In the United Kingdom, the professional body is the College of Health Care Chaplains, and while in the British Isles membership in these colleges is not always mandatory, membership is advantageous because the colleges are affiliated with a trade union (27–30).

There are health care providers who question the professional designation of chaplains (31). Arguments are often based on disputes concerning professional boundaries and the fact that chaplains usually have religious affiliations to which they are accountable and that are outside the jurisdiction of hospitals. Others argue that spirituality and religion are one and the same and that religion does not have a place in health care organizations. Issues of concern focus on whether chaplains violate organizational privacy policies if patient charts are read by chaplains either to counsel or to recruit patients. Opponents of chaplains as health care professionals also argue that chaplains are not bound by the same rules of confidentiality as other health care providers. Such arguments seem somewhat scurrilous. It is argued that chaplains under assumptions of priest-parishioner confidentiality are not obliged to reveal information about patients to other clinicians unless the patient gives permission or unless the information indicates that the patient is likely to harm himself or others. This latter argument against the role of chaplains appears to be sophistic, because one of the major problems of confidentiality in hospitals is that some clinicians record information about patients that is irrelevant to the health care problem and in some cases can even be considered defamatory.

Finally, another prevailing argument is that patients may not want to be visited by a chaplain (32). Again, if communications between patients and health care workers at intake are nondiscriminatory, then patients do not receive unwanted referrals. Those who argue against the professionalism of chaplains based on the premise of unwanted referrals fail to acknowledge the power differential that arises when patient autonomy is dismissed. Failure of health care professionals to refer patients to other colleagues constitutes a loss of patient autonomy. For example, do patients have the right to refuse a referral to psychology? If so, why not chaplaincy? Further, the issue of recruitment of referrals for spiritual care also appears to be related to power differentials and professional jealousies between various health care providers in hospital organizations. Conflicts over professional boundaries and the value of spiritual care and health do not enhance patient care.

Professional autonomy and accountability for the hospital chaplain involves following the organization's policies and the regulations of the chaplain's religious affiliations and maintaining the ethical and legal standards of contemporary society. Hospital chaplains must also ensure that community clergy visits also uphold the privacy and confidentiality policies of the institution. The environment in which chaplains and all health care providers work is fraught with many conflicts. Understanding and resolving conflicts leads to better care practices for patients.

Ethical Responsibilities: Theology versus Secularism

Because there is no longer an overriding moral imperative in contemporary society, it is critical that chaplains are members of hospital ethics committees. Their responsibilities are to assist in the drafting of consent to care, do not resuscitate codes, organ donation rules and regulations, as well as other health and policy issues. They clarify issues involving ethical dilemmas and value issues with staff members and senior hospital managers, and they assist in pragmatic solutions to problems. Chaplains ensure that human values are safeguarded in various aspects of institutional policies and behaviours. The chaplain faces many problems when the ethics concerning the value of human life and dignity are in conflict with the fiscal objectives of hospital administrators. Once again, chaplains can be faced with conflicts around professional boundaries, particularly with some bioethicists (33, 34). Most contemporary ethics committees value the contributions of both groups. Contemporary ethical dilemmas in medicine require philosophical, religious, and spiritual resolutions.

Chaplains are the chief advocates for patients and families, particularly when difficult ethical choices around end-of-life issues and consent to care must be made. They assist clinicians who must give patients and their families negative information about the patient's health and life expectancy and also act as "cultural brokers" between health care organizations and patients. Chaplains can also advise staff who may face ethical dilemmas when their personal moral codes seem to be in conflict with hospital policies (36, 37). Hospital chaplains, too, may find themselves torn between the obligations of their faith-based teachings and those of the secular state. As with other health care providers caught in such conflicts, the chaplain must then deal with the ethics and morality of either abandoning the patient or finding a source of reconciliation between conflicting ethical demands.

The Patient-Chaplain Relationship: Challenges

Many patients do not understand the role of chaplains in contemporary society (37–40). Individuals who do not have a religion-based spirituality may resist assistance from chaplains, who they believe may try to convert them or blame them for their lack of religious affiliation. However, if patients are given appropriate information about the various roles of health care providers, such reservations are dispelled. Instead of viewing the chaplain as a pseudo-professional, clinicians can point out to patients that the chaplain is not bound by the same rules of confidentiality and record keeping as the medical staff. Consequently, patients have a choice, and many find a safe place in which to discuss very personal concerns without fear of prejudice or recrimination. Further, chaplains do not present themselves as authority figures. The problems of power differentials that can exist between other health care professionals and patients, in which the clinician is the authority figure, do not exist between chaplain and patient in matters of health. The chaplain will be seen as the authority in matters of religion only if the patient has the same faith background as the chaplain and chooses to discuss theology.

In cases where patients have a religious belief system and perhaps are very angry with their misfortune, chaplains are able to give individuals permission to express their anger at God with the reassurance that they are still cared about. They are also able to administer religious sacraments when asked. Chaplains have an advantage over community clergy in that they can deal with problems from a nondenominational perspective in concert with advice from the rest of the health care team. Consequently, they can also help patients who hold secular beliefs cope with adversity through the wisdom of philosophical teachings. Further, although chaplaincy arose from the Christian religious tradition, the hospital chaplain uses the teachings of all religious and spiritual traditions to help individuals cope with illness and disease. At the same time, chaplains can also protect patients from unwanted proselytizing, both secular and religious.

As a liaison between patients, families, and medical staff, chaplains are sensitive to multicultural customs and have an extensive knowledge of health care institutional dynamics. Hospital chaplains often have extensive education and experience in crisis intervention methods. Although chaplains may receive compensation based on institutional agreements, most work many more hours and provide much more assistance than is contractually delineated.

Patient's responsibilities to chaplains are to understand that chaplains usually adhere to a personal moral imperative that is usually based on theology and that is often beyond the confines of organizational policies. Nevertheless, chaplains are accountable both to health care organizations, as part of a health care team, as well as to their faith groups. The relationship between chaplain and patient is one of interdependency because the patient also has a responsibility to the chaplain to adhere to the tenets of mutual respect, privacy, and confidentiality. Patients trust chaplains with the secrets of their souls and chaplains trust patients with the stories of their experiences (41).

The Role of the Chaplain

The chaplain-patient relationship is perhaps the most profound of the professional relationships because it is based solely on mutual trust—a trust that under no circumstances is betrayed. There is a sharing of the deepest understandings of self, personhood, and the ultimate reality of God. The following story illustrates the breadth and depth of understanding required of chaplains who comfort those who suffer.

A SECRET DIALOGUE WITH THE SELF

There is a person within us whom the outside world seldom sees. It is the "true self" of our dreams, expectations, or identity. I do not know where it comes from, as it sometimes seems to have little correlation with our abilities, work, or interests.

Years ago, I had a longstanding dream of owning a bar by the beach where I could spend my days in sunshine, hearing and sharing life stories with people who came in to the bar. But happily my life changed and so did my dream of myself.

Since I live in a northern country, my dream shifted to a small village near the ocean where I am part of a small northern fishing community and the people of that place. Ever since I moved to a home on the ocean, I have wanted a sea kayak. I belong in a big yellow one slicing through the open ocean. Now, in reality, I have trouble sitting in plush theatre seats through a whole concert performance. I have not been flexible enough to touch my toes in the last fifteen years, and I have no interest in working out to develop my aging body. I seldom have been out in the open water without getting seasick, and yet, I know I belong in a big yellow kayak slicing through the waves. This dream is essential to how I see myself.

The inability to make this dream come true is, at best, a very slight suffering, but it is an example of my hidden true self. I have been to dozens of stores and chatted with clerks about which kayak I should get. I have read reviews of twice as many kayaks on line and I even look in the classified ads in the newspaper for a used one. I still have not bought one. Yes, they are expensive, but that is not my deciding factor. The deciding factor is that I do not want to fail my identity.

There is less suffering in having an unfulfilled but "could be" realized dream than in a crushed reality of not maybe even liking kayaking or of being really lousy at it.

My story may seem to be too trivial to be of any real use to those with real suffering, except that it is an example of suffering without the fear that drives us away from people who suffer from loss of loved ones and/or from illnesses or injuries. My kayak has no basis in my life events; it is a delusion of expectations. My current survival does not depend on this idea of self. You can quite quickly judge me as "an old fart" and tell me to "get over it," or you can say, "If that's all you have to anguish about, you need a real life." If you are trying to be more supportive, you might even say, "You are more than kayaking . . .," but for me this story is the dream of my true self and all that is associated with being a free spirit, physically strong, and spiritually connected with people and my universe. It is possible for people to hear stories about the dream of kayaking because it doesn't make the listener afraid. But for those who suffer from illnesses or trauma, the response to their stories may illicit fear. The fear of others who may hear this type of suffering story is that they know that they, too, can become victims of such circumstances. Health care providers are keenly aware of how easily the events of their patients' lives can happen to them.

Managing suffering in medicine is a real challenge to chaplains and health professionals. Clinicians may feel the need to measure everything in an attempt to be in control of events. Theories are developed and tested, and the ethereal mysteries of suffering are given a score on a 10-point scale that ranges from 1, which means "get over it," to a catastrophic 10, "you are fucked." When such methods fail, the chaplain may find that, suddenly, there is more than one patient, and one patient may now be the health care provider him- or herself. As a result, suffering as separate from pain is often not addressed in medicine.

Suffering is intimately tied to what we believe about ourselves and the universe. I do believe that we all create some sense of order in our lives based on a conception of justice involving rewards and punishments owed to me for living a certain way.

In third grade, I remember actually doing my homework once. I was quite proud. It was complete and neat. I was sure I had done well. Well, the nun teaching the class was less impressed, and I got my usual "mercy mark." I thought that if I really worked at something, I would get A's. It wasn't fair, I deserved better. Though I doubt that the nun gave me a fair shake, I was suffering. I worked, and I didn't get my expected results. The world and I were not what I thought we were.

In October 1980, my sister's youngest son, Christian, died of spinal meningitis in a hospital in Florida. I had gone down to be with her and her husband. They had moved a few years before from New York City in order to improve the health of both their sons, who had northern allergies. Christian had also been born with two holes in his heart and had these surgically repaired when he was about one year old. He was doing well and was healthy, happy, and strong. One day he complained of a stiff neck, and later that day the doctor diagnosed it as meningitis. He was sent to a children's specialty hospital and was there a week before he died.

Now, I had been working as a hospital chaplain at a specialty children's hospital for several years and was no stranger to the arbitrariness of illness and death's selection of a child. I knew that life was fragile and there are no guarantees. My suffering after Christian's death was great because this was not supposed to happen to me. I had dedicated my life to God as a minister and worked where there was death all the time. God was supposed to keep these tragedies away from my family. We had a deal or, at least, I decided that we did. Yes. I grieved the loss of Christian and my sister's grief and suffering, but my suffering was secret. I am suffering because God broke a deal that I (we) had made. I knew that this was less than rational even back then, but a truth about my existence and work had been broken. I had difficulty returning to the children in the intensive care unit where I worked, not because they might die, but because I didn't have a good story to tell myself about why I was there.

How does one talk about these crazy delusional sufferings without getting two prescriptions from medical personnel or ending up being admitted for an emergency psychiatric consultation? I can just imagine the evaluation starting and ending with: "So John, you actually think that you had made a deal with God?"

How do you help those who suffer? The stories of individual suffering are private and idiosyncratic. Many people feel they will not be understood. Suffering is a process that involves one's dream of self, self-image, and identity. The process of suffering, in which individuals lose the central purpose of their lives and have considerable self-conflict and impaired personal relationships with others, the world, and themselves, is common to those who suffer. Suffering requires a belief system against which one claims justice and fairness. There is, on the part of the sufferer, a right way expected or owed.

To be useful to others, chaplains spend a lot of time understanding their own stories and sufferings.

"Suffering is inevitable: misery is optional."

Reverend John

The issue of suffering in spiritual care presents many challenges for the chaplain simply because the word *suffering* has myriad meanings. In medicine, we advocate for a definition in which suffering is a perception of threat to ideas of self and personhood. An individual's idea of self incorporates religious and spiritual teachings, and the definition of *suffering*, for medical care, does not usurp these teachings and beliefs. The definition removes the sense of rightness or wrongness of beliefs from medical care, which could be the case if the definition included specific religious and/or legal parameters. For the chaplain, idea of self must be explored more fully with patients than is possible with other health care providers.

As we have seen, the development of idea of self evolves from early childhood religious/spiritual teachings, information gleaned from society at large, and from personal secret dreams of individuals. Personhood involves personal standards of acceptability of behaviour of individuals based on factors such as culture, psychological life tasks, and spiritual/religious beliefs. Perceptions of threat include not only the possibility of destruction of one's current life but also regrets over past behaviour associated with the resolution of past traumatic events. Anticipated challenges of the present and future appear to be insurmountable. In addition to these concerns, which are likely to be germane to all persons, people with chronic illness must also confront the perception of loss of power due to physical and emotional impairments and/or disability.

Initially, chaplains spend considerable effort helping patients understand the nature of their changed present circumstances. For many there is a death of the idea of the old self, and patients may undergo all the grief and bereavement experienced with the physical death of a loved one. The chaplain is the person to whom one may consciously reveal the secrets of his or her soul without fear of being labeled as mentally ill. The challenge for the chaplain is to be ever alert for signs of psychological pathophysiology. When suspected, the chaplain must refer patients to psychologists and psychiatrists while still maintaining the sanctity of the chaplain-patient relationship. The chaplain is the guardian of the patient's secret self.

Patients may also confess to chaplains their perceptions of "sins" that they believe have resulted in their suffering. A discussion of the meaning of suffering is often explored from theological, cultural, and secular perspectives. Issues of hope, lost dreams, courage, and despair are addressed. Patients and chaplains may also explore the power of personal loneliness and perceptions of alienation from Christian and non-Christian existential perspectives. The stories patients tell chaplains may not be the same type of story they tell the medical personnel. They often tell chaplains stories of their concerns for restoration of their inner life, now and in the future, while what they tell medical staff may be about the nature of their current illness.

Unlike psychology and psychiatry, chaplains are not bound by expectations of care as determined by codes and models of adjustments, scales of well-being, or determinants of self-esteem. Individuals are not "fixed" by chaplaincy's approach to care. The role of the chaplain in suffering is to embrace those who may be considered "broken" by others and to walk with them through their emotional struggles for restoration of the self. In chaplaincy, there are no defined acceptable clinical outcomes. Chaplains do not prescribe medications. Patients can explore the "craziness" of the their perception of threat to their idea of self without fear of being put into psychological categories of mental illness and subsequently experiencing the stigma that still persists regarding this illness. They can discuss their failed dreams of personhood without the necessity of external measures of appropriateness and labels of depression. In short, patients can reveal themselves and be comforted and supported as they reconstruct their lives.

The role of the chaplain with those who suffer varies considerably throughout the patient-chaplain relationship. It takes many forms, such as advisor, counselor, father, friend, pastor, and mother, but it is governed by the overriding ethic that the patient is extremely emotionally vulnerable and that while the relationship is interdependent it is not equal. The chaplain is the professional and bears the responsibilities of professionalism. The ethics of professional integrity in such interdependent relationships are very complex and require constant vigilance. The therapeutic thrust of this interdependent relationship is that by sharing life experiences with those who suffer, the patient is reassured that he or she is still a viable and valued member of the society.

The focus of this discussion has been on the chaplain-patient relationship. The therapeutic skills of the chaplain often complement those of the social worker and/or psychologist, but it is the overriding relationship that determines the course of treatment. Usually, the patient, nurse, chaplain, psychologist, and social worker form a "working subteam" to help the patient with the resolution of specific problems. It is, however, the chaplain whom patients trust to protect them from perceived emotional and social abuse.

SUMMARY

The management of suffering begins with identification of the experience by physicians and nurses, who are the first persons to interact with patients often when illness and/or injury is in the acute stages. Following these initial assessments, care programs are implemented, and in the case of potentially chronic outcomes or disability, chaplains are the next professionals to meet the patient. This chapter advances the hypothesis that effective care depends on not only professional competency but also on health care providers and patients having the same expectations of care.

The discussion has also focused on system challenges imposed on health care professionals who first see the patient in a hospital setting. Issues of professionalism and personal autonomy and their relationship to professional accountability have been explored. It is argued that if patients have a basic understanding of these issues, then they will form realistic expectations of their care providers. The restrictions to care are discussed from an ethical perspective. The nature of ethical practice and its impact on the relationship between the patient, doctor, nurse, and chaplain show that knowledge of suffering as an entity separate and only sometimes related to pain is critical to effective care of those who suffer.

Each profession has specialized skills to address suffering, which allow for individual needs of patients based on personal power and cultural demands. The following chapter addresses the role of physiotherapists and social workers, who help integrate individuals who suffer into the greater community at large. Examples are presented from individuals who are either born with developmental deficits or are disabled due to illness and/or injury.

CHAPTER 13 QUESTIONS

1 What is the relationship between professional responsibilities, autonomy, and ethical practice of physicians who assist those who suffer?
2 What are the challenges to doctor-patient relationships in contemporary medicine?
3 What is the role of the doctor in the management of suffering?
4 What factors deter from the effective care of the patient?
5 What is the nature of the work environment of the nurse?

6 What specific skills do nurses possess to help patients who suffer?
7 What is the role of the chaplain in health care organizations?
8 What are the ethical responsibilities of the chaplain?
9 What distinct therapeutic skills do chaplains possess to help those who suffer?

14 Habilitation and Rehabilitation

The first health care professionals involved with patients are usually the physician, nurse, and sometimes the chaplain. Treatment objectives are to address the immediate physical problems and to identify those who suffer either with or without pain. Treatment planning may involve physiotherapy; social work; and in some instances psychology, occupational therapy, or vocational rehabilitation, as patients learn to control their new physical and emotional environments. Restoration of self-image and idea of self and resolution of personhood issues are the main treatment objectives. The focus of this chapter is on the habilitation and rehabilitation of individuals with chronic illness. The roles of the physiotherapist and social worker are used to show that modern medicine not only involves caring for people and curing disease but also fulfilling a social responsibility to help those who suffer survive and thrive.

Successful treatment outcomes depend on both patient and physiotherapist understanding the limitations that illness or injury has placed on the patient, recognizing the implications of professional obligations and boundaries on treatment outcomes, and having realistic expectations of each other's skills and abilities.

In previous chapters, the issue of suffering was discussed primarily from the perspective of chronic illness or injury. Chronic illness is commonly thought to occur when there is an experience of disease onset or traumatic injury. Chronic illness is also due to developmental disorders, birth injuries, or genetic abnormalities. Often the first clinician to deal with issues of rehabilitating patients with any of these disorders or rehabilitating individuals with acquired chronic impairments is the physiotherapist.

The purpose of this chapter is to (a) to explore the roles of the physiotherapist and social worker, who assist individuals who suffer either because of difficulties that prevent reentry into the community or obstacles that prevent full participation in the community, (b) describe the environmental constraints on health care providers who deal with the habilitation and/or rehabilitation of individuals with chronic illness or injuries in Western societies, and (c) discuss issues of professionalism, professional autonomy, and ethical practice, this time within the context of habilitation and rehabilitation and the goals of optimal care for those who suffer.

The Physiotherapist

Professional Responsibility and Autonomy

Few patients are aware of the environmental constraints placed on physiotherapists and the impact these constraints have on the therapist's professional responsibilities and professional autonomy. Consequently, patients may have limited expectations of the care available to them. The main objectives of physiotherapy are to help patients overcome physical impairments or disabilities and so restore ideas of self and personhood.

In physical therapy, successful habilitation or rehabilitation outcomes occur when there is an effective symbiotic relationship between patient and therapist. The patient has a basic understanding of the professional role of the physiotherapist and the therapist is aware not only of the patient's physical and potential emotional problems, but also of the patient's culture, religious/spiritual background, personality strengths and weaknesses, illness and wellness beliefs. Most importantly, the therapist must understand the nature of the patient's suffering.

In our current society there are many individuals who offer the application of modalities common to physiotherapy practice, but only individuals who are registered and licensed by their respective physiotherapy governing boards are legally able to call themselves physiotherapists. Physiotherapists undergo extensive academic and clinical training in universities and hospitals. Professional responsibility and personal autonomy are the hallmarks of the practice and are best understood from a historical perspective.

Historical Perspectives and Professional Constraints

Historically, physiotherapy practice dates back to 460 B.C. when practitioners Hippocrates and Hector first advocated massage and hydrotherapy to treat physical symptoms. Initially, physiotherapists worked solely under the direction of physicians, which may be the foundations of later attitudes that physiotherapy requires the supervision of medicine. However, the profession of physiotherapy practice as it is known today did not evolve from medicine but rather from four British nurses who formed the Chartered Society of Physiotherapy in 1894. Later, schools of physiotherapy were started in New Zealand in 1913 and in the United States in 1914. Because physiotherapy evolved from the profession of nursing and nursing's professional association was with medicine, the traditional practice of physiotherapy originally depended solely on physician referrals. Professional responsibility was based on personal integrity, and personal professional autonomy was limited.

After World War II, treatments were primarily exercise, massage, and spinal traction, which eventually evolved to include manipulation of the spine and extremity joints. Approaches to care eventually included the restoration of individuals' personhood as physiotherapists helped returning veterans from the two great wars to return to work and reintegrate into society after sustaining severe impairments and disabilities. As was the case with the profession of chaplaincy, the implementation of physical therapy practice into mainstream medicine was sometimes met with opposition from other health care providers who perhaps were concerned about professional boundaries. Although the implementation of schools of physiotherapy were initially met with opposition from some physicians and chiropractors who may have been concerned about intrusion into their territory of medical expertise, schools of physiotherapy were established in universities and community colleges throughout the world. Physiotherapy services expanded to include specialty areas such as cardio-respirology, neurology, rheumatology, orthopedics, and integumentary conditions. Physiotherapists formed professional governing and licensing organizations and are now regulated health care practitioners with full professional responsibility and autonomy. In Canada, for example, patients no longer need a referral from a doctor for physiotherapy treatment. Although modern-day physiotherapists are usually independent primary care clinicians in the areas of musculo-skeletal disorders, there is still a close relationship with medicine in all areas of care. Issues of personal integrity and autonomy are critical factors for both patients and physiotherapists (1–3).

Along with the freedoms of professional autonomy come responsibilities for standards of care. Originally physiotherapy was considered primarily an art, and its theories and treatment strategies were developed through inductive and deductive reasoning. Since the 1970s physiotherapy interventions have been based primarily on scientific evidence of efficacy. With the advent of a more scientific approach to care and the societal objective of containing health care expenditures, the art of physiotherapy, which includes care of the whole person physically, emotionally, and spiritually, is often diminished, as is the case in many areas of medical practice. The power of the relationship between physiotherapist and patient in the delivery of efficacious, cost-efficient health care delivery is well known (4).

The role of the physiotherapist in the management of chronic illness has changed considerably in the past twenty years. There are fewer rehabilitation hospitals and fewer in-patient physiotherapy departments. Instead there has been an influx of private, fee-for-service rehabilitation companies that employ myriad professionals, one of which may be a physiotherapist. Often these therapists work as independent contractors or as consultants. Full-time positions are no longer the norm. In such situations, patients may be seen by the physiotherapist only long enough to receive a manual treatment intervention and then the patient is seen by a kinesiologist or physiotherapy assistant to do exercises. Issues such as suffering and reintegration into the workplace may not be addressed until a crisis arises. Remediation of such events is very costly. Consequently, in many cases the therapist-patient relationship, which has been reported to be crucial to effective rehabilitation of the whole person, may not develop at all. Even in hospitals, the value of rehabilitation of the whole person can be ignored. Patients with neurological disorders, for example, are seen in hospital settings for very short periods of time and then referrals are usually made to long-term nursing care facilities where physiotherapy treatments may or may not be available. Physiotherapists struggle with organizational systems that fail to understand that management of the whole person and their presenting impairments will lead to a decrease in the development of permanent disabilities. The cost to health care systems due to disabilities is great both in fiscal and human terms. Many individuals with chronic illnesses do not have access to physiotherapy either because of fee-for-service billing practices or lack of public health care resources. As we have seen in chapter 2, these factors have a significant negative impact, not only on the restoration of personhood but also on the cost of health care delivery (5).

Further, outpatient care for individuals with neurological disorders is virtually nonexistent because of the amount of time required to provide care and the limitations on fees paid for such treatments. In the United States, Canada, and Australia, fee-for-service issues are seen to be barriers to care if patients are not insured or if insurance packages are insufficient. Current treatments are based primarily on statistical evidence of cause and effect. To meet these demands, the scope of physiotherapy practice is now defined as helping individuals prevent disability and restore physical function after illness and disease. Care of the whole person is often relegated to "old school" therapists, many of whom are no longer in the public health care arena, who now work as private practitioners. Most of these changes have been driven by economics and past responses to political pressures for physiotherapists to define professional boundaries (6–8).

The advent of managed care has also contributed to these changes in approaches to care, as managed care companies are usually fee-for-service clinics. Third-party payers, such as insurance companies, and government-based fee structures often limit care for those with chronic illnesses or disabilities. The management of pain is secondary to the management of the physical disorder, and measures of suffering are rarely included in patient assessments. Such fiscal restraints result in some patients being institutionalized rather than rehabilitated (9). It is important for patients to understand the nature of social systems' restrictions to care so that when they are referred to physiotherapists, they are able to understand the quality of care available within these constraints.

Ethical Considerations: The Partnership

In spite of the environmental constraints on physiotherapy practice, ethical clinical practice is the main objective of physiotherapy. In Canada, to maintain provincial licensing physiotherapists must pass tests relating to jurisprudence. Failure to pass these tests results in loss of a therapist's license to practice physiotherapy. Colleges of physiotherapy regulate and monitor professional performance.

In a study of professional values of 566 American physical therapists in 2005, issues of benevolence rated as the highest value of importance to therapists and power rated lowest. Critical issues were caring for others, empathy, justice, respect for others, professionalism, and accountability. Being willing to forgive others; working toward the welfare of others; being genuine, sincere, and truthful; and upholding ethical and legal standards were values held as most important for those tested. There were no differences based on age for either measures of benevolence or power, and items relating to social esteem and job security were associated with clinical competence (10–12).

There are many challenges to the integrity of individual physiotherapists, particularly when therapists must assess an individual's abilities and capabilities in cases involving litigation or return-to-work insurance claims. The potential for conflict of interest arises when physiotherapists receive additional financial compensation for evaluations of the performance of patients who are currently under their care. The various colleges of physiotherapy make it clear that the fiduciary responsibility is always to the patient. Other complications may arise when careless note taking, imprecise billing practices, or inappropriate commercial enterprise contradicts the rules of ethical practice. As with all other contemporary regulated health care providers, the therapist faces severe penalties or loss of license if found guilty of malpractice or inappropriate methods. Physiotherapists are also obliged to report competency deficiencies of colleagues to their respective colleges of physiotherapy (13). Patients need to clearly understand the factors that constitute ethical practice.

Contemporary health care is optimal when patients understand the qualifications, capabilities, and organizational restraints imposed on their health care. Failure to understand the nature of professional autonomy and the demands of ethical practice may result in experiences in which the patient feels victimized not only by health problems but also by social structures and the community at large.

The Patient-Physiotherapist Relationship

The relationship between physiotherapist and patient has long been one in which the therapist functions both as healer and teacher and the patient is the one who receives the healing and instruction (10). Usually, healing and instruction occurs in agreement with the patient's goals and desires to achieve both physical and emotional independence. This relationship is somewhat unique in contemporary medicine because it fosters the empowerment of patients who may feel a loss of personal power due to illness and/or injury and the experience of suffering.

Initially, the main thrust of the relationship is on improving physical abilities. The therapist and patient discuss the patient's goals. The therapist offers advice and assurance that he/she will help the patient achieve these goals if they are within the scope of ethical practice. A treatment plan is devised and agreed upon. The therapist tells the patient what he or she must do to achieve these objectives. Self-efficacy and confidence on the part of the patient are critical to successful habilitation or rehabilitation. The therapist and patient discuss the significance of the impairment to the individual's everyday life. For example, how does the impairment affect job performance? The responsibility of the patient is to honestly inform the therapist of any real limitations. Sometimes, in cases of litigation, inaccurate information is given because patients are afraid to get better because they fear that their legal case will be compromised. As stated in chapter 6, therapists' knowledge of the basic mechanisms of personal injury law helps dispel patient fears. Clearly, trust is a prime factor in the patient-physiotherapist relationship (14).

In cases of impaired neurological development, the relationship between patient and physiotherapist may span several years. In cases where there are developmental delays in children, the whole family is actively involved in the child's treatments. The therapist actually has many "patients" other than the child. In these situations, treatment contracts are complex, involving direct and in some cultural traditions extended family members. The therapist's first responsibility is still to the child. Accountability, in extreme cases, may supersede parental authority and may extend to the authority of the state. Regardless of the circumstances, the therapist must always advocate for the patient.

Personality traits between therapists and individuals must be compatible. The patient must be confident that, like all good teachers, when performance does not match physical and emotional capabilities, the physiotherapist will explore the reasons why. Unsuccessful relationships usually result when physiotherapists distance themselves from the personhood of the patient and focus solely on physical technique, statistical probabilities, and organizational restrictions. Patients need to feel that the therapist will advocate for them both within health care organizations and in the community at large and that any personal information given by the patient will be treated with respect and the utmost confidentiality. To ensure this process occurs, physiotherapy codes of ethical practice precisely define which information must be included in patients' charts. Hospital and clinic charts are legal documents, and care is taken to ensure that reporting is accurate and does not cause harm to the patient, particularly in cases involving litigation.

The Physiotherapist and Suffering

Some physiotherapists may feel ill equipped to assist patients with issues of suffering. This may be due to the fact that as patients give physiotherapists permission to physically touch them repeatedly in the course of treatments, perceptions of intimacy may arise in which individuals reveal considerably more private, personal information to the therapist than they perhaps would under other circumstances. Effective physiotherapy involves the challenge of maintaining a professional but empathetic relationship with patients while also determining what parts of the stories patients tell actually relate to the nature and effects of the illness or injury and which ones may be unrelated. Physiotherapists need to be very conscious of the dangers of incorrectly interpreting patient stories from a psychopathological perspective. Physiotherapy education addresses these issues, but the management of suffering per se is not usually part of the physiotherapy curriculum.

Because the thrust of physiotherapy is to restore physical abilities, some therapists feel ill equipped to deal specifically with issues of suffering, which is still regarded, by some, as either a psychological illness or the secondary component of pain (15, 16). Further, others believe that if physical performance is improved, then ideas of self and personhood will automatically follow. This assumption is not always true. For example, in cases of severe trauma and disability, the degree of physical impairment may be so marked that persons may never become the people they once were. Past ideas of self are lost forever, and self-image is dramatically changed. The world that the individual once knew no longer exists. In these cases, issues of suffering are of prime importance and may have a marked impact on physical therapy treatment outcomes. Failure to acknowledge and address suffering can lead to an escalation of patient complaints and result in impairments becoming disabilities (17).

Successful rehabilitation outcomes require considerable expertise and maturity on the part of the physiotherapist if inaccurate labeling of patient behaviour is to be avoided. Another challenge to be faced is the duality of the person-centered versus the authority-based medical model approach. Both models have the potential to do harm in rehabilitation because in each model the health professional is the person with power and the patient is the subordinate, so the establishment of trust is of paramount importance. The goal of the physiotherapist is to prevent or modify disability and restore personhood. Any perception of threat to idea of self and personhood must be addressed. Exercise for the sake of increasing strength, endurance, and range of joint motion will be of little value to patients who fear they will not be able to perform activities of daily living, or work, or pursue avocational activities.

In chapter 1, we heard the story of Marlene, the young woman who was to undergo dialysis for kidney failure. In her plea for cyberspace help, she justified her pleas when she said "I used to have dreams. . . ." The role of the physiotherapist is to help individuals pursue new dreams when past ideas of self and personhood are irreparably lost. Unfortunately, under current models of care in which the health professional "knows best," conflicts between the patient's dreams and goals and the therapist's goals may result in the patient being labeled as "not accepting his condition" or being in "denial."

In spite of the fact that care contracts established between therapists and patients do allow patients more personal power, physiotherapists always have absolute power in the therapeutic relationship because the patient is the one who experiences suffering and is vulnerable. The physiotherapist's validation of the patient's perceptions of threat to self and personhood helps the patient develop timelines in which such issues are the main focus for resolution and determines the patient's perceptions of final treatment outcomes. The patient's suffering is addressed, while the therapist-patient relationship is still maintained. The following story illustrates the importance of the therapist-patient relationship and suffering.

THE STORY OF ERIC

Eric was an old soldier in a veteran's hospital. His lungs had been damaged years ago when he was in the army. Years of smoking had also taken its toll, and Eric was now in acute respiratory distress. One day, the head nurse on the ward asked if the physiotherapist would come, immediately, to see Eric because he was refusing to let the nurses suction the infected secretions out of his lungs. Clare, a physiotherapist assigned to the Respiratory ward was young and sassy. Ordinarily, she conducted the morning fitness class for all the ambulatory patients on the ward. Eric was not one of the "regulars."

As she entered Eric's room and approached his bed, Clare was met with swearing and cursing coming from Eric and the gentle but firm coaxing of the somewhat frustrated nurse in charge of his care. Clare introduced herself and told Eric that she and he were going to get him to cough up his secretions; he responded with another stream of profanities. Clare, who could "swear like a soldier" herself, responded in kind, and doing so, she noticed a slight flicker of recognition in Eric's eyes. It was that recognition that happens between people when they recognize someone like themselves. Clare's empathetic and quick evaluation of Eric was critical because it allowed Eric to see that his fear and concerns were validated while at the same time being reassured that help was available. Clare continued with the treatments, and soon Eric attempted to help her. Finally, he settled down, and the nurse was able to suction the secretions and attend to Eric's other care needs. Clare left the room telling Eric that she expected to see him in the morning exercise class in the very near future. Professionally, she was very worried about Eric because his other vital signs were not good.

Later in the afternoon, the ward nurse called again. This time she said she was calling because Eric was insisting that she call the "big mouth" physiotherapist who had helped him that morning. On the second visit, as Clare approached Eric's bed she was greeted with a tired smile, and when the nurse caught Clare's glance, she winked. At this point

Eric's eyes sparkled and the three worked together to help him breathe more easily. In the first encounter between Clare and Eric, Clare was clearly the person with power. In the second visit, Eric was in charge. The shift in the power differential between Eric and Clare helped Eric maintain his idea of self as a competent and powerful person.

In the following days the medical team was able to help Eric further, and eventually, he was part of the morning exercise class. His new treatment objectives were to be able to walk to the little restaurant near where he lived and where he usually met his buddies for morning coffee. He and Clare planned a personal exercise program that would help achieve these objectives. Eventually, the day came when Clare and Eric went for a short walk outside the hospital grounds, and on return to the hospital, stopped in the hospital coffee shop for a coffee.

In Eric's case, the therapist-patient relationship, although somewhat unorthodox, contributed positively to his health care and is an example of how sometimes unique, personal, and professional the physiotherapist-patient relationship can be. In crises when patients believe their lives are threatened, they need to hear "first we are going to do this" and then "we will work on that," and most important, "I am not going away, we are in this together." Such an approach can be the beginning of patient-therapist trust. When individuals suffer, some people may respond better to a more formal, scientific, objective approach, but all methods are part of the role of the physiotherapist who understands the nature of suffering and applies appropriate suffering-specific strategies to care. Clare, with the help of the nurse, validated Eric's experience and empathized and helped restore his autonomy, idea of self, and personhood.

Restoration of idea of self and personhood are important therapeutic objectives in physiotherapy clinical practice. These objectives can be achieved when the therapist's role is consistently that of the non-knower and the patient, the knower, is asked to define what will determine success. In most cases of chronic illness and/or injury this method of care is successful, but when it is not, referrals to other health care providers are made. The therapist can assure the patient that even though the referral is made, the physiotherapist-patient relationship remains intact. Often patients fear being labeled as being mentally ill if they seek help resolving issues of suffering. If the physiotherapist-patient relationship is very strong, the physiotherapist may ask the patient for permission to discuss his or her problems with other health care providers, such as a psychologist or social worker, to obtain advice. If such permissions are not obtained, and advice is sought from team members without patient consent, the physiotherapist-patient relationship may be irreparably damaged even though no ethical boundaries have been broken.

Finally, the physiotherapist is also the patient's advocate in the workplace. Physiotherapists, with permission from the patient, may speak to employers, lawyers, and insurance company adjusters about the patient's abilities and limitations of physical performance. It is critical that physiotherapists remember that they are the guardians of the patient's stories of self and personhood. Physiotherapy reports must always be free from bias and be relevant only to the problems that can be addressed by the technical skills of the therapist. The physiotherapist's opinions about the validity of the individual's idea of self and personhood are only of importance to others if there is a direct connection between these concerns and the presenting impairment or disability.

The final steps of effective rehabilitation involve the physiotherapist and patient determining issues that need to be addressed with the help of a social worker to enable the patient to be integrated or reintegrated into society.

The Social Worker

Historical Profile

Historically, the profession of social work originated in works of charity in the United States and the United Kingdom and evolved in response to societal problems that occurred at various times of social change. These changes range from the upheavals at the dawn of the industrial age to post–World War II social transformations involving rapid economic growth to the present shifts in societal norms due, in part, to technological advances. Initially, in the United States the poor were seen to be a direct threat to the social order, and social workers became a part of the government policies with a main function of maintaining the status quo of commerce. In the late nineteenth and early twentieth centuries, individuals such as Jane Addams and Jessie Taft changed the face of professional social work as it embraced tenets of social reform and social justice. In medicine, after the American New Deal policies of 1930, social workers began to address public health and mental health concerns of both individuals and society at large (18).

In Britain, hospital social workers were known as almoners, and in 1964 the Institute of Almoners was renamed the Institute of Medical Social Workers. The complete amalgamation of social workers and hospital almoners in Britain occurred in 1970. Currently social workers in Britain are members of the British Association of Social Workers.

Professionalism and Professional Autonomy

Social work demands considerable professional responsibility and autonomy because it is often caught in conflicts between social policy and the needs of individuals. In 2000, the International Federation of Social Workers defined social work as: "A profession that promotes social change, problem solving in human relationships, and the empowerment and liberation of people to enhance well-being. Utilizing theories of human behaviour and social systems, social work intervenes at the points where people interact with their environments. Principles of human rights and social justice are fundamental to social work" (19).

Social workers' objectives are to address social issues at all levels of life. The role involves counseling, advocacy of individuals and groups, case work, and the development and implementation of social policy. Professional accountability is mandated by professional organizations of social work such as the International Federation of Social Workers, the National School Association of Social Workers in the United States, the Canadian Association of Social Workers, and the British Association of Social Workers. Social workers are responsible not only to their professional groups but also to the institutions that employ them (20–22).

Because of the broad scope of practice, professionalism in social work has many challenges. Determinations of an appropriate knowledge base, establishment of professional boundaries between psychiatry, psychology, and other helping professions, and determining proper boundaries between worker and client are key issues. Professionalism in social work may be challenged not only by social change and reform, but also, by power politics. The complexity of the competing factors demands that ethical practice in social work be precisely defined.

Ethics in Social Work: Conflicts

The Canadian Association of Social Workers code of ethics states that social workers are obliged to work in the best interest of their clients. "Best interest" means that the wishes, desires, motivations, and plans of the client are taken as the primary consideration in any intervention plan developed by the social worker and can be changed only when the client's wishes are documented to be unrealistic, unreasonable, and potentially harmful to self or others or otherwise determined inappropriate when considered in relation to a mandated requirement (23).

Social workers' actions must be taken with the belief that the client will benefit from the action. Further, the social worker must consider the client as an individual, a member of a family unit, a member of a community, and a person with distinct ancestry or culture. These factors are to be considered in any decision affecting the client.

Others argue that social workers are the custodians of the public values of a society and that social workers must guard the moral integrity of that society. Social workers are involved with social justice issues, access to health care, civil liberties, and the fair distribution of benefits, burdens, and economic considerations of the community at large. Social workers must provide accurate information to policy workers and must be prepared to stand up for what is morally and ethically sound even if it means sacrificing their job. Social workers are obliged to monitor their own competence and that of others (24).

Because social work has a dual responsibility, both to the individual as well as to the society at large, there is the potential for considerable misunderstanding of the role of the social worker. For example, in the area of disability, advocates of the personal tragedy theory of disability view disability as a negative life event in which individuals require professional and medical assistance. The problems are viewed as primarily medical and interventions focus on the individual. Others adhere to the social oppression theory of disability and argue that disability is not due solely to impairments but also to political inequality. The focus of treatment interventions are human rights, unemployment, housing, educational access, and transportation. Some proponents argue that medicine has made individuals second-class citizens, and a plethora of advocacy groups have arisen worldwide. These arguments seem to be professional power struggles, the ethics of which are questionable. When considering the experience of suffering, care must be taken to ensure that individuals who are ill are not adversely affected by such debates.

Further, postmodern medicine has adopted the view that individuals are solely responsible for their health, and patients are now commonly referred to as clients or customers. This change in perspective has important ramifications for the quality of health care delivery provided to individuals.

Client or Customer?

The issue of nomenclature was previously discussed in chapter 6, which addresses personal autonomy and power differentials in medicine. When examining the role of the social worker, the patient/client debate takes on another dimension. It is sometimes argued that calling individuals "clients" changes the nature of the fiduciary relationship between the health care provider and the person who is ill or impaired (25–27).

Clients become objects of political machinations in which their names and corresponding illnesses, injuries, impairments, or disabilities are irrelevant. There is a depersonalization of the person. In some instances, this approach serves the greater society well. Insurance adjusters may easily deny benefits to a client, and social workers can quite objectively determine that the client has not adjusted to his/her disability. If, on the other hand, individuals are considered to be patients, that is, someone seeking care, such decisions are not made so easily. Patients have fears and worries that are in common with the fears of the health care providers. Compassion and empathy become critical outcomes of effective social work interventions. Because of the duality of the social worker's role as social advocate/activist versus professional health care provider, ethical practice in the profession of social work is of paramount importance and fraught with many challenges. Few patients are aware of this duality and the potential complexities (28–30).

The Social Worker–Patient Relationship

To be an effective consumer of health care services or to be an informed patient is the social responsibility of all individuals. In health care, it is important for patients to determine how the social worker defines his or her role. If the social worker visits an individual based on the policy needs of the health care organization, then expectations are based on social issues rather than the person's private concerns. In most hospitals, social workers have a dual role, and informed individuals must have a basic understanding of the limits and boundaries of this role. Some social workers do psychological counseling, and others are more concerned with placement, the practicalities of returning to work after illness or injury, and social fiscal resources. Often it is the social worker who is the first health care professional to help a patient determine how to create a new idea of self and explore the possible dimensions of this changed idea throughout the many aspects of the individual's life.

Relationships that involve therapeutic counseling are based on trust and mutual respect. Relationships based on fiscal restraints or policy determinations can be filled with mistrust and apprehension on the part of the person with a chronic illness. Sometimes, social workers are also involved with the personal issues of health care providers, and such relationships are based not only on trust, respect, and confidentiality but also on the social work code of ethics, which requires social workers to be vigilant in assessing health care professionals' competencies. "In-house" relationships, that is, involving colleagues with whom one works, are extremely difficult.

The Social Worker and Suffering

Social workers who do personal counseling have the skills to address the many concerns relating to the perceptions of threat to idea of self and personhood. Psychotherapeutic assessments and interventions are based on habilitation in cases of devastating disability, and rehabilitation is the goal in less catastrophic situations. Issues of mutual trust, empathy, and compassion are in common with all other health care providers. Special skills focus on determining how to provide individuals evidence that their stories of suffering are validated. In many instances of suffering the social worker is the key to helping a person make effective life transitions. Social workers are skilled in matters of public policy and so are experts in helping people retrain for new jobs. Social workers assist patients in the formulation of a new idea of self, and because of their expertise in the machinations of society, they are able to help individuals pursue a new personhood that is acceptable to the patient as well as the community.

The challenge for the social worker is to find a balance between the practicalities of life and the fear sufferers have that they are no longer part of the world they once knew, in which they felt some degree of competency. Discussions revolve around fears of loss of rights, the escalation of responsibilities sufferers have to others in their lives, and the impact of suffering on family and friends. Social workers can help individuals find appropriate community resources for financial and employment concerns and access education and social services such as housing and child care resources. More importantly, the social worker can help with the emotional rehabilitation of individuals who now must live in a reality that is unfamiliar and untried.

The social worker also advocates for those who suffer by acknowledging the patient's vulnerability to political exploitation based on fiscal objectives both in health care organizations and the work place. Often those who suffer are unable to manage returning to their previous work because they now have a sense of the futility of human endeavors. Institutions usually do not understand the process of suffering and the social responsibility of society to those who suffer. Education of the patient and the community at large is one of the goals of the social worker who addresses suffering. The social worker can help with the restoration of ideas and beliefs of self and personhood from a secular perspective and can help individuals find new ways of navigating prevailing social customs and restraints. Because of their advanced clinical skills, social workers are able to discern the differences between sorrow and clinical depression in patients and are able to ensure that patients receive optimal care.

Often social workers are the greatest clinical resource for achieving the goals of transcultural health care delivery for those who suffer. This knowledge is critical to effective family consultations and patient advocacy. Sometimes the social worker is the only health care provider with whom a sufferer feels comfortable discussing the meaning of his/her changed life because social workers, unlike chaplains, for example, are seen to be outside the realm of religious and spiritual dogma. They are the health care providers who are often the most informed about social policy. Some patients may want to examine their changed idea of self and personhood from an exclusively secular, pragmatic perspective and believe that this approach is only possible with a social worker. Achieving the goals of habilitation and rehabilitation of individuals with chronic illness or disabilities depends to a large extent on the structural competencies of social workers and their interactions with multidisciplinary health care providers.

SUMMARY

This chapter has explored the roles of physiotherapists and social workers and their roles with those who suffer. The main thrust of the arguments presented is that patients are better served if they understand the challenges and limitations of health care providers. With such knowledge, patients have more personal power and autonomy in matters of their health. The relationships between health professionals and those who suffer have considerable impact on patients' ability to restore or modify ideas of self and to embrace changed aspects of personhood. Each health care professional has specific therapeutic skills that will facilitate effective habilitation or rehabilitation of individuals with developmental impairments, chronic illnesses, and/or chronic disability.

Efficacious, cost-effective health care delivery depends on appropriate referrals, comprehensive assessments, and relevant and effective treatment interventions. Successful reintegration of individuals into the community is more likely to occur when there are realistic expectations of physiotherapists and social workers based on patients' knowledge of the health care providers' specific workplace environment and the rules and regulations relating to professionalism, autonomy, and medical ethics. In turn, health professionals must understand the cultural, ethical, spiritual, and religious orientation of the patient. The expectations of the health care provider and the patient must be in concert. Suffering does not disappear with the discharge of the patient from the hospital, but rather may persist for a considerable time. The cause of suffering may never disappear, but the power of the experience may dissipate so that individuals may, at times, experience the joys of life. The challenge to health care providers is to be able to recognize suffering as a normal life experience that may or may not be related to pain and to discern when psychological depression is impacting on the patient's ability to restore ideas of self and personhood.

The next chapter deals with challenges patients experience as they reclaim aspects of personhood after the experience of suffering. Health care professionals need to understand that individuals may need further care after discharge from health care facilities. The nature and prevalence of a wounded psyche and the differences between surviving and thriving are explored.

CHAPTER 14 QUESTIONS

1. What is the historical evolution of the profession of physiotherapy in medicine?
2. What are the key professional values identified by physiotherapists?
3. What challenges to personal integrity face individual physiotherapists who treat those who have chronic illnesses?
4. What is the nature of an effective physiotherapist-patient relationship?
5. What is the historical evolution of the profession of social work?
6. What are the ethical conflicts faced by social workers?
7. How does the relationship between the social worker and patient differ from that of the nurse, chaplain, or physiotherapist who treats individuals who suffer?
8. What are the various roles the social worker may play in the management of suffering?

15 The Wounded Spirit

RECLAIMING PERSONHOOD

The arguments previously presented in this book have focused to a large extent on factors that are perceived as a threat to idea of self and how health care professionals may help patients restore their ideas of self and cope with suffering. Suffering involves a perception of threat not only to ideas of self but also to beliefs about personhood. Personhood issues involve how patients will manage work, leisure, family responsibilities, and involvement in their communities. Health care professionals need to remember that comprehensive care of those who suffer requires an awareness that even when issues impacting on idea of self are addressed and resolved, the reintegration of those who have experienced suffering into the community may be compromised because individuals who suffer are often left with a wounded spirit. Past attitudes in which health care professionals have labeled patients as "not accepting" their illness or disability are not useful and contribute to the experience of prolonged suffering. Such labeling occurred because health care providers did not understand the nature of the concept of a wounded spirit and its impact on health.

The purpose of this chapter is to outline how restoration of idea of self is vital to resolving suffering, and how individuals may reclaim their personhood. To provide effective care, health care professionals must have an understanding of (a) factors that constitute a wounded spirit, (b) the nature of a wounded spirit in individuals who suffer because of developmental disorders, and (c) the nature of the wounded spirit and chronic illness and how individuals may reclaim personhood through either paid or unpaid work. The discussion focuses not only on the challenges individuals face when attempting reintegration into society but also on the responsibility of the health care professionals. Examples are presented from patients who have epilepsy, arthritis, or cerebral palsy.

The Wounded Spirit

For those who suffer due to chronic illness, the term *wounded spirit* refers to the memory individuals have of who they once were and the knowledge that they will never again be that person or experience their lives in ways of the past. Dreams of the future may be drastically altered or nonexistent, and fundamental spiritual and/or religious beliefs may be challenged. In North American societies, where competition and productivity are highly valued social and personal goals, some individuals with chronic illness who are no longer able to meet previous life objectives may experience feelings of worthlessness. They may feel that they are no longer part of the greater society. The relationship between dreams and well-being is important. A popular French entertainer who survived a severe health trauma once commented that although his health crisis had subsided and life now had a new rhythm, great sadness was felt because he was still unable to dream of a new future self. Loss of trust in life and the future is a common state of the wounded spirit. Sorrow often accompanies past memories of a lost idea of self and personhood. Sometimes memories of past trauma may trigger feelings of fear and dread. Laura, the patient presented in chapter 2 whose family died tragically in a car accident wrote the following about trust and loss.

> . . . Fear of death, disease, and injury,
> Now become a fear of another beating rather than a fear of losing
> For all is lost . . .

Those who suffer often report living between two worlds. One world is that of everyday life, and the other is a world they inhabit when past memories of either trauma or hopes of thwarted ideas of self and personhood are remembered.

> . . . The world becomes quiet at night
> A time of restoration, faith that a new day
> Will dawn.
> Except for those of us who dwell in this hollow place.
> For us the night is a time for waiting and enduring.

Sometimes, the wounded spirit is expressed by patients as despair that they will never establish a new rhythm for their lives.

> . . . She tried to put the pieces together to form something new.
> Just to see if she could,
> Just to see what it would be like.
> But the pieces all belonged to someone else
> And she was left with bleeding hands . . .

It is important for patients, families, and health care providers to understand that the resurgence of such memories is "normal" and not an indication of pathological illness. In some instances, soothing a wounded spirit may require the help of a health care professional. Comfort of the patient is often a neglected component of modern health care delivery.

For those who are born with developmental deficits, suffering may never be related to their impairments and/or disabilities but rather to perceptions of threat to idea of self caused by societal attitudes. Environmental boundaries and restrictive government pension regulations are factors that may contribute to feelings of worthlessness and of not being part of the general society. The nature of the wounded spirit in these cases may be due to difficulties in simply trying to establish an independent idea of self and personhood. People with developmental limitations may be so bombarded with their practical limitations that dreams of self are unattainable luxuries.

One of the themes of this book is to challenge the reader to acknowledge and understand the experience of suffering in medicine as a unique entity, separate from and only sometimes related to pain. A second theme is to understand suffering outside the domain of palliative care. Some of the processes involved in suffering, such as loss, bereavement, and grief match those of the experiences of death and dying, only in suffering, it is the death of an individual's old dream of self and the inability to assimilate into a new and different life. Individuals may be faced with the realization that they may only be able to survive their suffering, but not thrive. Surviving suffering in chronic illness entails carrying on in spite of adversity, while thriving implies the ability to flourish, improve physically, be emotionally healthy, be creative, succeed, and prosper. Whether one thrives or merely survives is a function of the extent of disability, the personality of the individual, the personal external support systems, societal environments, and unexpected future life events. The need to survive and flourish is a desire of the individual, not the health care provider. It is the responsibility of health care professionals to help individuals actualize their desires or optimize the inevitable limitations.

Clinical experience shows that everyday life is enhanced when the relationship between restoration of idea of self and personhood is in balance and the changed idea of self and new personhood is acceptable to the individual. Sometimes such equilibrium may take an individual a lifetime to achieve or recognize. Unexpected current life events may trigger distressing memories of past experiences. Care of the wounded spirit is critical to achieve the societal goals of preventative medicine. Patients may again need the help of family doctors, social workers, pastors, psychologists, and sometimes psychiatry. Such occurrences are part of the process of maintaining the self and personhood after the experience of suffering. Failure to acknowledge and understand the dynamics of the wounded spirit may result in incomplete assessment of patient health care problems and an escalation of visits to physicians. Care of individuals also involves care of the family.

Restoring the rhythm of life after suffering due to chronic illness is complicated. For example, a study of families of patients with end-stage renal disease who were treated with renal dialysis showed that the family's strong sense of unity was correlated with early death of the patient. The authors of this study postulated that the high level of engagement of the family with each other and the patient may have resulted in the patient deciding to sacrifice himself to protect the family from further suffering (1). In other studies in which families received family counseling, outcomes were much more positive. This view was expressed in a study of families of individuals with hypertension. Those families who received family therapy demonstrated a 75% lower mortality (2).

Some of the problems that may arise in families with members who have a chronic illness are rigid family roles, unclear communication methods, poor problem-solving skills, blurred power boundaries, and unresolved past family conflicts. Often the patient may react more strongly to how the family responds to the situation than to the difficulties of the actual illness (3).

Many who experience suffering in medicine and are left with a wounded spirit have considerable difficulty healing these psychological wounds. In addition to the power differentials that exist in the medical system, which, as we have seen, can contribute to feelings of powerlessness in the patient, family power differentials are often forced to shift due to the chronicity of the illness. Sometimes marital roles change with the once-dominant person now being in a dependent role. In single-parent families, the children may be deprived of any parental figure and may even take on the role of the missing parent. The child faces additional suffering because his/her idea of self as a child is threatened or lost. In cases where the family member must be institutionalized, family members may believe that they have failed to manage or tolerate the patient's disability. Such families may undergo much personal guilt and be subjected to the disapproval of others in their communities. This fact is especially true when families belong to a culture in which family care of the ill is an important value. In such situations, individual family members may also experience the sorrow of a wounded spirit.

Systems theory has long argued that if one component of the family system changes, the whole system changes. In contemporary society, where the concept of family has much variability based on nonmarital unions, nonbiological extended families, and multicultural traditions, healing of the wounded spirit is very challenging. Because of this variability, precise problem identification is critical to successful problem resolution. To achieve this goal, health care providers have a useful measurement tool such as the MASQ, which quickly identifies those who are experiencing suffering so that suffering as an entity separate from pain is not overlooked and appropriate care is provided.

To help those whose spirit is wounded, clinicians and the community at large must recognize that the negative power of past memories of self and personhood is diminished if those who are part of the patient's world know that with the onset of chronic illness or injury individuals may feel that they have become "psychological refugees" in a world that is no longer familiar (4). As we have seen expressed by Laura at the beginning of this chapter, some sufferers believe they no longer fit in with the people and events of their past life and many struggle with feelings of not being "normal." While people with chronic illnesses or disabilities may soon learn that being different is also normal, unfortunately, the community they belong to often does not, but rather views people with chronic illness as broken.

The Wounded Spirit and Developmental Disorders

As a young physiotherapist, I worked in a school for disabled children. I made a point of doing therapy with the children outside the walls of the clinic. We would practice gait training as we walked along a neighboring street and, weather permitting, sometimes did exercises in a little park next to the clinic. On occasion we would meet people who made comments about how sad it was that "such a pretty little girl or charming little boy is so crippled." Later, the child and I would talk about the encounter and talk about what to say in response to such comments. These wee children knew that in addition to all the health challenges they had to manage, they also had the additional job of educating others so that people might understand that individuals with physical and emotional limitations were normal. We talked about the fact that all people have limitations but many of these limitations are not readily visible. While I hope that these "talks" helped these children as they got older, it became apparent that often the children did not interpret such remarks the same way I did. Usually, the children's responses were much more practical and direct. One little boy replied by saying "my mother said that I'm not supposed to talk to strangers," and another little girl was fascinated by the speaker's gold tooth and in all innocence asked, "Why do you have that shiny tooth?" While innocence offers some protection for children, often little attention is paid to the development of ideas of self and personhood as the child ages. In medicine, emphasis is usually on physical and emotional capabilities, as these constructs are related to "acceptable" behaviour and performance rather than to the development of dreams of self and personhood.

In patients with developmental deficits, grief is often experienced throughout life, as they continue to realize the extent of their physical limitations and lost opportunities because of their impairments. They may have to mourn the lost opportunities, the loss of what might have been if not for their impairments. They may be bereaved for considerable periods of time and have periods throughout their lives when they grieve the loss of what society deems as "normal." However, if health care professionals understand the process of suffering as separate from pain, then perceptions of threat to idea of self and personhood of both the patient and their families may be repeatedly addressed as the child ages. As mentioned in chapter 5 in the story of Robbie, the little boy whose mother had dyed his hair green, health care providers cannot assume that disability implies suffering. Robbie's ideas of self and self-image were not limited by the restrictions imposed on his physical capabilities due to his cerebral palsy. In retrospect, it seems that perhaps Robbie's mother was suffering, but instead of exploring this possibility, she was labeled by health care professionals as being mentally ill, and the possibility of the impact of suffering on emotional health was overlooked.

In cases of developmental deficits, patients and their families experience suffering. When one member of a family experiences suffering, responses to the experience affect all the other members of the family. In many instances in which children are born with developmental and/or genetic disorders, the family unit does not remain intact. Feelings of intense grief, guilt, and sorrow, when unaddressed, may result in dissolution of the family. More research is needed to determine the impact of these events on health and health care costs.

As children get older they have many other questions about their competency and normalcy. Physically challenged children have a history of questions and answers that are addressed over the years that aid in the development of idea of self and personhood. Families can be helped to understand that in spite of physical and/or emotional difficulties, their children still have the same psychological life development tasks to address as non-impaired persons do. Issues of trust, separation from parents, dichotomies between desires for independence versus dependency needs are examples of life tasks facing all children. Families need the reassurance that, although it may take their children longer, they will be able to achieve the goals of personhood. Independence may simply mean being able to dress oneself and perhaps attend the neighborhood school rather than a special private school for the disabled. Many of my former patients that I meet in later years have assumed the responsibility of educating others simply by the example of their very productive lives.

Some patients who were severely handicapped children later married and now have families, hold satisfying jobs, and are active members of their communities. Others live in supported environments and participate actively within these communities. Much can be learned from those who have experienced challenges from birth, and much of what we learn comes from welcoming people with disabilities into our lives in friendship.

The Wounded Spirit and Patients with a Chronic Illness

For individuals whose idea of self and personhood are threatened or changed due to the onset of chronic illness or injury, the process of integration back into their community is very different from that of children and adults who are born with developmental delays or disabilities. The resolution of suffering involves many experiences that in some ways are similar to the events that occur at times of death or dying.

Suffering due to chronic illness can involve the loss of overall health as well as a loss of strength and mobility. Consequently, patients are bereaved. Bereavement is the time that a person spends actively dealing with what is perceived as the threat of the actual loss of idea of self and personhood. Grief refers to the thoughts, feelings, attitudes, and psychological responses that occur within a person during bereavement. Mourning involves the public behaviours and ritual expressions of grief that a society deems appropriate and helpful for a person to practice during bereavement. Patients mourn the loss of their former idea of self and past activities and promises of personhood. In the case of suffering in medicine, patients are often abandoned or further traumatized because society may only accept certain ritual expressions as appropriate or suitable during this type of bereavement. Health care professionals may determine that crying and other expressions of sorrow are indicators of clinical depression rather than appropriate expressions of grief. Sometimes the patient becomes prematurely labeled with a psychological illness. Others in the community may determine that such expressions of grief indicate that the person does not want to accept their changed situations or are being manipulative for personal gain. It is important to realize that people may have to psychologically say goodbye to their old dreams of self and all that those dreams promised. Patients may not immediately know what the new idea of self will be or how this self will accomplish the tasks of everyday living.

Mourning may be an extended process for individuals with chronic illnesses because it takes a considerable length of time for health care professionals and patients to determine whether there will be any further improvement in the degree of impairment. Further, grief is a very normal response to such losses, and the memory of the extent of these losses may never be forgotten. The memories may linger but usually with much less power. At other times, grief may be enhanced as disabilities become worse due to ageing and/or other health problems that may arise over time. At best, such memories may fade to the point where they are simply poignant memories of the past.

The failure of health care practitioners to understand the dynamics of the wounded spirit, may result in its misinterpretation as a sign of psychological illness in the patient. The process of unresolved grief in chronic illness often revolves around health status and barriers to participation in community life. Work is central to a purposeful life in many cultures.

The Wounded Spirit: Reintegration into the Community

Work serves many purposes relating to personhood. When people work they meet other people, they help others in the workplace, and they get to know the self better. It can be argued that people have a "work instinct," and work is intricately bound to maintaining good health, effective family dynamics, satisfying leisure activities, sacred religious observation, and ethical participation in a community.

Work provides people with a sense of dignity. Work is perceived as a job, a career or a calling. Meaningful work is said to involve doing something that (a) has a social purpose and contributes to society, (b) has an element of moral correctness, (c) is enjoyable, at least in part, (d) provides one with a degree of autonomy and recognition for skills, and (e) provides the worker with the opportunity to have good relationships with others (5). Work allows one to excel and to exercise intelligence, imagination, and skill, key factors of personhood. It can be argued that some contemporary managers view workers as resources, and this attitude not only harms the individual but degrades society as a whole (5–7). If the thesis of work as a determinant of good health is accepted, then what is to be said of those whom society perceives as not working? How does the lack of recognized work affect the health of those who are retired or the elderly? What effect does work have on health when the above criteria of meaningful work are not possible? How do individuals attain a sense of self-worth when abilities and opportunities for meaningful work are not possible? (8).

As we have seen, those who suffer because of illness or injury do work; that is, they do something meaningful and useful in society. They work to preserve or maintain their idea of self and personhood. They work to find a new central purpose in life. They work often not merely to survive but to contribute. They work to resolve interpersonal discord with others and they work to overcome self-conflict. Resolution of these tasks enhances the quality of the individual's life and curbs health care expenditures. Clearly, these activities meet the criteria for work.

It is not only health care providers who have difficulties understanding the process of suffering as distinct from pain or the nature of the wounded spirit. Society at large often fails to understand suffering outside the contexts of palliative care or religious and spiritual teachings. Individuals and communities often fail to recognize how the law and spiritual and cultural traditions affect those who suffer. As a result, those who suffer may be seen to be the creators of their own misfortune and as a fiscal liability to society. In medicine, viewing suffering outside such constructs not only enhances the health status of patients but may also result in a decrease of pain. Much more research in the fields of biological and sociological science is needed to test these hypotheses. It is also critical to understand suffering from the perspective of personhood, particularly in the habilitation and rehabilitation of those with chronic illnesses or disabilities. My research team explored the concept of work. The results revealed the following information.

In our initial study (6) about suffering in chronic illness, a group of 81/122 patients, who had arthritis for a mean duration of 10.86 ± 11.14 SD years were assessed. Their mean age was 60.27 ± 13.35 SD years and 29% of the people were taking antidepressant medication. On admission to a day hospital program, 77% of the patients were very concerned about how they would manage life in the future. On discharge, only 45% had this same degree of concern. In these cases there was little or no change in the degree of impairment. The greatest change was that all people had an exercise program involving group and individual participation and access to the health care team as needed. People cared about them and rewarded them with praise for their efforts.

Patients also reported that life would be very difficult if their present support system was not available but most patients believed they would cope. People said that they would adapt to whatever change demanded. While most patients believed that others expected them to do their best, they sometimes felt more was expected than was possible. Many individuals also reported that they believed that others wanted them to be the same as they were in the past. Patients also wanted to be the same as they had once been. Often expectations of what constituted "doing my best" were different between patients and others. Patients wanted to be self-reliant, independent, and active. Only a very small number (less than 2%) did not have any expectations of themselves, most people expected "a lot" from themselves. When patients were asked how they saw themselves in the future, most people envisioned having their families and other supportive people around them. Again, many wanted to be active and independent and enjoying life.

An important finding was that nearly 50% of the people who on admission to the day hospital program said they feared becoming disabled did not have that fear on discharge. Aging was another concern, as was the belief that individuals would not make any further gains in rehabilitation. A few people said they had no thoughts about the future. Other issues of concern that were identified were loneliness, inability to work or return to work, financial stability, and self-image. Males were significantly more concerned that they would not be able to manage alone. Pain was not identified as a major issue by males or females. Clearly, there are many factors that contribute to prolonged suffering and result in a wounded spirit. Because of the advanced age of those studied, work consisted primarily of self-maintenance. In many cases, health care providers and health care systems become an intrinsic component of an individual's community life.

In younger people, the issue of work defined as doing something useful or meaningful in society is also of considerable concern. In a group of 113 people with epilepsy whose mean age was 41.56 ± 11.42 SD years, 43/113 were seizure free. Fifty-five (55/113) were diagnosed with complex partial seizures, 52/113 had tonic-clonic seizures and 6/113 were not classified. Fifty-six (56) individuals worked outside the home and 57 did not. Of those who worked, 12/56 had more than one seizure per month, 43/56 were seizure free, and in 1/56 case seizure frequency was unknown. Of those who did not work, 29/57 had more than one seizure per month,

24/57 were seizure free, and in 4/57 cases seizure frequency was unknown. None of the patients were on antidepressant medications. All were on anticonvulsant polytherapy. Of the total group, 49% had multiple medical disorders and 45% only had epilepsy. Nineteen percent (19%) of the people lived alone, 4% had no family contact, 36% had no formal job training, 35% were trained on the job, 50% currently had a paid job, and 80% of those with a paid job worked full time. Of those with a paid job, 52% were female. In total, 56/100 worked for monetary compensation. Thirty-five percent (35%) were on a disability pension, but of those with pain only 45% received a pension. Total suffering scores were significantly higher in the nonworking group as were measures of pain. Items that assessed self-efficacy or self-confidence were greater in those patients who worked. Reasons for the above results were explored further. The first issue was to determine if there were work belief differences between those who worked and those who did not.

Those who did not work were more likely to believe that one had to work to be considered "normal." They believed that their families did not want them to work outside the home for fear of sustaining injuries or injuring others. This concern was particularly true with female respondents. Males were more likely to believe one had to work to be considered "normal," and potential pension loss was of greater concern to males. Nonworkers also believed that they did not have enough education to get a job and could not get transportation to and from work if they did get work. They also believed that they would not be able to take their medication on time if working, and they were very concerned that they would lose their pension benefits if they had a job. They believed that seizures would negatively affect job performance. Nonworkers also believed that not having a job was the only barrier to independent living, while those who worked generally did not hold this view. The inability to work is a factor contributing to the development of a wounded spirit.

The resolution of suffering depends not only on restoration of ideas of self but also on the ability to structure or restructure issues of personhood. The examples above show that thriving after suffering is enhanced if individuals (a) have good family support, (b) work outside the home, (c) believe others care about them, (d) have a community of which they are a part and, (e) have confidence (self-efficacy) in their abilities. Individuals with disabilities or severe impairments who work are only allowed to earn a small amount of money before their disability pensions are decreased or terminated. These government rules are often insurmountable barriers to independent living. In the group of arthritis patients, many had such difficulties. Most people were unemployed either because of age or disability. Loss of loved ones, separation from family, and job loss due to retirement were all key factors of prime concern to health providers rehabilitating the elderly. Further, most of the elderly patients in the study were diagnosed with clinical depression and were managed with drug therapy. There was no evidence that the issue of a wounded spirit had been considered (9).

SUMMARY

This chapter explored the nature of the wounded spirit and factors that relate to the reclaiming of personhood after debilitating chronic illness or injury. The concept of a wounded spirit was briefly explored from the perspectives of individuals born with developmental limitations and those with acquired disabilities due to chronic illness. The reintegration of individuals with epilepsy into their community showed that work is a critical factor contributing to an individual's positive idea of self and the attainment of personal power (6, 8). An exploration of work indicates that work does not simply involve payment for tasks performed. Work occurs anytime someone does something that is useful and meaningful in society. In chronic illness, maintenance of the self and personhood benefit society from the perspectives of both social ethics and fiscal expenditures. Examples of work and work beliefs were presented from two distinct populations of persons with chronic illnesses. Results from a group of older patients who had arthritis were contrasted with a group of younger individuals with epilepsy. Many of the patients with arthritis were taking medications to treat depression. It may be that many people who were diagnosed as having clinical depression were actually expressing their suffering through sorrow and sadness.

In contemporary society there is much concern in the popular press about the over prescription of medications to patients, particularly the elderly. Understanding the differences between the process of suffering and the expression of the experience of suffering may help address this problem. Not only do many health care providers see suffering as a secondary component of pain, some also see sorrow, one of the expressions of suffering, and clinical depression as one and the same psychological illness. One of the major challenges to surviving suffering is the failure to understand the distinctions between sorrow and clinical depression and the impact of fear, anxiety, and loneliness on those who suffer. The following chapter addresses these issues and shows the power of human creativity to overcome these obstacles.

CHAPTER 15 QUESTIONS

1 What is the nature of a wounded spirit?
2 How do the challenges to restoring idea of self and personhood differ between those individuals who have developmental disabilities and those with acquired impairments or disabilities?
3 What is the nature of bereavement, grief, and mourning in individuals who suffer because of chronic illness?

4. How do individuals with developmental disorders experience bereavement, grief, and mourning?
5. What role does "work" play in the resolution of suffering?
6. What familial dynamics may contribute not only to suffering but also to its resolution?

16 Surviving and Thriving

Research confirms clinical observations that suffering and pain are separate and only sometimes related phenomena. In medicine, suffering is defined outside the context of, but not in opposition to, religious, spiritual, or political teachings. Suffering is a perception of threat to idea of self and personhood and has distinct and universal characteristics, the expressions of which are personal and idiosyncratic. In clinical practice, failure to make the distinction between the process of suffering and the personal expression of the experience can lead to the development of chronic health problems and even disability.

The influences of religious and spiritual teachings, medical and legal discourse, cultural traditions, and the conflicts between demands of psychological developmental tasks across the life span are examples of the myriad factors contributing to the experience of suffering. Key issues of concern, as determined from studies of over 300 patients with chronic illnesses such as arthritis, epilepsy, migraine headache, and spinal cord injuries, centre on the degree of concern that patients have that their illness or injury will have a negative effect on the challenges of ageing, their relationships with a partner, children, friends, personal life goals, work beliefs, job performance, and community involvement.

The importance of understanding the language of suffering and its relevance to patient power and autonomy has been shown, and strategies for care demand a multi- and interdisciplinary approach. Measures of suffering need to be included in patient assessments, and suffering-specific treatments are needed for optimal patient care as well as cost containment in health care delivery. Suffering is a life experience that impacts significantly on health and is a concern for all health care practitioners.

As we have seen in previous chapters, there are many societal beliefs and attitudes that can contribute to or escalate suffering. Failure to differentiate individuals' idiosyncratic expressions of suffering from mental illness also has adverse effects on health and well-being.

The purpose of this final chapter is to (a) delineate common misunderstandings of the differences between sorrow and depression and between depression and suffering, (b) discuss the influence of fear, anxiety, and loneliness, and (c) illustrate how facilitating personal creativity can help overcome these obstacles to surviving suffering and restore personal power.

Obstacles to Surviving and Thriving

Sorrow and Depression

The process of surviving suffering is a profound life experience, and many of the fundamental tasks essential for personal survival have been explored. We have seen that suffering is a much neglected and misunderstood concept in medicine because suffering is often related to pain but hardly ever considered in its own right. Suffering and sorrow are sometimes perceived as one and the same phenomenon. In the care of individuals with chronic illnesses, differentiation between the construct of suffering and that of sorrow is valuable. Sorrow is an expression of profound sadness, unhappiness, mournfulness, ruefulness, grief, heartache, or bereavement. It is a profound response to adversity that occurs in the human life experience. Even though patients who experience sorrow may have considerable difficulty managing everyday tasks, the element of hope that events will improve is not totally lost (1).

During the process of suffering, individuals may experience all or none of these phenomena in response to a loss of central purpose in their lives or because of impaired interpersonal relationships and feelings of self-conflict. Suffering and sorrow may erroneously be thought to be one and the same, but suffering is an experience to which sorrow may or may not occur as a response. Sometimes, sorrow is further mislabeled as clinical or major depression, but psychologists clearly identify clinical depression as a disease (2). While such classifications may be useful to science, the stigma of mental illness persists in contemporary society and may negatively impact not only on an individual's identity but also on ideas of self. One challenge to contemporary psychology/psychiatry is to accurately differentiate "normal" sadness or sorrow from clinical depression.

Depression has many meanings in contemporary society. Generally, depression is a term used when individuals have a pessimistic sense of inadequacy in which there is a despondent lack of activity as well as an accompanying loss of interest or pleasure in normal activities. In medicine, clinical depression is a mental disorder and is currently understood to be characterized by a broad spectrum of symptom type, severity, and course of illness. It is generally defined as "a disease with characteristic affective, cognitive and vegetative complaints which has a typical course and predictable response rate to treatment" (3). Symptoms and signs vary across the life span, and clinical depression is often associated with other physical and/or psychological conditions. The syndrome of depression includes both psychological and somatic symptoms (3–7). The diagnosis of clinical depression carries with it a social stigma as do various types of chronic illnesses such as epilepsy and other types of physical disability. Health care providers should not add to patients' health care burdens by incorrectly labeling sorrow as clinical depression.

Suffering is a normal life experience, not a disorder, and is defined as "a state of severe distress associated with events that threaten the intactness of the person" (8). This process of suffering continues until the perceived threat is removed or the integrity of the person is restored. Clinical depression falls within the medical dichotomy of mental vs. physical disorders.

Depression and Suffering

Suffering is a life experience in which there is a perception of threat to an individual's dream of self and how the individual believes he/she should behave in the face of adversity. Individuals who suffer lose their sense that life has a central purpose, and they experience considerable self-conflict and impaired interpersonal relationships. In chronic illness, some cases of prolonged and unrelieved suffering may lead to clinical depression and a failure to thrive if the patient believes that he/she is no longer able to be part of the community and has no emotional support from family or friends. In clinical depression, a variety of symptoms may occur that reflect a sad and/or irritable mood. Health care professionals label these symptoms as clinical depression when they deem them to have exceeded normal sadness or grief and the quality of the experience of depression is moribund in nature. That is, the individual has a feeling that he/she has little or no internal vital force left within the body and/or mind; there is no hope. Depressive signs are characterized not only by negative thought but by marked neuro-vegetative signs that indicate that there are changes in the brain causing a profound decrease in normal activity and engagement in life. Unresolved clinical depression may result in a failure to survive.

When considering the concept of thriving as opposed to surviving, it is important to understand the differences between suffering and clinical depression. There are many theories of the etiology of clinical depression. The literature reveals several theories dealing with biological factors such as neurotransmitters, hormones, and biological rhythms as well as genetic predisposition, environmental influences, and developmental events (5). Clinical depression is said to be multifactorial and is influenced by a combination of events such as life stressors and lack of social support. While those who suffer may also have life stressors and lack social support, the process of suffering is unique because suffering involves a perception of threat, and it is the patient, not the health care professional, who determines whether suffering is occurring or not. The expression of both suffering and clinical depression may be culturally bound, but the nature of the experiences is different (5–7).

Suffering may originate from any circumstance that the individual perceives as a threat to any aspect of his/her person. Threats originate from events that have an intense personal meaning to the individual and that the person labels and interprets as life threatening. Such perceptions of threat are highly personal. The same event can elicit different thoughts, emotions, and actions in different individuals. What causes suffering in one individual may be inconsequential in another. Paradoxically, in medicine, suffering can arise from the onset of disease as well as from treatments if individuals perceive these events as impacting on the wholeness of the person. Due to the vast and encompassing nature of suffering, anyone who is aware of themselves as an individual, a person, experiences suffering at some point in their lives. Conversely, not everyone will have an episode of clinical depression in their lifetime, despite biology, culture, or environment.

There are also significant differences in the diagnosis of suffering and depression. While both suffering and depression are subjective experiences, they are diagnosed in very different ways and by very different experts. When dealing with depression, medical nosologies such as the American Psychiatric Association's Diagnostic and Statistical Manual (currently DSM-IV-TR) or the World Health Organization's International Classification of Disease (ICD-10) are used. At least five of the following symptoms must simultaneously present for at least a period of two weeks to make a positive diagnosis. They are: depressed mood, anhedonia, loss of energy, loss of confidence or self-esteem, sleep disturbances, change in appetite, negative self-concept or guilt, difficulty in concentration, psychomotor agitation or retardation, and suicidal ideation. The subjective character of the diagnosis of clinical depression stems from the fact that there are no physiological tests to firmly indicate a biological disorder, but rather symptoms serve as the criteria for diagnosis. The diagnosis of depression is usually made by a physician, be it in primary care or by a specialist in psychiatry or psychology.

Determinations of suffering, on the other hand, are made by asking the expert, who in this case is the patient. Although some injuries, losses, or threats seem to be universal, they are still experienced by individuals in a particular place and time. Because one can only have indirect knowledge of another's suffering, the causes of suffering are idiosyncratic and cannot be anticipated. Currently, there are no biological markers and no formal diagnostic criteria (8, 9). The diagnosis of suffering is further confounded, as we have seen, by a lack of understanding of the language of suffering and the expectations of the nature of suffering in contemporary society.

Experts in the field (10) argue that it is necessary to have a deep understanding of patients as individuals if one is to grasp and relieve their suffering. Until recently, no systems or tools were available to help the clinician quickly identify those who suffer. A tool entitled the MASQ (Measuring and Assessing Suffering Questionnaire), discussed in chapter 9 of this book, has been developed to facilitate the recognition of suffering in patients with chronic illness or disabilities. The use of tools such as the MASQ not only facilitates the identification of suffering individuals by clinicians but also overcomes counteractive mechanisms sometimes utilized by patients who try to manage their own suffering.

Depression then is a mental disorder diagnosed by an expert clinician based on the signs and symptoms of patients. While suffering does have universal characteristics, it is a process that is diagnosed by the person who experiences it. Treatment objectives for depression and suffering are vastly different. While the construct of depression is more elaborately defined than the experience of suffering, the treatment of depression is more straightforward.

Conventional treatments for depression include pharmacology, psychotherapy, or a combination of both. There are myriad alternative treatments including exercise, acupuncture, massage therapy, yoga, transcranial magnetic stimulation, homeopathy, and vitamin therapies. These interventions vary in their degrees of success and relapse depending on the nature of the depression. Treatments are aimed at physiological, psychological, and environmental factors thought to be involved in the etiology of depression. In severe cases of clinical depression, the main treatment objective is survival rather than thriving. Many long-term drug therapy regimes inhibit patients' attempts to thrive because of drug side effects.

In essence, suffering is relieved when the nature of the perceived threat and its impact on the person is known. When the threat is removed or replaced in importance, suffering is resolved. For example, a dance instructor who is disabled because of severe arthritis may suffer not only because she believes her body is unattractive because of joint abnormalities caused by the disease but also because she is no longer able to dance professionally and consequently unable to earn a living. If health care providers listen to the story of her fears with "empathetic attentiveness" and engage in her attempts to restore her idea of self using "nondiscursive thinking," the patient may be helped to recognize elements impacting on her integrity and find a resolution to her suffering (10). We have discussed potential suffering treatment methodologies in considerable detail in previous chapters. Often patients who suffer are helped by simply assigning meaning to past behaviours or beliefs, while for others, a deep spiritual transcendence occurs. In the example of the dancer with severe arthritis, she may discover that she is more than her physical body. She might realize that throughout her life friends always commented on her infectious laugh and beautiful smile. Remembering that children always love her and gravitate to her mischievous personality and acknowledging her gifts of being an excellent teacher might help her resolve suffering. She may need professional assistance as well, and speaking with her doctor about using a variety of methods to modify pain may be of value. The patient might decide to teach children to dance as a way of restoring the central purpose of her life. In the process of determining a new purpose for her life, this individual might be able to restore past interpersonal relationships and learn new ways of relating to others. Issues of self-conflict may be restored by recognizing the full dimension of her idea of self rather than focusing solely on the idea of a physically beautiful dancer. This example shows how individuals who suffer can pass through stages of surviving as a person to thriving.

A challenge for health care providers is to recognize that suffering is not depression or pain but a distinct entity with universal measurable characteristics. Suffering may, in some cases, be directly related to pain, and in these situations pain control is the first priority of treatment. Prolonged unresolved suffering may lead to clinical depression, and in such cases immediate psychological and/or psychiatric care must be implemented, but many health care providers question whether what is labeled by patients as depression and/or pain is often actually unrelieved suffering. While injury to personhood can be expressed by a range of emotions including sadness, anger, and depression, the affect, that is, the outward expression of injury, is not the injury itself. Because of negative societal attitudes towards depression, individuals labeled with this problem may experience a profound stigma attached to their identity. They become known as "Mary, who is mentally ill." The challenge for such individuals is to not incorporate pathology into their idea of self. Patients are more than their symptoms. Recognition of the power of stigma is important because in some cases depression in chronic illness may actually be suffering that has not been addressed. Failure to understand the differences between clinical depression and suffering may affect the integrity of the person who still has inner unresolved conflicts. Clearly, differentiation of suffering as distinct from depression is critical to the effective health care management of individuals with a chronic illness or disability.

Fear, Anxiety, and Loneliness

When people survive suffering they may be left with a wounded spirit, and thoughts and feelings about old disappointments and sadness over lost dreams may resurrect. Surviving suffering demands an ability to restructure the idea of self and personhood and the ability and opportunity to reintegrate into the general community. Considerable courage is required to overcome the fear and anxiety generated by suffering in chronic illness. Not only do patients have to retrain their body to perform tasks in a variety of different ways, they must readjust every aspect of their life. The process of resolving suffering may involve times in which patients experience a great deal of fear and anxiety and times when they fear being overcome not only by a personal sense of loneliness but also the existential loneliness common to mankind. The question then arises as to how health care professionals may be of further assistance.

Individuals with unresolved suffering may believe that they are committed to a life in which they are cursed or helpless victims. To some clinicians, the idea of being cursed connotes primitive beliefs about witchcraft or the occult, and victimization may be interpreted by psychology as "catastrophizing" (5). Dismissive negative judgments about the patient's mental health capabilities may be made by health care professionals when individuals hold these views. Such professional attitudes seem incongruous when nearly every spiritual and religious tradition in the world acknowledges the existence and power of personal beliefs on health. Failure to know the patients as whole persons may result in an escalation of suffering because individuals have no one that can be trusted with their worries and fears. Consequently, patients are often lonely for someone who understands their fears outside the context of professionalism. There is profound longing and loneliness for simple human compassion and kindness over scientific expertise. Patients are lonely not only for the lost self but also for their lost world. Health care providers can help patients by simply sitting and listening, often to the same story being told over and over again. Understanding the need to blame someone or something for the patient's predicament is critical to the resolution of suffering. Eventually, with compassionate care, the individual realizes that sometimes bad things just happen and no one, especially the patient, is to blame. Sometimes patients are terrified that other catastrophic events will continue to follow the advent of illness and disability. They wait for the next bad event. A comforting presence and the simple reassurance that these fears are not uncommon and that both the clinician and patient will work together no matter what the future holds can make all the difference. Failure to address the fear and anxiety patients experience may result in further deterioration of health. Again, talking about the fears and taking action, perhaps through exercise or creative acts of writing about concerns, will help manage fear and anxiety. It is of considerable value if clinicians can, at times, relate their own personal experiences of fear and anxiety to patients and show how these issues can be resolved.

Individuals may also experience much anxiety due to conflicting cultural, religious, and social beliefs that they once held about their idea of self. While we have explored the ways various spiritual traditions address suffering, we have not addressed the belief of some that suffering is a life experience with an intrinsic value in human existence.

Some individuals may believe that their chronic illness or disability is a punishment or a curse from God for past bad behaviours, while others may believe that their suffering will bring rewards in an after life. Patients who hold these views may be overcome at times with a fear that their beliefs are false. These beliefs must be heard and respected. The role of the clinician now includes giving patients a "scientific blessing," which involves helping them understand that they are not responsible for their illness or disability. The probable scientific factors leading to the chronic nature of the illness or disability must once again be explained.

Health care professionals can reassure patients that all people experience these fears from time to time. Special psychological techniques used in stress management classes can help individuals regain a sense of control over their body, mind, and emotions.

When suffering is unresolved, clinicians must often reestablish new personal bonds of trust with patients, based on respect for patients' spiritual/religious beliefs, even if those beliefs are not values acknowledged by medicine per se. Kindness and compassion supersedes scientific expertise. Reassurance of the individual's worth as a human being and the uniqueness of the person as an individual may be of considerable value in assisting the patient's management of fears and anxiety about surviving suffering. Health care professionals must also have the courage and ability to acknowledge their own existential fears and to share their feelings and ideas with their patients while still maintaining a professional relationship. Patients must know that the bonds of trust between them and their health care provider will not be broken.

If we recall the story of Marron, the young woman who believed that she needed to go to a tribal medicine man to obtain a charm to protect her from a curse that she believed had been place on her, we remember that acceptance of that practice by the health care team was pivotal in her successful physical and emotional rehabilitation. Health care providers need to be open to the beliefs and cultural traditions that may be unfamiliar or contrary to the beliefs of the health care provider. Effective health professionals are willing to work with patients and families when beliefs are outside the usual boundaries of medicine (9).

To assist clinicians in achieving this goal, accurate objective clinical notes are required. Some professionals, such as nurses and chaplains, also do reflective journaling in which they document not only what individuals say verbatim but also what the health professional determines is the meaning of this information. Further, clinicians may choose to seek personal advice from their colleagues in social work, psychology, psychiatry, and chaplaincy when there are deep conflicts between patient and clinical beliefs. Reflective journaling also can assist the clinician to be sure that he or she is understanding the nature of the patient's story and to confirm troubling elements with the patient on subsequent visits.

The relationship between the patient with chronic illness and the health care provider may persist intermittently over the lifetime of the patient. Profession-specific problems will be addressed over the years. The issue of suffering may never arise again, but health care providers must always be on the alert for the reoccurrence of further suffering. Early detection depends on simply knowing the patient as a person, a factor sometimes forgotten in contemporary medicine, where successful treatments are determined by changes in technological tests rather than on the quality of health of the whole person. All of medicine's efforts to help with the resolution of suffering are in vain if an individual's creative impulse to survive and thrive is not respected and acknowledged.

Thriving after Suffering: Creativity and Power

Creativity is often thought of in terms of artistic abilities, but there are many fields of medicine, such as art therapy and cognitive behaviour therapy, that use the inherent creative impulse within all human beings as both a diagnostic and a therapeutic tool. When the health goal is to thrive rather than simply survive, imagination and intuition may serve patients well. Nearly every physiotherapist knows that complete rehabilitation of patients with chronic illness or disability involves more than improving physical performance. Rehabilitation is also a process in which the patient's creative abilities play an enormous part. For example, the most effective adaptive equipment has come about because patients with disabilities have discovered creative ways and methods to solve the myriad problems associated with activities of daily living. Many of these "discoveries" have been incorporated into commercial devices. The ability of patients to restructure ideas of self and create new lives and careers is remarkable. Because many associate creativity solely with artistic competence, the ability to thrive after suffering demands a clear understanding of the construct of creativity outside the parameters of the fine arts.

Much scholarly work has been done in the field of mental health and creativity, but much more work is needed in the area of creativity in everyday life, particularly with those who suffer after chronic illness. Definitions of creativity vary but generally include the idea of mental and social processes that generate new ideas or concepts or new associations between existing ideas or concepts. This process is thought to be driven by conscious or unconscious insight. Everyday creativity can be defined as "products, ideas or behaviours produced or occurring in day-to-day activities that are characterized by originality and their meaningfulness to others" (10, p. 620). In the area of social science research, creativity is seen to have four domains. They involve the creative process per se, which includes cognitive, behavioural, and environmental factors. Further, to be creative, one must have skills in a particular area and must have ideas or behaviours that are produced as a result of everyday occurrences and that are original and meaningful to others. The last component is that individuals must be open to being imaginative and intuitive and have the personality traits that permit them to act upon their creative impulses (11, 12).

When exploring unresolved suffering and/or the nature of the wounded spirit in those individuals who for the most part have survived suffering, emotional creativity is an issue that requires much more consideration and study. Highly creative people are said to be individuals who are able to recognize patterns of behaviour and events from the world around them and make connections between these events. Creative people are thought to be flexible thinkers who take risks and are open to challenging assumptions. Further, they are able to take advantage of chance events and see issues in new ways. These are qualities that are essential to the resolution of suffering. Factors such as personality, motivation, and cognitive style can also influence creative performance in everyday life.

To thrive after suffering from chronic illness, individuals must be able to define and redefine their problems and be able to choose appropriate strategies to resolve their difficulties. Individuals must be able to have insight into the fullness of problems (13–16). Some patients who survive suffering do not have enough insight to be able to deal creatively with everyday life, and they require assistance from health care professionals, family, and the community at large. Sometimes patients are put on drug therapy regimes that severely impact on their insight and awareness. In such cases, individuals may require help to be in touch with reality and make sense of the world around them in order to live fully. Creativity also demands an ability to be able to find more than one correct solution to a problem. Health care providers who have a sincere respect for individuals as whole persons may assist patients in clarifying issues throughout the course of normal conversations that occur during treatment sessions.

Family therapists have identified barriers to the creative process (17, 18). Individuals who have experienced suffering due to chronic illness may have a profound fear of failure, particularly if they believe they are "cursed" or are to blame for their illness. Patients who are unable to recognize their emotional, intellectual, and intuitive strengths or the strengths of others, particularly family members, may have difficulty finding creative ways of managing health-related life problems. Some people may be fearful of appearing silly, and others may not be able to change old ways of living, even though those ways may no longer work. Some patients may have difficulty accessing their imagination, but with the skilled help of professional health care providers, they may do so and may also access other personal resources. Societal factors such as stigma and stereotyping based on health status are also factors that prevent those who suffer because of chronic illness from finding creative solutions to everyday life challenges. In our exploration of suffering in individuals born with developmental delays, it is evident that individuals can learn to counteract overt stigma. Many patients overcome barriers by joining self-help or advocacy groups that work on behalf of disabled persons.

Throughout this book, we have seen the many challenges to the care of those who suffer. Effective health care delivery depends, first, on an understanding of suffering as an entity separate and only sometimes related to pain and, second, on developing the interventions to foster the habilitation or rehabilitation of those who suffer because of chronic illness or disability. Finally, the challenge of modern medicine is to provide client-centred, cost-effective health care within a context of respect and honor for the diverse beliefs and practices of individuals and the demands of contemporary society. If health care professionals recognize suffering as an entity separate from pain and acknowledge its impact on health, patients may not only survive the experience but also flourish and thrive. The stories and creative expressions of Robbie, Marron, Laura, Mr. Whitehead, and Marlene have confirmed the belief that both the art and science of medicine must be applied to help those who suffer manage suffering and enhance health.

SUMMARY

The failure to understand the differences between sorrow and depression can hinder the restoration of personhood and act as a barrier to the successful resolution of suffering. This chapter explored the issue of unresolved suffering and the expanded role of the health care provider with emphasis on the differences between the ability to survive and the desire to thrive. The inability to discern between sorrow and suffering and misdiagnosing sorrow as clinical depression lead to failure to survive and thrive after suffering. Fear, anxiety, and both personal and existential loneliness are also factors that hinder the resolution of suffering. Respecting individuals' religious, spiritual, or cultural beliefs about suffering and the rewards of exploring these issues with patients when there is a solid trusting, respectful relationship between health care provider and patient were discussed. Beliefs that suffering is caused by being cursed or because of past misdeeds may be driven by the fear that the person is no longer a valued member in the family or greater society. Individuals may have become "poor Harry" or "heroic John" rather than "my dear friend Harry" and "my clever friend John." The natural human creative impulse may assist people in restoring their sense of personal power and devising methods by which they not only survive but thrive after suffering.

Optimal care depends on the ease with which individuals are reintegrated into society. In addition to a direct "hands-on" approach to care, health professionals can encourage their respective professional organizations to not only protect the general public by ensuring its members are licensed but also inform the public of the need to understand the relationship between suffering and health. Professional colleges can also support patient advocacy groups and provide public education about the capabilities of those who are disabled or those who are living with chronic illness, and about the nature of suffering and the wounded spirit. In the past, such attempts have been presented from the perspective of compassion for the poor unfortunates. Current approaches would be better presented from the perspective of abilities and advantages to the integrity of society. The issue of suffering as an entity separate from pain, if incorporated into the undergraduate education of all health care professionals, would result in optimal health for individuals and the containment of health care delivery costs.

CHAPTER 16 QUESTIONS

1. What is the difference between sorrow and depression?
2. How is depression defined?
3. What is the treatment for depression?
4. What can be done to resolve sorrow?
5. What is the difference between depression and suffering?
6. How do fear, anxiety, and loneliness contribute to unresolved suffering?
7. What is the difference between depression and suffering in individuals with chronic illness and individuals who do not have a chronic illness?
8. How does the human creative impulse contribute to the individual's ability not only to survive but thrive after the experience of suffering?

Epilogue

Throughout time, every age has been defined by certain characteristics that have demarcated it from previous times. There have been the Dark Ages, the Renaissance, the Age of Enlightenment, the Industrial Age, and ages of disillusionment. Each age has marked a historical, philosophical, and sociological chapter in the history of humankind. Contemporary medicine, like most postmodern institutions, is responsive to the technological age. Like the husband who abandons his wife for a younger, more exciting mistress, medicine sometimes seems to be smitten by the sensuous lure of technology and statistics and appears to be in danger of abandoning the fragile, unpredictable human person, the patient. It is no longer acceptable to set aside the teachings of history and the scholars of the humanities in an uncritical devotion to the promises of science.

The challenge of contemporary medicine is to meet the current technological age with an intelligent desire to respond to change with integrity and a continued commitment to the enhancement of the human condition. Technology is not "a means unto itself," but rather simply a tool. The goal of medicine remains dedicated to the health and well-being of individuals and the society at large. Every age has left a legacy in philosophy, art, literature, music, and medicine. Every age has advanced the industrialization of society and pursued the objectives of scientific inquiry. Every age has taught horrific lessons about the impacts of war, illness, and disease and of humanity's neglect of its own kind.

When evaluating the problem of suffering in contemporary medicine, the problem of failure to clearly understand suffering as an entity separate and only sometimes related to pain, we may well agree with the poem written by William Wordsworth, in 1798:

I HEARD a thousand blended notes,
While in a grove I sate reclined,
In that sweet mood when pleasant thoughts
Bring sad thoughts to the mind.

To her fair works did Nature link
The human soul that through me ran;
And much it grieved my heart to think
What man has made of man.

Through primrose tufts, in that green bower,
The periwinkle trailed its wreaths;

And tis my faith that every flower
Enjoys the air it breathes.

The birds around me hopped and played
Their thoughts I cannot measure:—
But the least motion which they made
It seemed a thrill of pleasure.

The budding twigs spread out their fan,
To catch the breezy air;
And I must think, do all I can,
That there was pleasure there.

If this belief from heaven be sent,
If such be nature's holy plan,
Have I not reason to lament
What man has made of man?

It is important for patients to know that all is not lost. Our patients have taught us much about suffering outside the parameters of pain. From those under our care we now understand suffering as an experience with distinct universal and measurable characteristics. Suffering, in medicine, occurs when patients perceive a threat to ideas of self and personhood. Perceptions of threat occur during the course of medical and legal discourse associated with injury and disability. Conflicts that may arise when individuals are unable to meet the demands of developmental psychological life tasks because of limitations due to chronic illness can also result in suffering. Power differentials between medical professionals and patients, the loss of patient autonomy, and the impact of cultural differences and social norms are all key determinants that can escalate the process of suffering. The nature, power, and expression of suffering are determined by the patient.

Every age has been rescued by the compassion and creativity of human beings. In medicine, compassion takes the form of respect for patients as whole persons and acknowledgement of individuals as members of a caring community. Treatments for unresolved suffering and restoration of a wounded spirit are the responsibility of all health care providers. Because of the many technological resources available, medicine now has the ability to advance the art and science of medical practice to a higher level when assisting those who suffer. We have learned how to hear the unique language of suffering and understand the importance of listening to patients' stories, not just to identify physical illness but also to comprehend the power suffering has over patients, their families, and their communities. Every health care professional has special clinical skills that can be critical to the resolution of suffering in persons with chronic illness. Suffering can no longer be regarded solely as the secondary component of pain. In respect for our patients, it seems fitting then to conclude this book with a poem from my patient Laura. The powerful images in this poem remind us of the profoundly intimate relationship between the soul, the self, and the all encompassing experience of the loneliness of suffering. The poem also reenforces the call to all health care professionals for help. Patient-centred cost-effective care demands the recognition of suffering as a phenomenon separate from pain and the implementation of suffering-specific treatment strategies into clinical practice.

SOUL MATES

Dark secret Lover, Black eyes envelop my soul,
Stealing the light.
Down, down, I sink,
Spiraling into your being.

Passionate lover, all embracing,
Muscular arms enfold, grasping my breath.
With frenzied hands, our bodies cling together,
Limbs entangled.

My soul, a coldness so profound,
That I blaze with its fire.
Constant lover, Ever faithful.
Dark eyes flashing in the silent night.

The nothingness of a Sunday afternoon.
You, my dear companion,
Hand clasped in mine.
Your arm around my shoulder.

We wander,
Through the greenness of my life.
Only I call your name,
Dear devoted loneliness.

Only I see your eyes turn to yellow spheres.
Your tongue of flames,
Pierce through my soul.
Dear, secret lover!

My loneliness, my constant heart,
My own true love.
Secret lover,
My soul, My soul, My love.

APPENDIXES

Appendix A

SHORT FORM (COMPLETE)

DATA SUMMARY (RAW SCORES)

MEASURING AND ASSESSING SUFFERING QUESTIONNAIRE

NAME: ______________________ DATE: __________

ASSESSOR: ______________________

Likert-Type Scale: (1 - 5). 5 = Worst Response.

I. GRAND TOTAL SCORES

PART A PAIN	PART B SUFFERING	PART C WORK BELIEFS	PART D SELF-EFFICACY
Max. Pain (5)	Max. Distress (5)	Negative Beliefs (5)	No Confidence (5)
(4)	(4)	(4)	(4)
(3)	(3)	(3)	(3)
(2)	(2)	(2)	(2)
(1)	(1)	Positive Beliefs (1)	Total Confidence (1)
Patient's score:	Patient's score:	Patient's score:	Patient's score:
Date:	Date:	Date:	Date:

COMMENTS: ______________________

ASSESSOR SIGNATURE: ______________________

<u>SHORT FORM</u> *(SUFFERING COMPONENT ONLY)

<u>DATA SUMMARY</u> (RAW SCORES)

<u>MEASURING AND ASSESSING SUFFERING QUESTIONNAIRE</u>

NAME: ______________________ DATE: ______________

ASSESSOR: ______________________

Likert-Type Scale: (1 - 5) 5 = Worst Response.

I. GRAND TOTAL SCORE

II. SUBSET SCORES

	<u>PART B</u> SUFFERING	**<u>SECTION I</u>** RELATIONSHIPS	**<u>SECTION II</u>** IDEA OF SELF	**<u>SECTION III</u>** RESPONSE TO ILLNESS	**<u>SECTION IV</u>** COPING
Max. Distress (5)					
(4)					
(3)					
(2)					
No Distress (1)					
	Patient's score: Date:	Patient's score: Date:	Patient's score: Date:	Patient's score: Date:	Patient's score: Date:

COMMENTS: ______________________

ASSESSOR SIGNATURE: ______________________

DATA SUMMARY (RAW SCORES)

LONG FORM

MEASURING AND ASSESSING SUFFERING QUESTIONNAIRE

NAME: ____________________ DATE: __________

ASSESSOR: ____________________

Likert-Type Scale: (1 - 5). 5 = Worst Response.

I. GRAND TOTAL SCORES

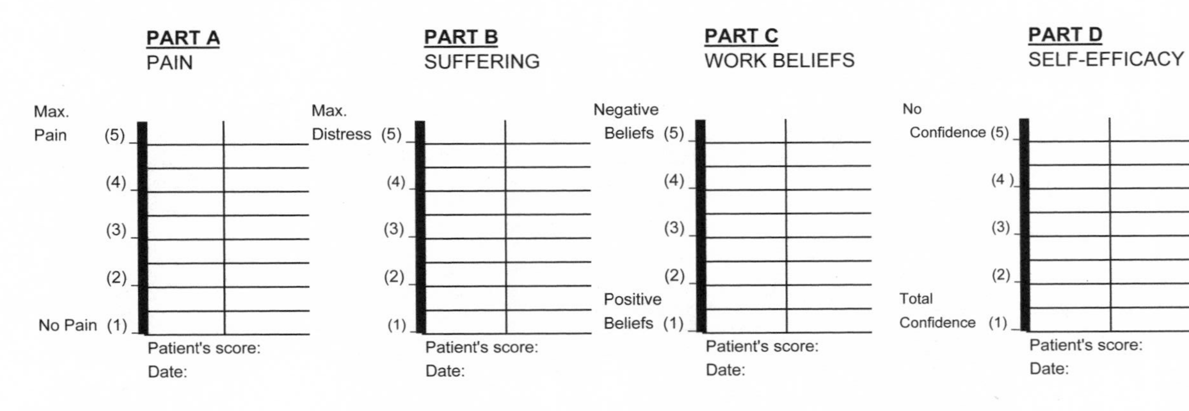

PART A
PAIN

Max. Pain (5)
(4)
(3)
(2)
No Pain (1)

Patient's score:
Date:

PART B
SUFFERING

Max. Distress (5)
(4)
(3)
(2)
(1)

Patient's score:
Date:

PART C
WORK BELIEFS

Negative Beliefs (5)
(4)
(3)
(2)
Positive Beliefs (1)

Patient's score:
Date:

PART D
SELF-EFFICACY

No Confidence (5)
(4)
(3)
(2)
Total Confidence (1)

Patient's score:
Date:

COMMENTS: ____________________

II. SUBSET SCORES

LONG FORM

PART A
1. PAIN

NAME: ____________________

INTENSITY

Max. (5)
(4)
(3)
(2)
Min. (1)

Patient's score:
Date:

COPING

Max. (5)
(4)
(3)
(2)
Min. (1)

Patient's score:
Date:

*** Please note: the higher the score the more negative the response.**

COMMENTS: ____________________

PART B
2. SUFFERING

SECTION I
RELATIONSHIPS

Max. Distress (5)
(4)
(3)
(2)
No Distress (1)

Patient's score:
Date:

SECTION II
IDEA OF SELF

(5)
(4)
(3)
(2)
(1)

Patient's score:
Date:

SECTION III
RESPONSE TO ILLNESS

(5)
(4)
(3)
(2)
(1)

Patient's score
Date:

SECTION IV
COPING

(5)
(4)
(3)
(2)
(1)

Patient's score:
Date:

COMMENTS: ____________________

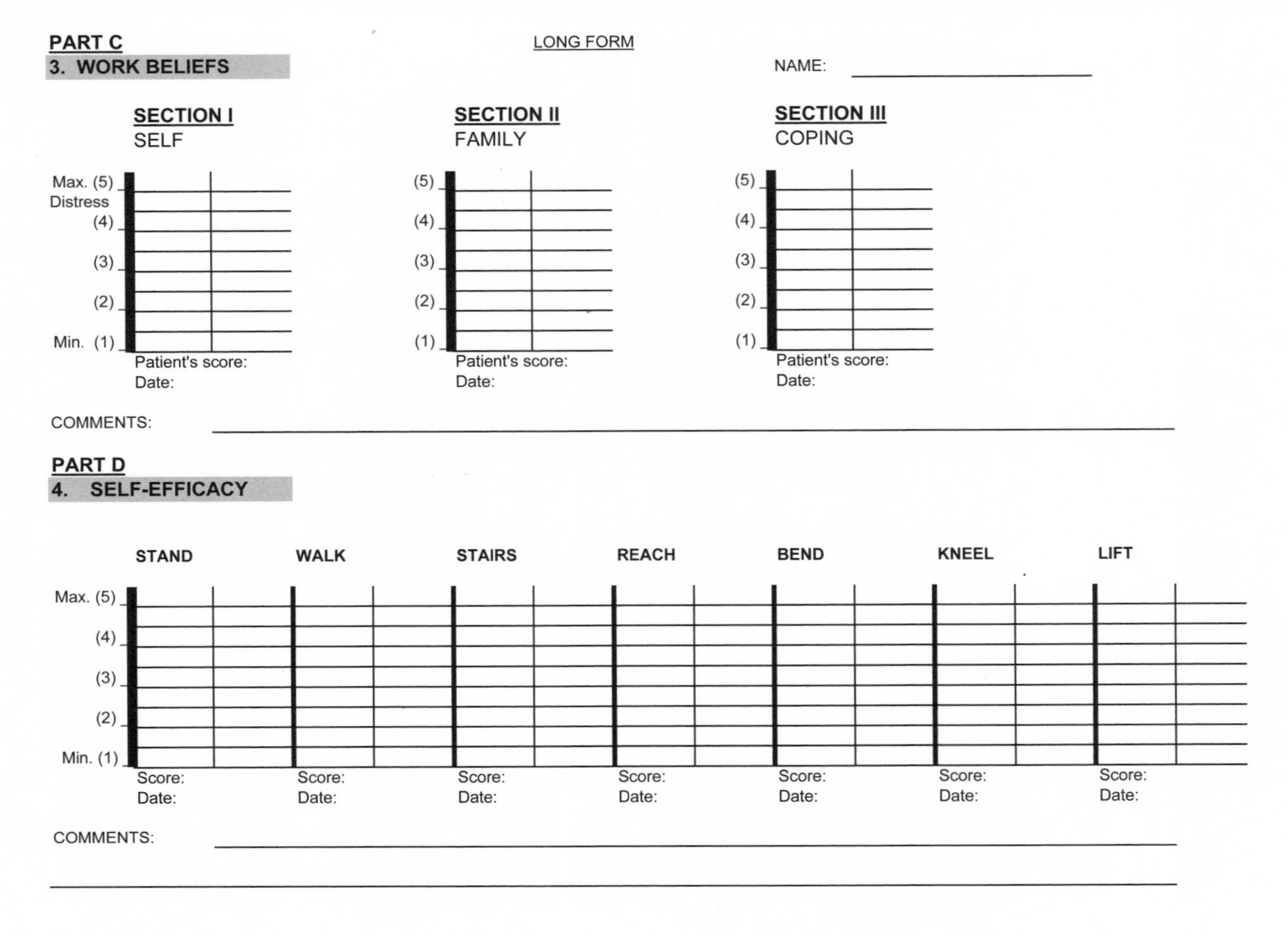

PART C
LONG FORM

3. WORK BELIEFS

NAME: ____________

SECTION I
SELF

Max. (5)
Distress
(4)
(3)
(2)
Min. (1)

Patient's score:
Date:

SECTION II
FAMILY

(5)
(4)
(3)
(2)
(1)

Patient's score:
Date:

SECTION III
COPING

(5)
(4)
(3)
(2)
(1)

Patient's score:
Date:

COMMENTS: ____________

PART D

4. SELF-EFFICACY

	STAND	WALK	STAIRS	REACH	BEND	KNEEL	LIFT
Max. (5)							
(4)							
(3)							
(2)							
Min. (1)							
	Score: Date:	Score: Date:	Score: Date:	Score: Date:	Score: Date:	Score: Date:	Score: Date:

COMMENTS: ____________

LONG FORM

NAME: ______________________

	CARRY 1		CARRY 2	
Max. (5)				
(4)				
(3)				
(2)				
Min. (1)				
	Score:		Score:	
	Date:		Date:	

COMMENTS: ____

____

____

SHORT FORM (COMPLETE)

NORMATIVE DATA SUMMARY (Z SCORES)

MEASURING AND ASSESSING SUFFERING QUESTIONNAIRE

NAME: ______________________ DATE: __________

ASSESSOR: ______________________

- Z SCORE:	LESS DISTRESS.
0 Z SCORE:	DISTRESS LEVEL COMPARABLE TO MEAN OF ESTABLISHED GROUP.
+ Z SCORE:	MORE DISTRESS.

CALCULATIONS: $Z = \frac{(\bar{x} - X)}{SD}$

NOTE:
$\bar{x}$ = patients' mean score
X = mean of sample subscore
SD = standard deviation of sample

Likert-Type Scale: (1 - 5). 5 = Worst Response.

I. TOTAL SCORES

Z-score: The number of Standard Deviation Units above or below the mean.

Z-score	PAIN	SUFFERING	WORK BELIEFS	SELF-EFFICACY
(5)				
(4)				
(3)				
(2)				
(1)				
Mean (0)				
(-1)				
(-2)				
(-3)				
(-4)				
(-5)				
	Patient's score: Date:	Patient's score: Date:	Patient's score: Date:	Patient's score: Date:

COMPARISON GROUPS:

	PAIN	SUFFERING	WORK BELIEFS	SELF-EFFICACY
Arthritis:	$\bar{x}$ = 2.89 ± 0.597 SD	$\bar{x}$ = 3.27 ± 0.655 SD	N/A	N/A
Epilepsy:	$\bar{x}$ = 3.51 ± 0.631 SD	$\bar{x}$ = 2.31 ± 0.837 SD	$\bar{x}$ = 4.02 ± 1.01 SD	$\bar{x}$ = 2.40 ± 0.451 SD

COMMENTS: ______________________

ASSESSOR SIGNATURE: ______________________

SHORT FORM * (SUFFERING COMPONENT ONLY)

NORMATIVE DATA SUMMARY (Z SCORES)

MEASURING AND ASSESSING SUFFERING QUESTIONNAIRE

NAME: ______________________ DATE: ____________

ASSESSOR: ______________________

- Z SCORE:	LESS DISTRESS.
0 Z SCORE:	DISTRESS LEVEL COMPARABLE TO MEAN OF ESTABLISHED GROUP.
+ Z SCORE:	MORE DISTRESS.

CALCULATIONS: $Z = \frac{(\bar{x} - X)}{SD}$

NOTE:
x̄ = patients' mean score
X = mean of sample subscore
SD = standard deviation of sample

Likert-Type Scale: (1 - 5). 5 = Worst Response.

I. TOTAL SCORES Z-Score: The number of Standard Deviation Units above or below the mean.

PART B (total subscale scores)
2. SUFFERING

Z-scores	TOTAL SUFFERING	RELATIONSHIPS	IDEA OF SELF	RESPONSE TO ILLNESS	COPING
(5)					
(4)					
(3)					
(2)					
(1)					
Mean (0)					
(-1)					
(-2)					
(-3)					
(-4)					
(-5)					
	Patient's score:	Patient's score:	Patient's score:	Patient's score:	Patient's score:
	Date:	Date:	Date:	Date:	Date:

COMPARISON GROUPS:					
Arthritis:	x̄ = 3.27 ± 0.655 SD	x̄ = 3.29 ± 0.952 SD	x̄ = 4.01 ± 0.742 SD	x̄ = 3.01 ± 0.808 SD	x̄ = 2.78 ± 0.724 SD
Epilepsy:	x̄ = 2.31 ± 0.837 SD	x̄ = 2.25 ± 1.19 SD	x̄ = 2.56 ± 1.15 SD	x̄ = 2.39 ± 0.82 SD	x̄ = 2.04 ± 0.74 SD

COMMENTS: ______________________

ASSESSOR SIGNATURE: ______________________

LONG FORM

NORMATIVE DATA SUMMARY (Z SCORES)

MEASURING AND ASSESSING SUFFERING QUESTIONNAIRE

NAME: ______________________ DATE: __________

ASSESSOR: ______________________

- Z SCORE:	LESS DISTRESS.
0 Z SCORE:	DISTRESS LEVEL COMPARABLE TO MEAN OF ESTABLISHED GROUP.
+ Z SCORE:	MORE DISTRESS.

CALCULATIONS: $Z = \frac{(\bar{x} - X)}{SD}$

NOTE:
x̄ = patients' mean score
X = mean of sample subscore
SD = standard deviation of sample

Likert-Type Scale: (1 - 5). 5 = Worst Response.

I. TOTAL SCORES

Z-score: The number of Standard Deviation Units above or below the mean.

Z-score

	PAIN	SUFFERING	WORK BELIEFS	SELF-EFFICACY
(5)				
(4)				
(3)				
(2)				
(1)				
Mean (0)				
(-1)				
(-2)				
(-3)				
(-4)				
(-5)				
	Patient's score: Date:	Patient's score: Date:	Patient's score: Date:	Patient's score: Date:

COMPARISON GROUPS:

	PAIN	SUFFERING	WORK BELIEFS	SELF-EFFICACY
Arthritis:	x̄ = 2.89 ± 0.597 SD	x̄ = 3.27 ± 0.655 SD	N/A	N/A
Epilepsy:	x̄ = 3.51 ± 0.631 SD	x̄ = 2.31 ± 0.837 SD	x̄ = 4.02 ± 1.01 SD	x̄ = 2.40 ± 0.451 SD

COMMENTS: ______________________

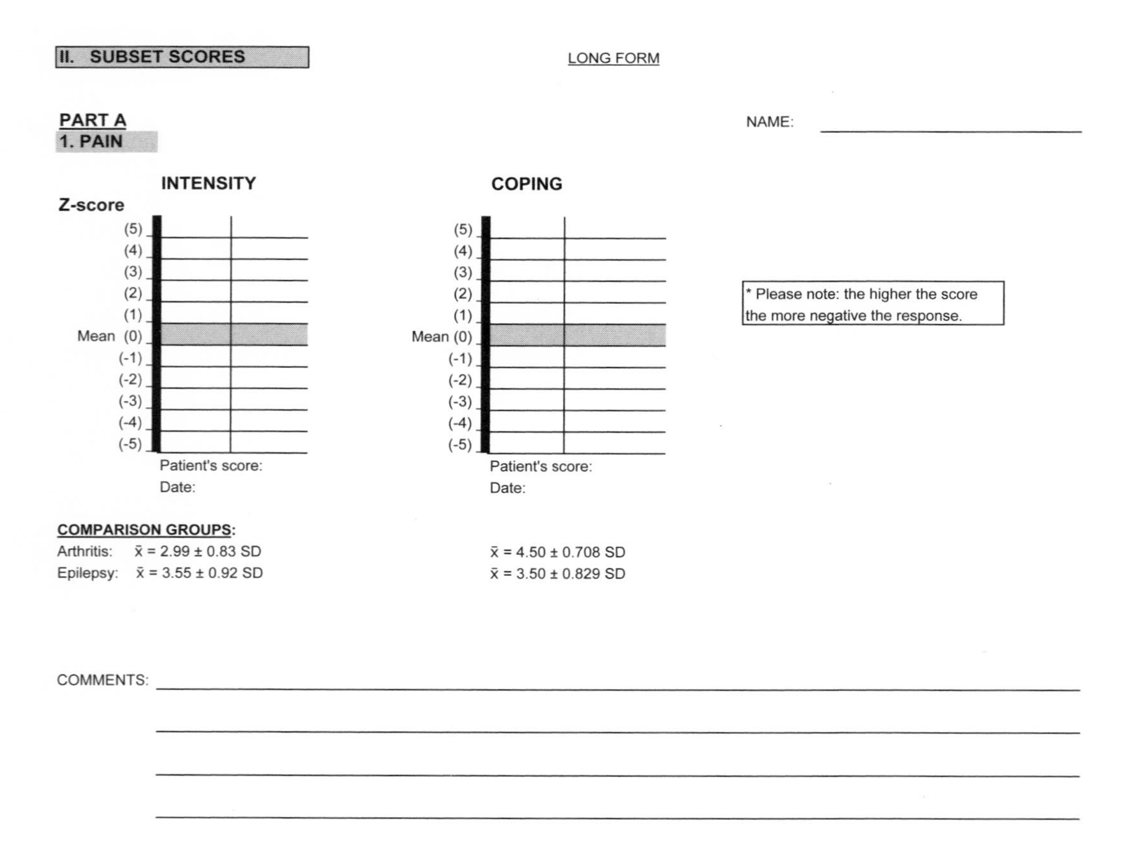

II. SUBSET SCORES

LONG FORM

PART A

1. PAIN

NAME: ______________________

Z-score	INTENSITY	COPING
(5)		
(4)		
(3)		
(2)		
(1)		
Mean (0)		
(-1)		
(-2)		
(-3)		
(-4)		
(-5)		
	Patient's score:	Patient's score:
	Date:	Date:

* Please note: the higher the score the more negative the response.

COMPARISON GROUPS:

	INTENSITY	COPING
Arthritis:	$\bar{x}$ = 2.99 ± 0.83 SD	$\bar{x}$ = 4.50 ± 0.708 SD
Epilepsy:	$\bar{x}$ = 3.55 ± 0.92 SD	$\bar{x}$ = 3.50 ± 0.829 SD

COMMENTS: ______________________

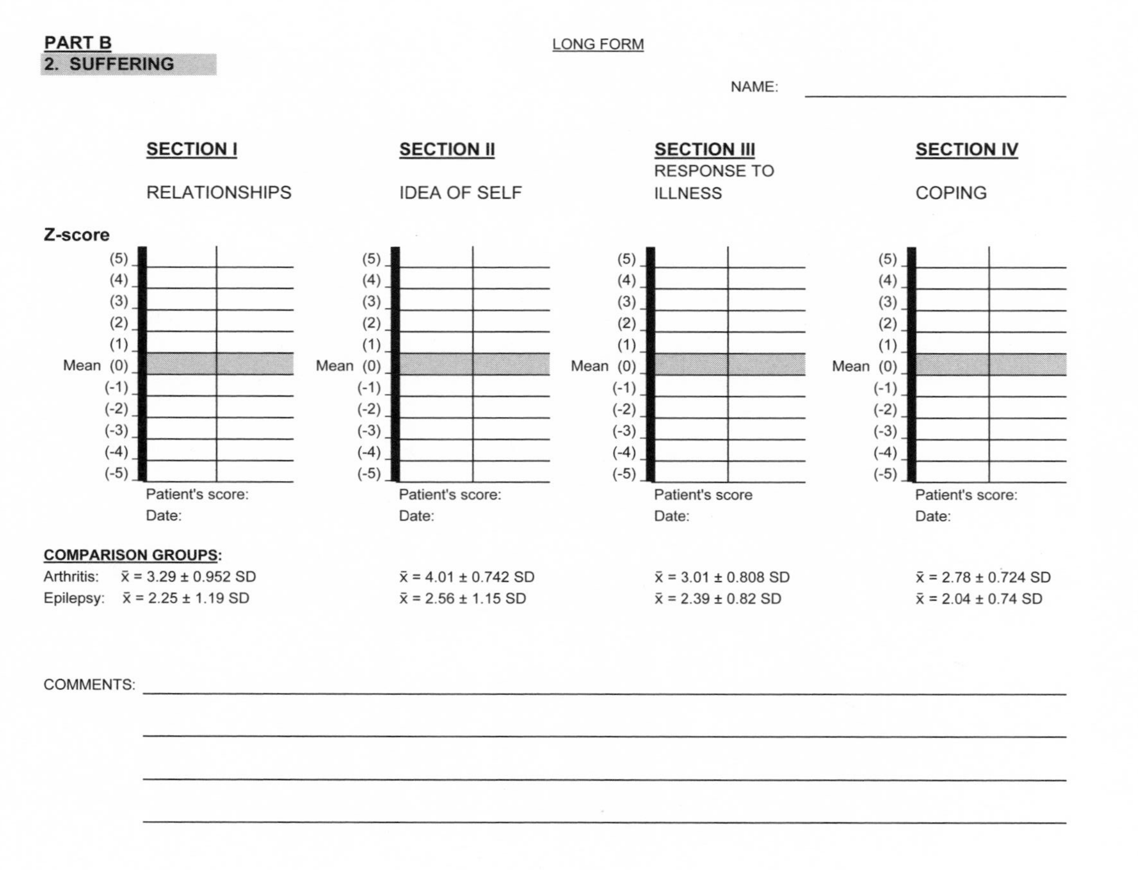

PART B
2. SUFFERING

LONG FORM

NAME: ____________________

	SECTION I	SECTION II	SECTION III	SECTION IV
	RELATIONSHIPS	IDEA OF SELF	RESPONSE TO ILLNESS	COPING

Z-score

(5)
(4)
(3)
(2)
(1)
Mean (0)
(-1)
(-2)
(-3)
(-4)
(-5)

	SECTION I	SECTION II	SECTION III	SECTION IV
	Patient's score:	Patient's score:	Patient's score	Patient's score:
	Date:	Date:	Date:	Date:

COMPARISON GROUPS:

	SECTION I	SECTION II	SECTION III	SECTION IV
Arthritis:	$\bar{x}$ = 3.29 ± 0.952 SD	$\bar{x}$ = 4.01 ± 0.742 SD	$\bar{x}$ = 3.01 ± 0.808 SD	$\bar{x}$ = 2.78 ± 0.724 SD
Epilepsy:	$\bar{x}$ = 2.25 ± 1.19 SD	$\bar{x}$ = 2.56 ± 1.15 SD	$\bar{x}$ = 2.39 ± 0.82 SD	$\bar{x}$ = 2.04 ± 0.74 SD

COMMENTS: ____________________

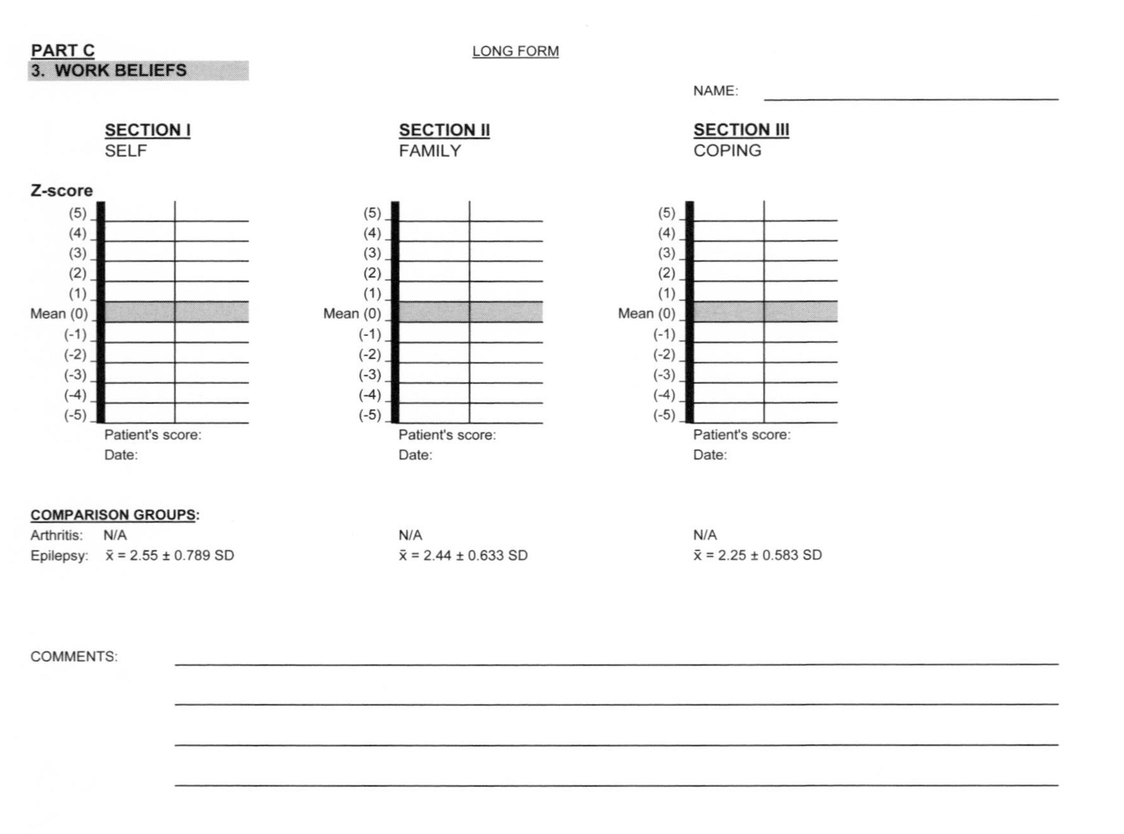

PART C

3. WORK BELIEFS

LONG FORM

NAME: ____________________

	SECTION I SELF	SECTION II FAMILY	SECTION III COPING
Z-score			
(5)			
(4)			
(3)			
(2)			
(1)			
Mean (0)			
(-1)			
(-2)			
(-3)			
(-4)			
(-5)			
	Patient's score:	Patient's score:	Patient's score:
	Date:	Date:	Date:

COMPARISON GROUPS:

Arthritis:	N/A	N/A	N/A
Epilepsy:	$\bar{x}$ = 2.55 ± 0.789 SD	$\bar{x}$ = 2.44 ± 0.633 SD	$\bar{x}$ = 2.25 ± 0.583 SD

COMMENTS: ____________________

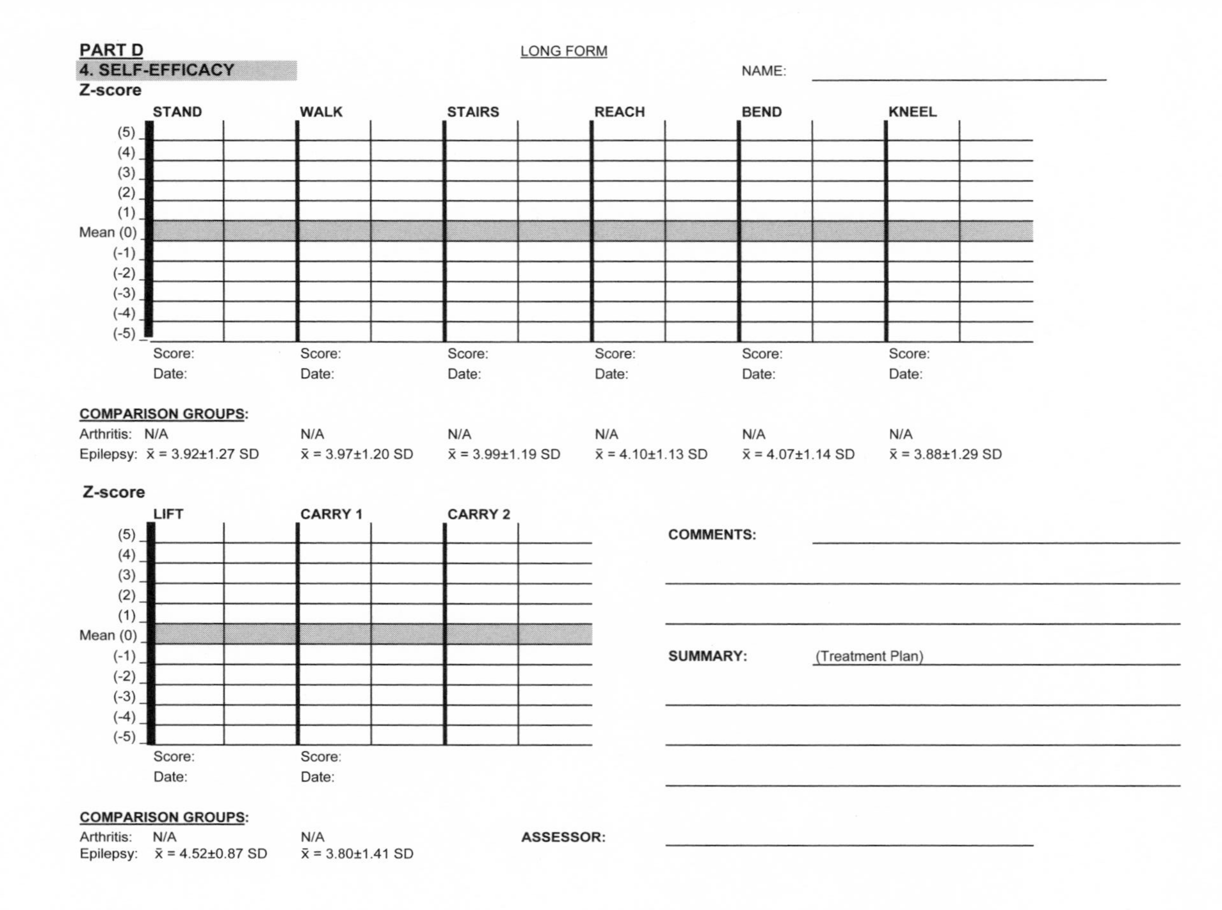

PART D LONG FORM

4. SELF-EFFICACY

NAME: ______________________

Z-score

	STAND	WALK	STAIRS	REACH	BEND	KNEEL
(5)						
(4)						
(3)						
(2)						
(1)						
Mean (0)						
(-1)						
(-2)						
(-3)						
(-4)						
(-5)						
	Score:	Score:	Score:	Score:	Score:	Score:
	Date:	Date:	Date:	Date:	Date:	Date:

COMPARISON GROUPS:

	STAND	WALK	STAIRS	REACH	BEND	KNEEL
Arthritis:	N/A	N/A	N/A	N/A	N/A	N/A
Epilepsy:	$\bar{x}$ = 3.92±1.27 SD	$\bar{x}$ = 3.97±1.20 SD	$\bar{x}$ = 3.99±1.19 SD	$\bar{x}$ = 4.10±1.13 SD	$\bar{x}$ = 4.07±1.14 SD	$\bar{x}$ = 3.88±1.29 SD

Z-score

	LIFT	CARRY 1	CARRY 2
(5)			
(4)			
(3)			
(2)			
(1)			
Mean (0)			
(-1)			
(-2)			
(-3)			
(-4)			
(-5)			
	Score:	Score:	
	Date:	Date:	

COMMENTS: ______________________

SUMMARY: (Treatment Plan) ______________________

COMPARISON GROUPS:

Arthritis:	N/A	N/A
Epilepsy:	$\bar{x}$ = 4.52±0.87 SD	$\bar{x}$ = 3.80±1.41 SD

ASSESSOR: ______________________

REFERENCES

Chapter 1

1 *Oxford compact English dictionary*. Ed. C. Soanes. Oxford: Oxford University Press, 2000.

2 Cassell, E. *The nature of suffering and the goals of medicine*. 2nd ed. Oxford: Oxford University Press, 2004.

3 Clarke, B. M., A. R. M. Upton, C. M. Castellanos, and M. Schmuck. "Measuring and assessing suffering in arthritic patients." In *Spirituality and health: Multidisciplinary explorations*, ed. A. Meier, T. O'Connor, and P. VanKatwyk. Waterloo, ON: Wilfred Laurier University Press, 2005. 227–241.

4 Chapman, C. R. "Suffering: The contributions of persistent pain." *Lancet* 353, no. 9171 (1999): 2233–2237.

5 Shaver, W. A. "Suffering and the role of abandonment of self." *Journal of Hospice and Palliative Nursing* 4, no. 1 (2002): 46–53.

6 Vanhooft, S. *The meaning of suffering. Hastings Centre Report* 28, no. 5 (1998): 13–19.

7 Chapman, C. R., and J. Garvin. "Suffering and its relationship to pain." *Journal of Palliative Care* 9, no. 2 (1993): 5–13.

8 Stratton-Hill, J. R. C. "Suffering as contrasted to pain, loss, grief, despair, loneliness." In *The hidden dimensions of illness: Human suffering*, ed. P. L. Stark and J. P. McGovern. New York: League for Nursing Press, 1992. 69–80.

9 Erikson, K. "The alienation of suffering: The idea of caring." *Scandinavian Journal of Caring Science* 23 (1992): 119–123.

10 Clarke, B. M. "Pain, suffering and physiotherapy." *Physiotherapy Canada* 50, no. 2 (1998): 112–117.

11 Erikson, K. "Understanding the world of the patient, the suffering of human beings: The new clinical paradigm for nursing to caring." *Advanced Practice Nurse Quarterly* 3 (1997): 8–13.

12 Clarke, B. M. "The impact of suffering in physiotherapy practice: Cost containment." *Physiotherapy Canada* 52, no. 1 (2000): 25–32.

13 Egnew, T. R. "Suffering, meaning and healing: Challenges in contemporary medicine." *Annals of Family Medicine* 7, no. 2 (2009): 170–175.

14 Bannister, D. "Knowledge of self in psychology for physiotherapists." In *Psychology for physiotherapists*, ed. E. Naomi Dunkin, A. J. Chapman, and A. Gale. London: The British Psychology Society & Macmillan Press Ltd., 1981. 174–194.

15 Gaddow, G. "Suffering and interpersonal meaning." *Journal of Clinical Ethics* 2, no. 2 (1991): 103–107.

16 Pullman, D. "Human dignity and the ethics and esthetics of pain and suffering." *Theoretical Medicine* 23 (2003): 75–94.

17 Mackay, R. C. "What is empathy?" In *Empathy and the helping relationship*. New York: Springer Publishing, 1990. 3–12.
18 Sobel, R. "The myth of the control of suffering." *Journal of Medical Humanities* 17, no. 4 (1996): 255–259.
19 Thomas, S. L. H. "Why did it happen to me?" *Journal of Religious Studies* 26 (1990): 323–334.
20 Clarke, B. M., A. R. M. Upton, and C. M. Castellanos. "Pain and suffering: Measuring the suffering component." In *Proceedings of the 11th World Congress on Pain* (Aug. 21–26, 2005, Sydney, Australia), ed. H. Flor, E. Kalso, and J. O. Dostrovsky. Seattle, WA: IASP Press, 2006. 204, Abstract 550-P156.
21 Clarke, B. M., A. R. M. Upton, and C. M. Castellanos. "Work beliefs and work status of people with epilepsy." In *Proceedings of the 26th International Epilepsy Congress* (Aug. 28–Sept. 1, 2005, Paris, France). *Epilepsia*, 46, suppl. 6 (2005): 129, Abstract P292.
22 Clarke, B. M., A. R. M. Upton, and C. M. Castellanos. "Internal barriers to work: Practice implications." In *Proceedings of the Canadian Physiotherapy Congress* (May 26–29, 2005, Victoria, BC). Abstracts, 10.

Chapter 2

1 Gadon, G. "Suffering and Interpersonal Meaning." *Journal of Clinical Ethics* 212 (1991): 103–107.
2 Clarke, B. M., A. R. M Upton, and C. Castellanos. "Suffering: Measuring the immeasurable." In *Central neuropathic pain: Focus on post stroke pain*, ed. J. L. Henry, A. Panju, and K. Yshpal. Seattle, WA: IASP Press, 2007.
3 Clarke, B. M., A. R. M. Upton, C. Castellanos, and M. Schmuck. "Measuring and assessing suffering in arthritic patients." In *Spirituality and Health: Multidisciplinary explorations*, ed. A. Meir, T. O'Connor, and P. VanKatwyk. Waterloo, ON: Wilfred Laurier University Press, 2005. 227–241.
4 Wissler, R. L., D. L. Evans, A. J. Hart, M. M. Morry, and M. J. Saks. "Explaining pain and suffering awards: The role of injury characteristics and fault attribution." *Law and Human Behavior* 21, no. 2 (1997): 108–207.
5 Sebok, A. J. "How Germany views U.S. tort law: Duties, damages, dumb luck and the differences between the two countries." *Findlaw's Writ*, July 23, 2001. http://writ.news.findlaw.com/sebok/20010723.html (accessed November 21, 2007).
6 Koziol, H. "Comparative law—a must in the European Union: Demonstrated by tort law as an example." *Journal of Tort Law* 1, no. 3 (2007): 1–10.
7 Clarke, B. M., A. R. M. Upton, K. Kamath, T. Al-Harbi, and C. Castellanos. "Transcranial magnetic stimulation for migraine: Clinical effects." *Journal of Headache and Pain* 7, no. 5 (2006): 341–346.
8 Norman, G., and D. Streiner. *Biostatistics: The bare essentials*. Hamilton, ON: B.C. Decker Inc., 2000.

9 Clarke, B. M. "The impact of suffering in physiotherapy practice: Cost containment issues." *Physiotherapy Canada* 52, no. 1 (2000): 25–31.
10 Gracovetsky, S. A., A. Marriot, M. P. Richards, N. M. Newman, and S. Asselin. "The impact of inefficient clinical diagnosis on the cost of managing low back pain." *Journal of Health Care Management* 17 no. 3 (1997): 31–33.
11 Watkins E., P. C. Wollan, J. Melton, and B. P. Yawn. "Silent sufferers." *Mayo Clinic Proc.* 81 (2006): 167–171.
12 Tang, N. K. Y., and C. Crane. "Suicidality in chronic pain: A review of the prevalence, risk factors and psychological links." *Psychological Medicine* 36, no. 5 (2006): 575–586.

Chapter 3

1 Wordsworth, W. Poems of the imagination: XXXIII. In *The poetical works of William Wordsworth in six volumes, Vol. 2, a new edition*, ed. Edward Moxon. London: Dover Street, 1857, 308.
2 Hafiz. "Now is the time." In *The gift: Poems by Hafiz*, trans. Daniel Ladensky. New York: Penguin Compass; 1999. 16–161.
3 Rawlinson, M. C. "The sense of suffering." *Journal of Medicine and Philosophy* 11, no. 1 (1986): 39–62.
4 Freud, S. "Civilization and its discontent." In *Sources of Suffering*, trans. J. Strachey. New York: Norton, 1962.
5 Kant, I. *Groundwork of the metaphysic of morals*, trans. H. J. Paton. New York: Harper, Torchbooks, 1956.
6 Cohen, A. *Everyman's Talmud: The major teachings of the rabbinic sages.* New York: Schocken Books, 1995.
7 Mohrman, M. E., and M. J. Hanson. *Pain seeking understanding: Suffering, medicine, faith.* Cleveland, OH: The Pilgrim Press, 1999.
8 Louw, D. J. *Meaning in suffering: A theological reflection on the cross and the resurrection for pastoral care and counseling.* International Theology Series, vol. 5. New York: Peter Lang Publishing, 2000.
9 Perkins, J. *The suffering self: Pain and narrative representation in the early Christian era.* London: Routledge, 1995.
10 Balkan, D. *Disease, pain, and sacrifice.* Chicago: University of Chicago Press, 1968.
11 Cassell, E. J. "Recognizing suffering." *Hastings Centre Report* 21, no. 3 (1991): 24–31.
12 Lindholm, L., and K. Erikson. "The dialectic of health and suffering: An ontological perspective on young people's health." *Qualitative Health Research* 8, no. 4 (1998): 513–525.
13 Mellor, P. A. "Self and suffering: The deconstruction and reflexive definition in Buddhism and Christianity." *Religious Studies* 27 (1991): 46–53.
14 van Hooft, S. "The meaning of suffering." *Hastings Centre Report* 28, no. 5 (1998): 13–19.

15 Giddens, A. *The constitution of society: Outline of the theory of structuration*. Berkeley: University of California Press, 1984.
16 Weil, S. "The love of God and affliction." In *The Simone Weil Reader*, ed. G. A. Panichas. New York: David McKay Co., 1977.
17 Levinas, E. "Useless suffering." In *The provocation of Levinas: Rethinking the other*, ed. R. Bernasconi, and D. Wood. London: Routledge; 1988.
18 Fichter, J. H. *Religion and pain*. New York: Crossroad Publishing Co., 1981.
19 Cohen, H. *Reason and hope: Selections from the Jewish writings of Herman Cohen*. New York: Norton, 1971.
20 Prakish, N. "Medical ethics in India." *Journal of Medicine and Philosophy* 13 (1988): 231–255.
21 Prakish, N. *Health and medicine in Hindu tradition: Continuity and cohesion*. New York: Crossroad Publishing Co., 1989.
22 Patel, H. G., P. Oliver, and B. Ram. "The need for cultural sensitivity." In *Caring for Hindu patients*, ed. D. Thakrar, R. Das, and A. Sheikh. Oxford: Radcliffe Publishing, 2008. 41–53.
23 Engler, S. H. "Vicissitudes of the self according to Psychoanalysis and Buddhism: A spectrum model of object relations development." *Psychoanalysis and Contemporary Thought* 6 (1983): 29–72.
24 Christensen, L. W. "Suffering and the dialectical self in Buddhism and relational psychoanalysis." *The American Journal of Psychoanalysis* 59, no. 1 (1999): 37–57.
25 Rubin, J. B. "The emperor of enlightenment may have no clothes." In *The couch and the tree: Dialogues in psychoanalysis and Buddhism*, ed. A. Molino. New York: North Point Press, 1998.
26 Engler, J. "Therapeutic aims in psychotherapy and meditation: Developmental stages in the representation of the self." In *Transformations of consciousness*, ed. W. K. Engler and D. Brown. Boston: Shambhala, 1986.
27 Scotton, B. W. "Treating Buddhist patients." In *Handbook of religion and mental health*, ed. H. Koenig. San Diego, CA: Academic Press, 1998.
28 Molino, A. *The couch and the tree: Dialogues in psychoanalysis and Buddhism*. New York: North Point Press, 1998.
29 Wei-Ming, T. "Pain and suffering in Confucian self-cultivation." *Philosophy East and West* 34, no. 4 (1984): 379–388.
30 Antes, P. "Medicine and living the tradition of Islam." In *Healing and restoring: Health and medicine in the world's religious traditions*, ed. L. E. Sullivan. New York: Macmillan Publishing Co.; 1989.
31 Renard, J. *Seven doors to Islam: Spirituality and the religious life of Muslims*. Berkeley: University of California Press; 1996.
32 Cragg, K., and R. M. Speight. *The house of Islam*. Belmont, CA: Wadsworth Publishing Co., 1988.

33 Winter, T. J. "The Muslim grand narrative." In *Caring for Muslim patients*, ed. A. Sheikh and A. R. Gatrad. 2nd ed. Oxford: Radcliffe Publishing, 2008, 25–35.
34 Ahmed, A. A. "Health and disease: An Islamic framework." In *Caring for Muslim patients*, ed. A. Sheikh and A. R. Gatrad. 2nd ed. Oxford: Radcliffe Publishing, 2008. 35–45.
35 Hultkrantz, A. "Health, religion and medicine in Native North American traditions." In *Healing and restoring: Health and medicine in the world's religious traditions*, ed. L. E. Sullivan. New York: Macmillan Publishing Co., 1989.
36 Waldram, J. *Aboriginal health in Canada: Historical, cultural and epidemiological perspectives*. Toronto, ON: University of Toronto Press, 1995.
37 Primeaux, M. H. "American Indian health care practices: A cross-cultural perspective." *Nursing Clinics of North America* 12, no. 1 (1977): 55–65.
38 Mbiti, J. S. *African religions and philosophy*. 2nd ed. Portsmouth, NH: Heinemann, Oxford, 1990.
39 Good, C. M. *Ethnomedical systems in Africa: Patterns of traditional medicine in rural and urban Kenya*. New York: The Guilford Press, 1987.
40 Mabunda, M. M. "Perceptions of disease, illness and healing among selected black communities in the Northern Province, South Africa." *South African Journal of Ethnology* 24, no. 1 (2001): 11–16.
41 Harley, G. W. *Native African medicine*. London: Frank Cass and Co. Ltd., 1970.
42 Ademuwagun, Z. A., J. A. Ayoade, I. E. Harrison, and D. M. Warren. *African therapeutic systems*. Crossroads Press; 1979.
43 MacKay, I. R. "Humanism and the suffering of the people." *Internal Medicine Journal* 33, no. 4 (2003): 195–202.
44 Belkin, G. S. "Moving beyond bio-ethics: History and the search for medical humanism." *Perspectives in Biology and Medicine* 47, no. 3 (2004): 372–385.
45 Talbot, J. A., and D. B. Mallot. "Professionalism, medical humanism and cultural bio-ethics: The new wave—does psychiatry have a role? *Journal of Psychiatric Practice* 12, no. 6 (2006): 384–390.

Chapter 4

1 Giger, J. N., and R. E. Davidhizar. "Introduction to transcultural nursing." In *Transcultural nursing*, ed. J. N. Giger and R. E. Davidhizar. 3rd ed. New York: Mosby, 1999. 3–19.
2 Plawecki, H. M., T. R. Sanches, and J. A. Plawecki. "Cultural aspects of caring for Navajo Indian clients." *Journal of Holistic Nursing* 12, no. 3 (1994): 291–306.
3 Spector, R. "Cultural diversity in health care and illness." *Journal of Trans Cultural Nursing* 13, no. 3 (2002): 197–199.
4 Lenninger, M. "The theory of culture and ethno nursing research methods." In *Transcultural nursing*, ed. M. Lenninger and M. R. McFarland. 3rd ed. New York: McGraw-Hill, 2002. 71–116.

5 Kymlicka, W. *Multicultural citizenship: A liberal theory of minority rights*. Oxford: Oxford University Press, 1995.
6 James, M. R. "The normative consequences of identity construction." In *Deliberative democracy and the plural polity*. Lawrence: University Press of Kansas, 2004.
7 Wochel, S. "The rightful place of human rights: Incorporating individual, group and cultural perspectives." In *The psychology of rights and duties: Empirical contributions and normative commentaries*, ed. N. L. Finkel and F. M. Moghaddam. Washington, DC: American Psychological Association, 2005. 197–220.
8 Harre, R. O. M. "An ontology for duties and rights." In *The psychology of rights and duties: Empirical contributions and normative commentaries*, ed. N. L. Finkel and F. M. Moghaddam. Washington, DC: American Psychological Association, 2005. 223–239.
9 Srivastana, R. H. *The health care professional's guide to cultural competence*. Toronto, ON: Mosby/Elsevier, 2007.
10 Helman, C. G. *Culture, health and illness*. 5th ed. Oxford: Oxford University Press, 2007.
11 Purnell, L. "The Purnell model for cultural competence." *Journal of Trans Cultural Nursing* 13, no. 3 (2002): 193–196.
12 Moore, P. J., S. Spernak, and E. Chung. "Patients' rights and physicians duties: Implications for the doctor–patient relationship and the quality of care." In *The psychology of rights and duties: Empirical contributions and normative commentaries*, ed. N. L. Finkel and F. M. Moghaddam. Washington, DC: American Psychological Association, 2005.
13 Haskell, T. L. "Taking duties seriously: To what problems are rights and duties the solution." In *The psychology of rights and duties: Empirical contributions and normative commentaries*, ed. N. L. Finkel and F. M. Moghaddam. Washington, DC: American Psychological Association, 2005. 243–252.
14 Lenninger, M. "Culture care assessments for congruent competency practices." In: *Transcultural nursing*, ed. M. Lenninger and M. R. McFarland. 3rd ed. New York: McGraw-Hill, 2002. 117–143.

Chapter 5

1 Erikson, E. *The life cycle completed*. New York: W.W. Norton & Co., 1982.
2 Ogbu, J. "Origins of human competence: A cultural ecological perspective." *Child Development* 52, no. 2 (1981): 413–429.
3 Berry, J. W., and J. Sam. "Acculturation and adaptation." In *Handbook of cross-cultural psychology*. Vol. 3, *Social psychology*, ed. J. W. Berry, M. H. Segall, and C. Kagitcibasi. 2nd ed. Boston: Allyn & Bacon, 1997. 291–326.
4 Hume, D. *A treatise of human nature*. Oxford: Clarendon Press, 2000.
5 Piaget, J. *Equilibrium of cognitive structures*. Chicago: University of Chicago Press, 1985.
6 Bandura, A. "The evaluation of social cognitive theory." In *Great minds in*

management: The process of theory development. New York: Oxford University Press, 2005.

7 Green, M., and J. Piel. *Theories of human development: A comparative approach*. 22nd ed. New York: Allyn & Bacon, 2010.

8 Ho, M. K., J. Rasheed, and M. N. Rasheed. *Family therapy with ethnic minorities*. London: Sage Publishing Co., 2003.

9 Dasen, P. "Theoretical frameworks in cross cultural development in psychology: An attempt at integration." In *Cultural perspectives in human development: Theory and applications*, ed. T. S. Saraswath. London: Sage Publications Co., 2003. 129–159.

10 Bronfenbrenner, U. "Ecological systems theory." *Annals of Child Development* 6 (1989): 185–246.

11 Harkness, S., and C. M. Super. *Parents' cultural belief systems: Their origins, expressions and consequences*. New York: Guilford Press, 1996.

12 Harkness, S., and C. M. Super. "The cultural construction of child development." *Ethos* 11, no. 4 (1983): 221–231.

13 Kagitcibasi, C. "Human development: Cross-cultural perspective." In *Advances in psychological science*. Vol. 2, *Development: Personal and social aspects*, ed. J. Adair, D. Belanger, and K. L. Dion. London: Psychology Press, 1997. 475–494.

14 Carter, B., and M. McGoldrick. *The expanded family life cycle: Individual, family and social perspectives*. 3rd ed. Boston: Allyn & Bacon, 1999.

15 Becvar, D. S., and R. J. Becvar. *Family therapy: A systematic integration*. 4th ed. Boston: Allyn & Bacon Press, 2000.

16 Gladding, S. T. *Counseling: A comprehensive profession*. Upper Saddle River, NJ: Merrill Prentice Hall, 2009.

17 Reiss, D., S. Gonzales, and N. Kramer. "Family process, chronic illness and health." *Archives of General Psychiatry* 43, no. 8 (1986): 795–804.

18 Georgas, J., S. Christakopoulou, Y. H. Portinga, R. Goodwin, A. Angleitner, and N. Charalambous. "The relationship of family bonds to family structure and function across cultures." *Journal of Cross Cultural Psychology* 28, no. 3 (1997): 303–320.

19 Tromdorff, G. "Future orientation and socialization." *International Journal of Psychology* 18, no. 1 (1983): 318–406.

20 Austrian, S. G. (ed.). *Development theories through the life cycle*. 2nd ed. New York: Columbia University Press, 2008.

Chapter 6

1 Conklin, W. E. *The phenomenology of modern legal discourse: The judicial production and the discourse of suffering*. Brookfield, VT: Ashgate Publishing Co., 1998.

2 Rothman, D. J. "The origin and consequences of patient autonomy: A 25-year perspective." *Health Care Analysis* 9, no. 3 (2001): 255–264.

3 Tauber, A. I. "Historical and philosophical reflections on patient autonomy." *Health Care Analysis* 9, no. 3 (2001): 299–319.

4 Neutel, C. I. "The concept of autonomy in a pluralistic society." *Pharmacoepidemiology and Drug Safety* 10, no. 5 (2001): 463–466.
5 Blackhall, L. J., S. T. Murphy, G. Frank, V. Michel, and S. Azen. "Ethnicity and attitudes toward patient autonomy." *Journal of the American Medical Association* 274, no. 10 (1995): 820–825.
6 Elliot, A. C. "Health care ethics: Cultural relativity of autonomy." *Journal of Transcultural Nursing* 12, no. 4 (2001): 326–380.
7 Englehardt, H. T. "The many faces of autonomy." *Health Care Analysis* 9, no. 3 (2001): 283–297.
8 Cassell, E. J. "Consent or obedience? Power and authority in medicine." *New England Journal of Medicine* 352 (2005): 4.
9 Bergma, J. "Identity, problem solving and autonomy." In *Doctors and patients: Strategies in long-term illness*, ed. J. Bergsma and M. Commers. Dordrecht, Netherlands: Kluwer Academic Publishers, 1997. 43–71.
10 Polder, J. J., and H. Jochemsen. "Personal autonomy in the health care system." Netherlands: Kluwer Academic Publishers, 477–491.
11 Hoogland J., and H. Jochemsen. "Professional autonomy and the normative structure in medical practice." *Theoretical Medicine and Bioethics* 21, no. 5 (2000): 457–475.
12 Bannister, D. "Knowledge of self." In *Psychology for physiotherapists*. Ed. E. Naomi Dunkin, A. J. Chapman, and A. Gale. London: The British Psychological Society & Macmillan Press Ltd., 1981. 174–194.
13 Johnson, T. S. *Professions and power*. London: Macmillan, 1986.
14 Nosse, L. J., and L. Sagiv. "Theory-based study of the basic values of 565 physical therapists." *Physical Therapy* 85, no. 9 (2005): 834–850.
15 Karny, E. "Core values and attitudes of occupational therapy practice." *American Journal of Occupational Therapy* 47 no. 12 (1993): 1085–1086.

Chapter 7

1 Rackman, H. "Aristotle, Athenian constitution." *Classical Review* 50 (1936): 22–23.
2 Keatings, M., and B. O'Neil. *Ethical and legal issues in Canadian nursing*. 2nd ed. Toronto, ON: W. B. Saunders, 2000.
3 Conklin, W. *The phenomenology of modern legal discourse: The juridical production and the disclosure of suffering*. Brookfield, VT: Ashgate Publishing Co., 1998.
4 Caulfield, T. A., and B. V. Tigerstrom. *Health care reform and the law in Canada: Meeting the challenge*. Edmonton: University of Alberta Press, 2002.
5 Guenther, E. "What's the truth got to do with it? The burden of proof instruction violates the presumption of innocence." *Wisconsin Defender* 13, no. 3 (Fall 2005): 1–5.
6 Gibson, E. "Is there a privacy interest in anonymized personal health information?" *Health Law Journal*, special edition (2003): 97–112.

7 Singer, J. A. "Have doctors forsaken their ethics?" *Foundation for Economic Education* (April 1995).
8 Henderson, A. "Power and knowledge in nursing practice: The contributions of Foucault." *Journal of Advanced Nursing* 20, no. 5 (1994): 935–939.
9 *The Oxford Dictionary of Law*, ed. E. Martin. Oxford: Oxford University Press, 1997.
10 Henderson, S. "Power imbalance between nurses and patients: A potential inhibitor of partnership in care." *Journal of Clinical Nursing* 12, no. 4 (2003): 501–508.
11 Sines, D. "The arrogance of power: A reflection on contemporary mental health nursing practice." *Journal of Advanced Nursing* 20, no. 5 (1994): 894–903.
12 Guinn, D. E. "Honour the patient's wishes." *Annals of Thoracic Surgery* 74, no. 5 (2002): 1431–1432.
13 *Some aspects of medical treatment and criminal law*. Report no. 74. Law Reform Commission of Canada, 1986. 1–9.
14 "Ethical issues: Health research with human subjects." *Canadian Bar Association Law Review* (July 2001). 6.
15 Cassell, E. J. The nature of suffering: Physical, psychological, social and spiritual aspects. In *The hidden dimensions of illness: Human suffering*, ed. P. L. Starck and J. P. McGovern. New York: National League for Nursing Press, 1992. 1–10.
16 Stratton-Hill, C., Jr. "Suffering as contrasted to pain, loss, grief, despair, loneliness." In *The hidden dimensions of illness: Human suffering*, ed. P. L. Starck and J. P. McGovern. New York: National League for Nursing Press, 1992. 69–80.
17 van Hooft, S. "The meaning of suffering." *Hastings Center Report* 28, no.5 (1998): 13–19.
18 Kahn, D. L., and R. H. Steeves. "The experience of suffering: Conceptual clarification and theoretical definitions." *Journal of Advanced Nursing* 11, no. 6 (1986): 623–631.

Chapter 8

1 Beecher, H. K. "The measurement of pain." *Pharmacology Review* 9 (1957): 59–209.
2 Erikson, K. "The alienation of suffering: The idea of caring." *Scandinavian Journal of Caring Sciences* 23 (1992): 119–123.
3 Erikson, K. "Understanding the world of the patient, the suffering of human beings: The new clinical paradigm from nursing to caring." *Advanced Practice Nurse Quarter* 3 (1997): 8–13.
4 Cassell, E. *The nature of suffering and the goals of medicine*. 2nd ed. Oxford: Oxford University Press, 2004.
5 van Hooft, S. "The meaning of suffering." *Hasting Centre Report* 28, no. 5 (1998): 13–19.
6 Chapman, C. R., and J. Gavin. "Suffering and its relationship to pain." *Journal of Palliative Care* 9, no. 2 (1993): 5–13.
7 Chapman, C. R. "Suffering: The contributions of persistent pain." *Lancet* 353, no. 9171 (1999): 2233–2237.

8 Stratton-Hill, C., Jr. "Suffering as contrasted to pain, loss, grief, despair, loneliness." In *The Hidden dimensions of illness: Human suffering*, ed. P. L. Stark, and J. P. McGovern. New York: League for Nursing Press, 1992. 69–80.

9 Loeser, J. D., and R. Melzack. "Pain: An overview." *Lancet* 353, no. 9164 (1999): 1607–1609.

10 Clarke, B. M. "Pain, suffering and physiotherapy." *Physiotherapy Canada* 50, no. 2 (1998): 112–117.

11 Clarke, B. M. "The impact of suffering in physiotherapy practice: Cost containment." *Physiotherapy Canada* 52, no. 1 (2000): 25–32.

12 Clarke, B. M., A. R. M. Upton, and C. M. Castellanos. "Pain and suffering: Measuring the suffering component." In *Proceedings of the 11th World Congress on Pain* (Aug. 21–26, 2005, Sydney, Australia), ed. H. Flor, E. Kalso, and J. O. Dostrovsky. Seattle, WA: IASP Press, 2006. 204, 550-P156.

13 Clarke, B.M., A. R. M. Upton, and C. M. Castellanos. "Work beliefs and work status of people with epilepsy." In *Proceedings of the 26th International Epilepsy Congress* (Aug. 28–Sept. 1, 2005, Paris, France). *Epilepsia* 46, suppl. 6 (2005): 129, P292.

14 Clarke, B.M., A.R. M. Upton, and C. M. Castellanos. "Internal barriers to work: Practice implications." In *Proceedings of the Canadian Physiotherapy Congress* (May 26–29, 2005, Victoria, BC). Abstracts, 10, AL102 .

15 Clarke, B. M., A. R. M. Upton, C. Castellanos, and M. Schmuck. "Measuring and assessing suffering in arthritic patients." In *Spirituality and health: Multidisciplinary explorations*, ed. A. Meier, T. O'Connor, and P. VanKatwyk. Waterloo, ON: Wilfred Laurier University Press, 2005. 227–241.

16 Ware, J. E., M. Kosinski, and S. D. Keller. "A 12-item short form health survey." *Medical Care* 34, no. 3 (1996): 220–233.

17 Ware, J. E., K. K. Snow, M. Kosinski, and B. Gandek. *SF-36 Health Survey: Manual and interpretation guide*. Boston: The Health Institute, New England Medical Center, 1993.

18 Melzack, R. "The McGill Pain Questionnaire: Major properties and scoring method." *Pain* 1, no. 3 (1975): 277–299.

19 William, R. M., and A. M. Myers. "Functional abilities confidence scale: A clinical measure for injured workers with acute back pain." *Physical Therapy* 78, no. 6 (1998): 624–634.

20 Streiner, D. L., and G. R. Norman. *Health measurement scales: A practical guide to their development and use*. Oxford: Oxford University Press, 1989.

21 Cronbach, L. J., C. Goldine, H. N. Glesser, and R. Nageswari. *Dependability of behavioural measurement: Theory of generalizability for scores and profiles*. New York: John Wiley & Sons, 1972.

22 Cohen, J. "Weighted Kappa: Nominal scale agreement with provision for scaled disagreement or partial credit." *Psychological Bulletin* 70 (1968): 213–220.

23 Norman, G. R., and D. L. Streiner. *Biostatistics: The bare essentials*. St. Louis, MO: Mosby Year Books, 1994.

Chapter 9

1. Wade, D. T. "Assessment, Measurement and Data Collection Tools." *Clinical Rehabilitation* 18, no. 3 (2004): 233–237.
2. Williams, J. I., and C. D. Naylor. "How should health status measures be assessed? Cautionary notes on procrustean Frameworks." *Journal of Clinical Epidemiology* 45, no. 12 (1992): 1347–1351.
3. Austin, P. C. "A comparison of methods for analyzing health related quality-of-life measures." *Value in Health* 5, no. 4 (2002): 329–337.
4. Naliboff, B. D. "Choosing outcome variables: Global assessment and diaries." *Gastroenterology* 126, suppl. 1 (2004): S129–S134.
5. Melzack, R. "The McGill Pain Questionnaire: Major Properties and Scoring Methods." *Pain* 1, no. 3 (1975): 277–299.
6. Melzack, R. "The short-form McGill Pain Questionnaire." *Pain* 30, no. 2 (1987): 191–197.

Chapter 10

1. O'Connor, P. J. "Normative data: Their definition, interpretation and importance for primary care physicians." *Family Medicine* 22, no. 4 (1990): 307–311.
2. Estabrooks, C. A. "Measuring knowledge utilization in health care." *International Journal of Policy, Evaluation, and Management* 1, no. 1 (2003): 3–26.
3. Haynes, B., and A. Haines. "Barriers and bridges to evidence based clinical practice." *British Medical Journal* 317, no. 7153 (1998): 273–276.
4. Sackett, D. L., W. M. C. Rosenberg, J. A. M. Gray, and R. B. Haynes. "Evidence medicine: What it is and what it isn't." *British Medical Journal* 312, no. 7023 (1996): 71-2.
5. Haynes, R. B. "Loose connections between peer reviewed clinical journals and clinical practice." *Annals of Internal Medicine* 113, no. 9 (1990): 724–728.
6. Sackett, D. L., and R. B. Haynes. "On the need for evidence-based medicine." *Evidence Based Medicine* 1 (1995): 5.
7. Gray, J. A. M., R. B. Haynes, D. L. Sackett, and G. H. Guyatt. "Transferring evidence from health care research into medical practice: Developing evidence based clinical policy." *Evidence Based Medicine* 2 (1997): 36–38.
8. Maher, C. G., C. Sherrington, M. Elkins, R. D. Herbert, and A. M. Moseley. "Challenges for evidence based physical therapy: Accessing and interpreting high-quality evidence on therapy." *Physical Therapy Journal* 84, no. 7 (2004): 644–654.
9. Haynes, R. B., P. J. Deveraux, and G. H. Guyatt. "Physician's and patient's choices in evidence based practice." *British Medical Journal* 324, no. 735 (2002): 1350.
10. Clarke, B. M., A. R. M. Upton, and C. Castellanos. "Suffering: Measuring the immeasurable." In *Central neuropathic pain: Focus on post stroke pain*, ed. J. Henry, A. Panju, K. Yashpal. Seattle, WA: IASP Press, 2007. 249–260.

Chapter 11

1 Clarke, B. M., A. R. M. Upton, and C. Castellanos. "Suffering: Measuring the immeasurable." In *Central neuropathic pain: Focus on post stroke pain*, ed. J. Henry, A. Panju, K. Yashpal. Seattle, WA: IASP Press, 2007.
2 Clarke, B. M., A. R. M. Upton, C. Castellanos, and M. Schmuck. "Measuring and assessing suffering in arthritic patients." In *Spirituality and health: Multidisciplinary explorations*, ed. A. Meir, T. O'Connor, and P. VanKatwyk. Waterloo, ON: Wilfred Laurier University Press, 2005.
3 Norman, G., and D. Streiner. *Biostatistics: The bare essentials*. Hamilton, ON: B. C. Decker Inc., 2000.
4 Clarke, B. M. "The role of the physiotherapist in the management of epilepsy." *Physiotherapy Canada* 46, no. 2 (1994): 98–104.
5 Scheuer, M. L. "Medical aspects of managing seizures and epilepsy." In *Recent advances in epilepsy*, vol. 5, ed. T. A. Pedley, and P. S. Meldrum. New York: Churchill Livingstone, 1992.
6 Clarke, B. M., A. R. M. Upton, and C. Castellanos. "Work beliefs and work status in epilepsy." *Epilepsy and Behavior* 9, no. 1 (2006): 119–125.
7 Clarke, B. M., A. R. M. Upton, and C. M. Castellanos. "Internal barriers to work: Practice implications." In *Proceedings of the Canadian Physiotherapy Congress* (May 26–29, 2005, Victoria, BC, Canada), Abstract. 10, AL102.
8 Goadsby, P. J. "The pathophysiology of headache." In *Wolf's headache and other head pain*, ed. R. B. Lipton, and S. Solomon. Oxford: Oxford University Press, 2001.
9 Headache Classification Committee of the International Headache Society. The international classification of headache disorders. 2nd edition. *Cephalalgia* 24, suppl. 1 (2004): 8–160.
10 Clarke, B.M., A. R. M. Upton, M. V. Kamath, T. Al-Harbi, and C. Castellanos. "Transcranial magnetic stimulation for migraine: Clinical effects." *Journal of Headache and Pain* 7, no. 5 (2006): 341–346.
11 Wachtel, P. "The contextual self." In *Trauma and self*, ed. C. B. Strozier and M. Flynn. Lanham, MD: Rowman and Littlefield Publishers Inc., 1996.
12 Luckmann, J. *Transcultural communication in health care*. Albany, NY: Delmar, 2000.

Chapter 12

1 Clarke, B. M., A. R. M. Upton, and C. Castellanos. "Suffering: Measuring the immeasurable." In *Central Neuropathic Pain: Focus on post stroke pain*, ed. J. Henry, A. Panju, and K. Yashpal. Seattle, WA: IASP Press, 2007. 249–260.
2 Clarke, B. M., A. R. M. Upton, M. V. Kamath, T. Al-Harbi, and C. Castellanos. "Transcranial magnetic stimulation for migraine: Clinical effects." *Journal of Headache and Pain* 7, no. 5 (2006): 341–346.
3 Clarke, B. M., A. R. M. Upton, and C. Castellanos. "Work beliefs and work status in epilepsy." *Epilepsy and Behavior* 9, no. 1 (2006): 119–125.

4 Clarke, B. M. "The impact of suffering in physiotherapy practice: Cost-containment issues." *Physiotherapy Canada* 52, no. 1 (2000): 25–32.

5 Clarke, B. M. "Pain, suffering and physiotherapy." *Physiotherapy Canada* 50, no. 2 (1998): 112–122.

6 Clarke, B. M., A.R. M. Upton, C. Castellanos, and M. Schmuck. "Measuring and assessing suffering in arthritic patients. In *Spirituality and health: Multidisciplinary explorations*, ed. A. Meir, T. O'Connor, P. VanKatwyk. Waterloo, ON: Wilfred Laurier University Press, 2005.

7 O'Connor, J. "Good stories from there develop good care here: A therapeutic perspective." In *Coping with final tragedy*, ed. D. R. Counts and D. A. Counts. Amityville, NY: Baywood Publishing Co. Inc., 1991.

8 Johnson, T. S. *Professions and power*. London: Macmillan, 1986.

9 Reed, F. C. *Suffering and illness: Insight for caregivers*. Philadelphia: F. A. Davis Co., 2003.

10 Ignatieff, M. *The needs of strangers*. New York: Viking, 1985.

11 Sunwolf, F., R. Lawrence, and L. Keranen. "Story perceptions: Healing effects of storytelling in the practice of medicine." In *Narratives, health and healing: Communication theory, research and practice*, ed. M. Hartnel, P. M. Japp, and C. S. Beck. Mahwah, NJ: Lawrence Erlbaum, 2005.

12 Kosko, J., T. P. Klassen, T. Bishop, and L. Hartling. "Evidence-based medicine and the anecdote: Uneasy bedfellows or ideal couple?" *Pediatrics and Child Health* 11, no. 10 (2006): 665–668.

13 Tauber, A. I., "Historical and philosophical reflections on patient autonomy." *Health Care Analysis* 9, no. 3 (2001): 299–319.

14 Platt, F. W., and V. F. Keller. "Empathetic communication: A teachable and learnable skills." *Journal of General Internal Medicine* 9, no. 4 (1994): 220–226.

15 Cassell, E. J. "Diagnosing suffering: A perspective." *Annals of Internal Medicine* 131, no. 9 (1999): 531–534.

16 Bannister, D. "Knowledge of self." In *Psychology for physiotherapists*, ed. E. Naomi Dunkin, A. J. Chapman, and A. Gale. London: The British Psychological Society and Macmillan Press Ltd., 1981.

17 Wilber, K. *Integral Psychology: Consciousness, spirit, psychology, therapy*. London: Shambhala, 2000.

Chapter 13

1 Englehardt, H. T. "The many faces of autonomy." *Health Care Analysis* 9, no. 3 (2001): 283–297.

2 Hoogland, J., and H. Jochemsen. "Professional autonomy and the normative structure of medical practice." *Theoretical Medicine and Bioethics* 21, no. 5 (2000): 457–475.

3 Tauber, A. I. Historical and philosophical reflections on patient autonomy." *Health Care Analysis* 9, no. 3 (2001): 299–319.

4 Rohtman, D. J. "The origins and consequences of patient autonomy: A 25-year perspective." *Health Care Analysis* 9, no. 3 (2001): 255–264.

5 Hall, M., and C. E. Schneider. "Patients as consumers: Courts, contracts and the new medical market place." *Michigan Law Review* 106 (2008): 644–689.

6 Moore, P. J., S. Spernak, and E. Chung. "Patients' rights and physicians' duties: Implications for the doctor-patient relationship and the quality of health care." In *The psychology of rights and duties: Empirical and normative commentaries*, ed. N. J. Finkel and F. M. Moghaddam. Washington, DC: American Psychological Association, 2005. 179–195.

7 Worchel, S. "The rightful place of human rights: Incorporating individual, group, and cultural perspectives." In *The psychology of rights and duties: Empirical and normative commentaries*, ed. N. J. Finkel and F. M. Moghaddam. Washington, DC: American Psychological Association, 2005. 197–220.

8 Haskell, T. L. "Taking duties seriously: To what problems are rights and duties the solution." In *The psychology of rights and duties: Empirical and normative commentaries*, ed. N. J. Finkel and F. M. Moghaddam. Washington, DC: American Psychological Association, 2005. 243–252.

9 Dworkin, R. *Taking rights seriously*. Cambridge: Cambridge University Press, 1997.

10 Whitney, S. N., L. B. McCullough, E. Fruge, A. L. McGuire, and R. J. Volk. "Beyond breaking the bad news: The role of hope and hopefulness." *Cancer* 113, no. 2 (2008): 442–445.

11 Brown, A. E., S. N. Whitney, and J. D. Duffy. "The physicians' role in the assessment and treatment of spiritual distress at the end of life." *Palliative and Supportive Care* 4, no. 1 (2006): 81–86.

12 Talseth, A., and F. Gilje. "Unburdening suffering: Responses of psychiatrists to patients' suicide deaths." *Nursing Ethics* 14, no. 5 (2007): 620–635.

13 Summerfield, D. "The invention of post traumatic stress disorder and the social usefulness of a psychiatric category." *British Medical Journal* 322, no. 7278 (2001): 95–98.

14 Sensky, T. "Suffering." *International Journal of Integrated Care*, suppl. (Jan. 2010): 10.

15 Stringer, B., B. Van Meijel, W. De Vree, and J. Van Der Bijl. "User involvement in mental health care: The role of nurses." *Journal of Psychiatric and Mental Health Nursing* 15, no. 8 (2008): 678–683.

16 H. E. McHaffie. "HIV and Aids: The nursing response and some ethical challenges." *Nursing Ethics* 1, no. 4 (1994): 224–232.

17 Mathes, M. M. "Ethical challenges and nursing." *Medsurg Nursing* (Feb. 2000).

18 Polder, J. J., and H. Jochemsen. "Professional autonomy in the health care system." *Theoretical Medicine and Bioethics* 21, no. 5 (2000): 477–491.

19 Rabetoy, C. P., and B. C. Blair. "Nephrology nurses' perspectives on difficult ethical issues and practice guidelines for shared decision making. *Nephrology Nursing Journal* 34, no. 6 (2007): 599–629.

20 Hanssen, I. "An intercultural nursing perspective on autonomy." *Nursing Ethics* 11, no. 1 (2004): 28–41.
21 Larsson, I. E., M. J. Sahlsten, B. Sjostrom, C. S. Lindencrona, and K. A. Plos. "Patient participation in nursing care from a patient perspective: A grounded theory study." *Scandinavian Journal of Caring Sciences* 21, no. 3 (2007): 313–320.
22 Ferrell, B. R., and N. Coyle. *The nature of suffering and the goals of nursing*. Oxford: Oxford University Press, 2008.
23 Shonefeld-Ringel, S. "A re-conceptualization of the working alliance in cross cultural practice with non-western clients: Integrating relational perspective and multicultural theories." *Clinical Social Work Journal* 29, no. 1 (2001): 53–63.
24 Young-Mason, J. *The patient's voice: Experiences of illness*. Philadelphia: F. A. Davis Company, 1997.
25 McEvoy, L., and A. Duffy. "Holistic practice: A concept analysis." *Nursing Education in Practice* 8, no. 4 (2008): 412–419.
26 Barnum, B. S. *Spirituality in nursing: From traditional to New Age*. 2nd ed. New York: Springer Publishing Co., 2003.
27 Vandercreek, L., and L. Buron. *Professional chaplaincy: Its role and importance in health care*. New York: Association of Professional Chaplains, 2001.
28 Canadian Council on Health Services Accreditation. *Achieving Improved Measurement (AIM) Program*. Ottawa, ON: 1999. Sections 13.3 and 14.9.
29 Carey, R. G. "Chaplaincy, components of total patient care in hospitals?" *Journal of the American Hospital Association* 47, no. 14 (1973): 166–172.
30 Standards of the Association for Clinical Pastoral Education's Code of Professional Ethics. Part 2 Standard 102.1. http://www.acpe.edu, 2007 (accessed March 5, 2009).
31 Carey, R. D. "Change in perceived need value and role of the hospital chaplains." In *Hospital ministry: The role of the chaplain today*, ed. E. H. Lawrence. New York: Crossroad Publishing Co., 1985.
32 Fitchett, G., P. Meyer, and L. A. Burton. "Spiritual care: Who requests it? Who needs it?" *Journal of Pastoral Care* 54, no. 2 (2000): 173–186.
33 Daly, G. "Ethics and economics." *Nursing Economics* 18, no. 4 (2000): 194–201.
34 Gibbons, J. L., and S. L. Miller. "An image of contemporary hospital chaplaincy." *Journal of Pastoral Care* 43, no. 4 (1989): 355–361.
35 Gibbons, J. L., J. Thomas, L. Vandercreek, and A. K. Jessen. "The value of hospital chaplains: Patients' perspectives." *Journal of Pastoral Care* 45, no. 2 (1991): 117–125.
36 Simmonds, A. L. "The chaplain's role in bioethical decision-making." *Health Care Management Forum* 7, no. 4 (1994): 5–17.
37 Salladay, S. A. "Secularizing spiritual care." *Journal of Clinical Nursing* 25, no. 4 (2008): 222–223.
38 Lee, S. J. C. "In a secular spirit: Strategies of pastoral medical education." *Health Care Analysis* 10, no. 4 (2002): 339–356.
39 Piderman, K. M., D. V. Marek, S. M. Jenkins, S. M. Johnson, M. E. Johnson, J. F.

Buryska, and P. S. Mueller. "Patients' expectations of hospital chaplains." *Mayo Clinic Proceedings* 83, no. 1 (2008): 58–65.

40 Engelhardt, H. T. Jr. "The dechristianization of Christian hospital chaplaincy: Some bioethics reflections on professionalism." *Christian Bioethics* 9, no. 1 (2003): 139–160.

41 Monteith, W. G. "Professionalization and disclosure: An outsider's viewpoint." *Scottish Journal of Health Care* 9, no. 1 (2006): 31–32.

Chapter 14

1 Trizenberg, H. L., and C. M. Davis. "Beyond the code of ethics: Educating physical therapists for their role as moral agents." *Journal of Physical Therapy Education* 14, no. 3 (2000): 48–58.

2 Jensun, G. M, J. Gwyer, K. F. Shepherd, and L. M. Hack. "Expert practice in physiotherapy." *Physical Therapy* 80, no. 1 (2000): 28–43.

3 Griener, G. G. "Moral integrity of professions." *Professional Ethics* 2, nos. 3/4 (1993): 15–38.

4 Nosse, L. J., and S. Lilach. "Theory-based study of the basic values of 565 physical therapists." *Physical Therapy* 85, no. 9 (2005): 834–850.

5 Turner-Stokes, L. "Politics, policy and payment: Facilitators or barriers to person centered rehabilitation?" *Disability and Rehabilitation* 29, nos. 20/21 (2007): 1575–1582.

6 Fabrice, G., C. Lefevre, M. Cammeli, B. Pachoud, J. F. Ravaud, and A. Lepege. "Why is rehabilitation not fully person-centered and should it be more person-centered?" *Disability and Rehabilitation* 29, nos. 20/21 (2007): 1616–1624.

7 Sullivan, M. J. L., and C. Main. "Service, advocacy and adjudication: Balancing the ethical challenges of multiple stake holder agendas in the rehabilitation of chronic pain." *Disability and Rehabilitation* 29, nos. 20/21 (2007): 1590–1603.

8 MacLeod, R., and K. M. McPherson. "Care and compassion: Part of person-centered rehabilitation, inappropriate response or a forgotten art?" *Disability and Rehabilitation* 29, nos. 20/21 (2007): 1589–1595.

9 Robbins, H., R. J. Gatchel, C. Noe, N. Gajraj, P. Polatin, M. Deschner, A. Vakharia, and L. Adams. "A prospective one-year outcome study of interdisciplinary chronic pain management: Compromising its efficacy by managed care policies." *Anesthesia and Analgesia*. 97, no. 1 (2003): 156–162.

10 Greenfield, B. H. "The meaning of caring in five experienced physical therapists." *Physiotherapy Theory and Practice* 22, no. 4 (2006): 175–187.

11 Freiburger, J. K., and G. Holmes. "Physical therapy use by community based older people." *Physical Therapy* 85, no. 1 (2005): 19–33.

12 Cross, S. and J. Sim. "Confidentiality within physiotherapy: Perceptions and attitudes of clinical practitioners." *Journal of Medical Ethics* 26, no. 6 (2000): 447–453.

13 Rotarius, T., E. Hamby, and T. A. Feroldi. "How physical therapists perceive physicians: A stakeholder analysis." *Health Care Manager* 20, no. 4 (2002): 19–26.

14 Busch, H., S. Goransson, and B. Melin. "Self-efficacy beliefs predict sustained long-term sick absenteeism in individuals with chronic musculo-skeletal pain." *Pain Practice* 7, no. 3 (2007): 234–240.
15 Clarke, B. M., A. R. M. Upton, C. Castellanos, and M. L. Schmuck. "Measuring and assessing suffering in arthritic patients." In *Spirituality and health: Multidisciplinary explorations*, ed. A. Meier, T. O'Connor, and P. L. VanKatwyk. Waterloo, ON: Wilfred Laurier University Press; 2005.
16 Clarke, B. M., A. R. M. Upton, and C. Castellanos. "Suffering: Measuring the immeasurable." In *Central neuropathic pain: Focus on post stroke pain*, ed. J. Henry, A. Panju, and K. Yashpal. Seattle, WA: IASP Press, 2007.
17 Clarke, B. M. "Pain, suffering and physiotherapy." *Physiotherapy Canada* 50, no. 2 (1998): 112–122.
18 Agnew, E. N. *From charity to social work: Mary E. Richardson and the creation of an American profession*. Urbana: University of Illinois Press, 2004.
19 Hick, S. *Social work in Canada*. Toronto, ON: Thompson Educational Publishing, 2003. 15.
20 Oliver, M. *The politics of disablement*. London: Macmillan Educational Ltd., 1991.
21 Webb, S. A. "The politics of social work: Power and subjectivity." *Clinical Social Work* 1, no. 2 (2000).
22 Hasenfeld, Y. "Power in social work practice." *Social Service Review* 61, no. 3 (1987): 469–483.
23 Ehrenreich, J. H. *The altruistic imagination: A history of social work and social policy in the United States*. Ithaca, NY: Cornell University Press; 2001.
24 Manning, S. S. *Ethical leadership in human resources: A multidimensional approach*. Boston: Pearson Education, 2003.
25 Wing, P. C. "Patient or client? If in doubt, ask." *Canadian Medical Association Journal* 157, no. 3 (1997): 287–289.
26 Cowles, L. A. *Social work in the health field*. 2nd ed. New York: The Haworth Social Work Practice Press, 2003.
27 Rudebeck, C. "The body as lived experience." In *Medical humanities companion*, vol. 1, ed. M. Evans, R. Ahlzen, I. Heath, and J. MacNaughton. New York: Radcliffe Publishing, 2008. 27–43.
28 Health Canada. "Health law and ethics in relation to the use of complimentary and alternative health care and natural health related products: An invitational roundtable, 2001." http://www.hc-sc.gc.ca. (accessed December 30, 2002).
29 Raisa D., N. Kraetschmer, S. Urowitz, and N. Sharpe. "Patient, consumer, client or customer: What do people want to be called?" *Health Expectations* 8, no. 4 (2005): 345–351.
30 Lackey, J. F. *Accountability in social services: The culture of paper programs*. New York: Haworth Press, 2006.

Chapter 15

1 Reiss D., S. Gonzales, and N. Kraemer. "Family process, chronic illness and death." *Archives of General Psychiatry* 43 (1986): 795–804.
2 Moritsky, D. E. "Five-year blood pressure control and mortality following health education for hypertensive patients." *American Journal of Public Health* 73 (1983): 153–162.
3 Sholevar, G. P, and R. Perkel. "Family systems intervention and physical illness." *General Hospital Psychiatry* 12 (1990): 363–372.
4 O'Connor, J. A. "Good stories from there develop good care here." In *Coping with the final tragedy*, ed. D. R Counts and D. A. Counts. Amityville, NY: Baywood Publishing Co., 1991. 253–277.
5 Morin, E. M. "The meaning of work in modern times." Tenth World Conference on Human Resources Management, Rio de Janeiro, Brazil, August 20, 2004. www.hec.ca/estelle.morin (accessed April 20, 2009).
6 Clarke, B. M., A.R. M. Upton, and C. Castellanos. "Work beliefs and work status in epilepsy." *Epilepsy and Behavior* 9 (2006): 119–125.
7 Clarke, B. M, A. R. M. Upton, C. Castellanos, and M. L. Schmuck. "Measuring and assessing suffering in arthritic patients." In *Spirituality and health: Multidisciplinary explorations*, ed. A. Meier, T. O'Connor, and P. L. VanKatwyk. Waterloo, ON: Wilfred Laurier University Press, 2005.
8 Kome, P. *Wounded workers: The politics of musculoskeletal injuries*. Toronto, ON: University of Toronto Press, 1998.
9 Black, H. K. *Soul pain: The meaning of suffering in later life*. Society and Ageing series, ed. J. Hendricks. Amityville, NY: Baywood Publishing Co., 2006.

Chapter 16

1 Keedwell, P. *How sadness survived: The evolutionary basis of depression*. New York: Radcliffe Publishing, 2008.
2 Viguer, A., and A. Rothchild. "Depression: Clinical features and pathogenesis." In *Disorders across the life span*, ed. K. I. Shulman, M. Tohen, and S. P. Kutcher. New York: John Wiley & Sons, Inc., 1996.
3 Kleinman, A., and B. Good (eds.). *Culture and depression: Studies in anthropology and cross-cultural psychiatry of affect and disorder*. Berkeley: University of California Press, 1985.
4 Robertson, M. M., and C. L. E. Katona (eds.). *Perspectives in psychiatry*. Vol. 6, *Depression and physical illness*. Toronto, ON: John Wiley and Sons, Inc., 1997.
5 Davison, G. C, and J. M. Neale. *Abnormal psychology*. 6th ed. New York: John Wiley and Sons, Inc., 1994.
6 Becker, J., and A. Kleinman (eds.). *Psychological aspects of depression*. Mahwah, NJ: Lawrence Erlbaum, 1991.

7 Brown, G. W., and T. Harris. *Social origins of depression: A study of psychiatric disorders in women*. New York: The Free Press, 1978.

8 Richards, R. Everyday creativity, eminent creativity, and health: "Afterview for CRJ special issue on creativity and health." *Creativity Research Journal* 3 (1990): 300–326.

9 Toombs, S. K. *The meaning of illness: A phenomenological account of the different perspectives of physician and patient*. Boston: Kluwer Academic Publishers, 1992.

10 Richards, R. Creativity, everyday. In *Encyclopedia of mental health*, ed. H. S. Friedman. San Diego, CA: Academic Press, 1998

11 Cropley, A. J. "Creativity and mental health in everyday life." In: *Eminent creativity, everyday creativity and health*, ed. M. A. Runco and R. Richards. Greenwich, CT: Ablex Publishing Co., 1997. 231–246.

12 Csikszentmihalyi, M. *Flow: The psychology of optimal experience*. New York: Harper Perennial; 1990.

13 Hoyer, W. J., and J. M. Rybash. "Characterizing adult cognitive development." *Journal of Adult Development* 1, no. 1 (1994): 7–12.

14 Lubart, T. I., and R. J. Sternberg. "Life span creativity: An investment theory approach." In *Creativity and successful aging: Theoretical and empirical approaches*, ed. C. E. Adams-Price. New York: Springer Publishing Co., 1998. 21–42.

15 Sinnott, J. D. "Creativity and post formal thought: Why the last stage is the creative stage." In *Creativity and successful aging: Theoretical and empirical approaches*, ed. C. E. Adams-Price. New York: Springer Publishing Co., 1998. 43–72.

16 Runco, M. A. "A longitudinal study of exceptional giftedness and creativity." *Creativity Research Journal* 12, no. 2 (1999): 161–164.

17 Carson, D. K. "The importance of creativity in family therapy: A preliminary consideration." *The Family Journal* 7, no. 4 (1999): 326–334.

18 Nesbit, S. G. "My breast cancer: An occupational therapist's perspective." *Occupational Therapy in Mental Health* 22, no. 2 (2006): 51–67.

INDEX

Clarke, Beverley M.

On suffering: pathways to healing and health / Beverley M. Clarke.

p.; cm.

Includes bibliographical references and index.

ISBN 978-1-61168-028-7 (cloth: alk. paper)—

ISBN 978-1-61168-005-8 (pbk.: alk. paper)—

ISBN 978-1-61168-010-2 (e-book)

1. Pain—Psychological aspects. 2. Pain—Physiological aspects. 3. Pain—Treatment. I. Title.

[DNLM: 1. Stress, Psychological—etiology. 2. Stress, Psychological—therapy. 3. Chronic Disease. 4. Empathy. 5. Pain. 6. Professional–Patient Relations. WM 172]

RB127.C54 2011

616′.0472—dc22 2011004794